I0867031

CHILDREN AND YOUNG PEOPLE'S RESPONSE TO PARENTAL ILLNESS

A HANDBOOK OF ASSESSMENT AND PRACTICE

CHILDREN AND YOUNG PEOPLE'S RESPONSE TO PARENTAL ILLNESS

A HANDBOOK OF ASSESSMENT AND PRACTICE

Edited by

David Morley
University of Oxford, UK

Xiaoming Li
University of South Carolina, USA

Crispin Jenkinson
University of Oxford, UK

CRC Press
Taylor & Francis Group
Boca Raton London New York

CRC Press is an imprint of the
Taylor & Francis Group, an **informa** business

CRC Press
Taylor & Francis Group
6000 Broken Sound Parkway NW, Suite 300
Boca Raton, FL 33487-2742

First issued in hardback 2017

Version Date: 20160322

ISBN-13: 978-1-78523-007-3 (pbk)
ISBN-13: 978-1-138-46147-5 (hbk)

Library of Congress Cataloging-in-Publication Data

Names: Morley, David, 1967 September 7- , editor. | Li, Xiaoming, 1956 November 30- , editor. | Jenkinson, Crispin, 1962- , editor.
Title: Children and young people's response to parental illness : a handbook of assessment and practice / [edited by] David Morley, Xiaoming Li, Crispin Jenkinson.
Description: Boca Raton : Taylor & Francis, 2017. | Includes bibliographical references and index.
Identifiers: LCCN 2016012715| ISBN 9781785230073 (pbk. : alk. paper) | ISBN 9781498778718 (e-book)
Subjects: | MESH: Child of Impaired Parents--psychology | Parent-Child Relations | Parenting--psychology | Child | Adolescent
Classification: LCC RJ499.3 | NLM WS 105.5.F2 | DDC 618.92/89--dc23
LC record available at http://lccn.loc.gov/2016012715

Visit the Taylor & Francis Web site at
http://www.taylorandfrancis.com

and the CRC Press Web site at
http://www.crcpress.com

Contents

Editors

David Morley, PhD, is a senior research scientist in the Health Services Research Unit in the Nuffield Department of Population Health at the University of Oxford. He has published widely on the impact of parental illness, with a particular focus on the offspring of people with Parkinson's disease. Dr Morley also has significant interests in outcomes measurement and has contributed to the development of a number of instruments.

Xiaoming Li, PhD, is professor and endowed chair of Health Promotion, Education and Behavior at the Arnold School of Public Health, University of South Carolina, Columbia, South Carolina. He has worked with an interdisciplinary team of psychologists, anthropologists, sociologists, physicians and other healthcare professionals for over 20 years in the areas of mental health and HIV research in both US and international settings. Professor Li's research interests include the impact of parental HIV on children's well-being and issues of parental disclosure of adverse events, including HIV infection.

Crispin Jenkinson, DPhil, is a professor and unit director of the Health Services Research Unit at the University of Oxford. He is also a senior research fellow of Harris Manchester College, Oxford. Professor Jenkinson's research interests include quality of life and health status measurement, the evaluation of patient experiences of medical care, and methodology. He also has extensive experience in developing and validating outcome measures.

Acknowledgement

We wish to acknowledge the significant contribution of Sarah Dummett, University of Oxford, whose patience, proofreading skills and keen eye for detail were invaluable in the preparation of this text.

Contributors

Shuang Bi
Department of Psychology
University of Kentucky
Lexington, Kentucky, USA

Elaine Book
Pacific Parkinson's Research Centre
University of British Columbia
Vancouver, British Columbia, Canada

Peilian Chi
Department of Psychology
University of Macau
Taipa, Macau, China

Emily Crain
Wellesley Centers for Women
Wellesley College
Wellesley, Massachusetts, USA

Lauren R. Gilbert
Department of Psychology
University of Kentucky
Lexington, Kentucky, USA

Tracy R.G. Gladstone
Wellesley Centers for Women
Wellesley College
Wellesley, Massachusetts, USA

Eric A. Haak
Department of Psychology
University of Kentucky
Lexington, Kentucky, USA

Crispin Jenkinson
Health Services Research Unit
Nuffield Department of Population Health and Harris Manchester College
University of Oxford
Oxford, UK

Peggy S. Keller
Department of Psychology
University of Kentucky
Lexington, Kentucky, USA

Laura Kelly
Nuffield Department of Population Health
University of Oxford
Oxford, UK

Rikke Kieffer-Kristensen
Department of Psychology
University of Copenhagen
Copenhagen, Denmark

Xiaoming Li
Department of Health Promotion Education & Behavior
Arnold School of Public Health
University of South Carolina
Columbia, South Carolina, USA

Cynthia W. Moore
Department of Psychiatry (Division of Child and Adolescent Psychiatry)
Massachusetts General Hospital
Boston, Massachusetts, USA

David Morley
Health Services Research Unit
Nuffield Department of Population Health
University of Oxford
Oxford, UK

Kenneth Pakenham
School of Psychology
University of Queensland
Brisbane, Queensland, Australia

Shan Qiao
Department of Health Promotion Education & Behavior
Arnold School of Public Health
University of South Carolina
Columbia, South Carolina, USA

Paula K. Rauch
Department of Psychiatry
Massachusetts General Hospital
Boston, Massachusetts, USA

Dominik Sebastian Sieh
Department of Clinical Psychology
Leiden University
Leiden, Netherlands

Anne Visser-Meily
Brain Center Rudolf Magnus
Center of Excellence for Rehabilitation Medicine
University Medical Centre Utrecht
Utrecht, Netherlands

CHAPTER 1

Children's and young people's response to parental illness: introduction and overview

David Morley and Crispin Jenkinson

The past few decades have seen a fundamental change in the way that the impact of illness is assessed. The evaluation of healthcare interventions now increasingly includes systematic attempts to incorporate patient-based reports of outcome. Patient-reported outcomes have become central to the measurement of health and well-being (Black and Jenkinson, 2009). This is in stark contrast to only a few decades ago, when assessments were based primarily on clinical judgements and so-called 'objective' assessments of disease progression in terms of mortality and morbidity. Furthermore, there is increasing recognition that the consequences of illness are not solely confined to those diagnosed with a given condition (Firth, 2006). The burgeoning literature related to the carers of affected individuals is a testament to this. The importance of identifying and meeting the needs of carers, particularly in light of an ageing population, is now regarded as essential in achieving optimal goals for healthcare and healthy living (Morley et al., 2012). Historically, however, the effects on the offspring of those diagnosed with debilitating, sometimes life-threatening, conditions have been less well recognised. Without question, this has begun to change, and investigations into children's and young people's responses to parental illness have gained significant momentum over the past two to three decades.

Current research highlights the multifaceted response of children to parental illness. Many of these responses have the potential to be challenging in terms of, for example, children's emotional and physical well-being, their peer relationships and hopes for the future. What is also clear is that not all responses are negative and that positive outcomes can emerge. Many children adapt positively to parental illness, and this can afford the opportunity for personal growth in terms of, for example, the development of independence and empathy. Some such responses may be specific to a particular condition; others may be more generic when children are confronted with adapting to their parent's health status.

This book aims to expand on the issues raised above and provide an up-to-date account of how a broad and diverse range of parental conditions might affect children's and young people's well-being. It should be noted from the outset that the focus is not on young carers as classically defined, where children provide excessive or inappropriate levels of care (ADASS et al., 2012). Rather, the emphasis is on children and young people, most likely not engaged in a primary caregiving role, but nevertheless experiencing a range of challenges as a consequence of their parent's condition. The term 'child' throughout this text is intentionally broad and is used as an overarching term to refer to children of all ages, be they very young, in their adolescent years or, indeed, adult children of affected parents.

The text commences with a number of dedicated chapters that focus on a single-parental condition where a sufficient and coherent body of evidence has emerged. These conditions include multiple sclerosis, Parkinson's disease, acquired brain injury, depression, alcoholism, cancer, and HIV/AIDS. Each of these chapters is structured to provide an overview of the literature, an evaluation of any relevant interventions and an 'in practice' section that provides some basic guidance for readers in terms of best practice when addressing the impact of a given condition. Finally, each chapter makes recommendations for future research in the given parental condition. What is notable about many of these conditions is their rapidly changing nature due to advances in medical science. Indeed, while life expectancy has increased throughout much of the world, so has the number of people with long-term conditions. Conditions that were until relatively recently regarded as experienced in the last years of life have now become illnesses that are experienced over many years and, in some cases, decades of life. For example, 50% of people diagnosed with cancer now live in excess of 10 years post-diagnosis (Cancer Research UK, 2011) and, as a result of antiretroviral treatment, HIV/AIDS is now considered a controllable, treatable chronic condition (Drewes et al., 2013). Such profound changes in disease trajectories are likely to have significant implications for children's adjustment. Rather than dealing with impending death and, ultimately, the loss of a parent, children now often face a very different set of challenges as treatment regimens change the nature of diseases from terminal to chronic, or even curable. Research has tended to highlight these medical breakthroughs, but they bring with them challenges, both for those with long-term illnesses and for those who live alongside them.

As the chapters clearly demonstrate, not all parental conditions have received the attention that their potential impact on children might warrant. Consequently, a further chapter focusing on such conditions, where initial but limited research has been conducted, is also presented. These include amyotrophic lateral sclerosis/motor neurone disease, arthritis, chronic back pain, chronic pain, epilepsy, inflammatory bowel disease, leprosy, obsessive-compulsive disorder, schizophrenia and spinal cord injury. Broader issues are subsequently introduced, including the issue of parental disclosure, with specific reference to HIV/AIDS. What is clear from the current literature is that how and when children are informed of the parental condition can have a significant bearing on their consequent adjustment (Qiao et al., 2013). A chapter advocating a family-centred approach to parental illness is also presented. Increasingly, family-centred approaches are recommended in a range of clinical environments and conditions (Kuo et al., 2012), and such an approach makes intuitive sense where parental illness enters the family unit. The chapter also introduces a new assessment tool, the Screening Instrument for Adolescents of Parents with Chronic Medical Condition, which has the potential for significant uptake in the field. The book closes with a chapter focusing on issues of assessing how parental illness impacts upon children. The principles of sound scientific measurement are discussed, along with a range of considerations in the development and administration of measurement tools. The final chapter includes an appendix with a brief outline of some commonly used measures that have been incorporated in the assessment of parental illness.

This book highlights the very different demands placed on children that can be caused by a variety of conditions and underlines the importance of research into this often neglected aspect of illness. The intention is not only to bring together research in the area and heighten awareness of the potential impact of parental illness on children, but also to stimulate further research efforts. Although the primary focus is children's responses to their parent's condition, the challenges of parenting, for both the affected and unaffected parent, are also frequently highlighted. Without question, parental illness is very much a 'family affair' and what will become apparent is that no individual member of the family unit should be viewed in isolation.

REFERENCES

ADASS, ADCS and The Children's Society. (2012). Working together to support young carers and their families. www.childrenssociety.org.uk/sites/default/files/tcs/report_hidden-from-view_young-carers_final.pdf (accessed November 2015).

Black, N., Jenkinson, C. (2009). Measuring patients' experiences and outcomes. *British Medical Journal*, 339, 202–205.

Cancer Research UK. (2011). www.cancerresearchuk.org/health-professional/cancer-statistics (accessed November 2015).

Drewes, J., Gusy, B., Rüden, Uv. (2013). More than 20 years of research into the quality of life of people with HIV and AIDS: A descriptive review of study characteristics and methodological approaches of published empirical studies. *Journal of the International Association of Providers of AIDS Care*, 12(1), 18–22.

Firth, P. (2006). Patients and their families. *Recent Results in Cancer Research*, 168, 61–71.

Kuo, D.Z., Houtrow, A.J., Arango, P., Kuhlthau, K.A., Simmons, J.M., Neff, J.M. (2012). Family-centered care: Current applications and future directions in pediatric health care. *Maternal and Child Health Journal*, 16(2), 297–305.

Morley, D., Dummett, S., Peters, M., Kelly, L., Hewitson, P., Dawson, J., Fitzpatrick, R., Jenkinson, C. (2012). Factors influencing quality of life in caregivers of people with Parkinson's disease and implications for clinical guidelines. *Parkinson's Disease*, 2012, 190901.

Qiao, S., Li, X., Stanton, B. (2013). Disclosure of parental HIV infection to children: A systematic review of global literature. *AIDS Behavior*, 17, 369–389.

CHAPTER 2

Parental multiple sclerosis

Kenneth Pakenham

INTRODUCTION

Multiple sclerosis (MS) is a chronic degenerative disease of the central nervous system and is the most common neurological disorder among young adults in the Western world (Leary et al., 2005). The aetiology of MS remains largely unknown, clinical symptoms vary widely (e.g. cognitive impairment, pain, sexual dysfunction, fatigue, loss of bowel or bladder control, mobility and visual impairments, and emotional changes). There is currently no cure and often only minimal symptomatic relief (Rao et al., 1992). MS is a complex illness with an unpredictable course that has profound physical and psychosocial impact on most, if not all, areas of a person's life. Not surprisingly, people with MS have a higher prevalence of emotional disorders relative to other patient groups with comparable degrees of physical disability, and report lower quality of life than community comparison groups (Pakenham, 2012). The onset of MS typically occurs between 20 and 40 years of age, a time of life often associated with establishing a family. MS also occurs in women more frequently than in men, and mothers commonly take on a greater role in caring for children. MS can cause impairment and disruption in many areas of family functioning, particularly parenting (Pakenham et al., 1997; Power, 1985). Understandably, many parents with MS are concerned about the impact of their illness on their children and report difficulties associated with parenting (e.g. Braham et al., 1975). Data suggests that some of these children are 'at risk' and that parents with MS and their children require targeted support.

THE CHALLENGES OF PARENTING WITH MS

Parenting tasks and roles can be disrupted by MS relapses and symptoms, particularly mood disturbance, cognitive impairment, fatigue and mobility problems. For example, mothers with MS and their children (6–20 years of age) have reported lower maternal physical affection during a relapse than when symptoms were stable (Deatrick et al., 1998). Limited mobility can cause difficulties in transporting children and participating in family activities. Fatigue is one of the most commonly reported MS symptoms (Pakenham, 2012). Given the energy demands of parenting, chronic fatigue can greatly limit child-rearing activities (Pakenham et al., 2012). Other parenting challenges include relinquishing parental tasks (e.g. meal preparation) to other family members, managing perceived stigma associated with being a 'disabled parent', being dependent on children and finding family activities that can accommodate MS-related disabilities (Kikuchi, 1987; Pakenham et al., 2012). The loss of full and consistent engagement in family activities is one of the most common and disconcerting difficulties reported by parents with MS (Pakenham et al., 2012). External stressors such as financial difficulties and lack of formal support can compound difficulties related to the disabilities produced by MS.

Given the parenting limitations that can occur with MS, in dual-parent households the 'healthy' parent often takes on additional parenting responsibilities. Both the parent with MS and the parent without MS offer important and unique parenting contributions (Steck et al., 2001). However, the increased parenting workload of 'healthy' parents presents a range of difficulties that are similar to those reported by the parent with MS (Pakenham et al., 2012).

Despite the challenges of parenting with MS, parents can develop compensatory strategies, access resources and strengthen family bonds that enable effective parenting. This is supported by evidence from a study of 145 parents with MS and 91 partners which found that, compared to norms, both the MS parent and the healthy partner were significantly higher in parenting efficacy, although lower in parenting satisfaction (Sturgess, 2012). In addition, healthy partners reported higher family cohesion and lower family conflict compared to norms. Both parents seek out and utilise an array of resources within the nuclear and extended family, formalised services and the broader community (Pakenham et al., 2012).

One of the most common family-level coping strategies for dealing with parental illness is the redistribution of roles among family members. Not only does the 'healthy' parent assume extra duties and tasks, but also the children. Power (1985) found that families with a parent with MS that exhibited a willingness to share household and caregiving responsibilities were more cohesive and functioned better than families in which all members did not contribute equally. While it might be expected that family members will work together and take on extra family responsibilities when a parent is ill, the extent to which children should assume more adult responsibilities and tasks is controversial. In single-parent and economically disadvantaged families, children are more likely to take on higher levels of family responsibilities because of the absence of another parent and a lack of financial resources to access services.

YOUTH CAREGIVING

Children of parents with MS often take on a range of family caregiving tasks and responsibilities. Although a degree of caregiving during childhood is normative and is in fact valued and encouraged as part of the developmental process, the level of caregiving undertaken by children of parents with a serious medical condition is sometimes exaggerated and may not be congruent with their age and level of maturity. This is particularly the case for some children of a parent with MS. Several studies show that on average these children undertake higher levels of family responsibilities and caregiving tasks than children of 'healthy' parents (Pakenham and Bursnall, 2006; Yahav et al., 2005).

Some researchers have conceptualised the caring roles among children in the context of parental illness as 'parentification' or a pathological role reversal (Chase, 1999). Although extensive role reversal may occur in extreme cases, for most families caring does not mean children internalise the same sense of accountability that parents have for their children's welfare. Parent-child relationships are reciprocal and interdependent by nature, and regardless of some role adaptation, children report viewing their parents as parents. Youth caregiving may be more accurately conceptualised as a form of functional adaptive coping in the context of adversity rather than a pathological role reversal.

The caregiving tasks undertaken by children of a parent with MS have been assessed by the Youth Activities of Caregiving Scale (YACS; Ireland and Pakenham, 2010), and have been shown to fall into four broad categories: instrumental (e.g. paying bills and managing money), social-emotional (e.g. keeping the parent happy, safe and occupied), personal-intimate (e.g. assisting with toileting and dressing) and domestic-household care (e.g. preparing meals and shopping) (Pakenham and Cox, 2012a). These represent the core domains of young caregiving in the general literature (Pakenham, 2009). Interestingly, there are relatively high levels of agreement between the child's reports of their caregiving activities and the reports of both the parent with

MS and the 'healthy' parent regarding the child's caregiving (Pakenham and Cox, 2012a). The corroboration of child caregiving activities by parents provides important validation of the care and support provided by children in the context of parental MS.

Qualitative and quantitative studies suggest that, as with adult caregiving (Pakenham, 2005), youth caregiving is associated with both costs and rewards. Potential costs associated with youth caregiving include isolation, restrictions on school, social and recreational activities, stress and psychological problems (e.g. Pakenham and Bursnall, 2006; Pakenham and Cox, 2012a; Turpin et al., 2008). One study showed that higher levels of instrumental care and social-emotional care were the strongest predictors of poorer youth adjustment over a 12-month period (Pakenham and Cox, 2012a).

The rewards associated with youth caregiving include self-perceived maturity, increased confidence in caring and strengthened relationships (Pakenham et al., 2006; Pakenham et al., 2007). Interestingly, the personal-intimate care dimension of youth caregiving was found to be associated with better youth adjustment over 12 months (Pakenham and Cox, 2012a). This link may be due to the selection of better-adjusted children to undertake personal-intimate caregiving. It is also possible that providing personal care strengthens attachment between parent and child and involves personally rewarding care tasks (Ireland and Pakenham, 2010). Although this research showed that the effects of each caregiving dimension on youth adjustment varied, when scores across all the dimensions were summed, a higher overall caregiving load was predictive of poorer youth adjustment (Pakenham and Cox, 2012a).

As might be expected, greater youth caregiving is associated with higher levels of parental MS disability, disease severity, unpredictable symptoms and parental mental health problems, and less choice in caregiving (Pakenham and Bursnall, 2006; Pakenham and Cox, 2012a). In addition, consistent with findings from the broader youth caregiving literature, girls tend to report higher levels of caregiving than boys (e.g. Pakenham and Cox, 2012a). However, the few studies that have examined youth caregiving in the context of parental MS have not used other parental illness comparison groups, so it is not clear whether these patterns of findings are specific to MS.

EFFECTS OF PARENTAL MS ON CHILDREN

A common methodology used to determine the extent to which children of a parent with MS are at greater risk for mental health problems than children of 'healthy' parents is to compare such children with peers who have healthy parents, or with norms. A meta-analysis of such studies concluded that children of chronically ill parents were at risk for elevated internalising and externalising behaviour problems (Sieh et al., 2010). However, overall the effect sizes were small, suggesting that while parental illness is associated with poorer youth adjustment, it does not appear to be the main explanatory variable of such outcomes. A recent large-scale population-based study, which addressed some of the methodological problems of prior comparison studies, also found that children of a parent with a chronic medical condition were at greater risk for mental health problems than their peers with 'healthy' parents were (Pakenham and Cox, 2014a). However, consistent with the meta-analysis, effects sizes were small. This study also showed that children in a family with a non-parent ill family member present were at greater risk of mental health problems compared to their peers from 'healthy' families. The adverse effects of family illness remained after accounting for type of illness (physical illness, mental illness and alcohol/drug problems), demographics and youth caregiving responsibilities. Overall, findings showed that the risk for youth mental health difficulties increases with the addition of the following factors: presence of an ill parent (vs an ill non-parent family member), mental illness or a substance misuse problem (relative to family physical illness), elevated youth caregiving responsibilities and a range of demographics (e.g. single-parent household and reduced access to services).

There are two reviews of research on the effects of parental MS on children (Bogosian et al., 2010; Razaz et al., 2014). Both reviews included quantitative predictive and comparison studies, and qualitative research. Bogosian et al. (2010) concluded that parental MS has a negative impact on children. However, authors of the second, more recent, review were more circumspect about the potential adverse effects of parental MS, because of the poor quality of the studies, mixed findings and evidence of positive effects. Examination of the studies that have compared children of a parent with MS to children who have 'healthy' parents or norms shows that there are few such studies, and none of the comparison studies reviewed by these authors were published in the past five years. These studies also suffered a range of methodological limitations including small samples, and lack of control of the effects of potentially important confounding background variables (e.g. dual vs single parent, family size, and the presence of other ill family members).

A recent comparison study addressed many of the limitations of these studies and compared 126 children of a parent with MS to a matched control group of children from healthy parents where no other family member had an illness (Pakenham and Cox, 2014b). The control group was matched on eight demographics. Overall, results from this study did not support prior research findings, suggesting pervasive marked adverse impact of parental

MS on youth. Results showed that, compared to youth from healthy families, youth of a parent with MS did not report greater problems with respect to health, somatisation, prosocial behaviour, behavioural-social difficulties, caregiving experiences, attachment and family functioning. Comparisons within two developmental age ranges showed that there was a trend for pre-adolescents of a parent with MS to report more problems than adolescents, relative to their respective control participants. In fact, adolescents reported lower peer relationship problems than control adolescents reported, suggesting a positive impact of parental MS on youth in this age group.

The absence of marked adverse impact of parental MS was also evident in a retrospective population-based study of developmental outcomes in five-year-old children of a parent with MS (Razaz et al., 2015). Children of a parent with MS did not differ on developmental outcomes from children of unaffected parents. However, in the experimental group, children of parents with mental health morbidity, and those with longer duration of exposure to parental MS, were at higher risk for early childhood developmental vulnerability in the social and physical health domains, respectively. Although these two recent studies showed no marked adverse effects of parental MS on children, compared to peers with healthy parents, it should be noted that comparisons were based on group means and conceal those few children who have elevated mental health problems and/or who are at risk of future psychological morbidity. The challenge for researchers is to identify the characteristics that will enable identification of these at-risk children.

There are several explanations that may account for the overall lack of differences between children of a parent with MS and their peers with healthy parents evident in these two recent studies and several prior studies (De Judicibus and McCabe, 2004; Steck et al., 2007). It is possible that compensatory strategies and resources at the individual youth and family levels may mitigate the adverse effects of MS on family, such that youth of a parent with MS become indistinguishable from youth with healthy parents. Regarding family coping in response to illness, family members can pull together to provide support, thereby becoming more cohesive (Rolland, 1999). In addition, parents with MS and their partners access a wide range of parenting resources (Pakenham et al., 2012) and develop parenting strategies to manage difficulties (Parker White et al., 2009). At the individual youth level, children have been shown to rely on numerous adaptive coping strategies and resources that serve as protective factors in the context of dealing with parental MS (Pakenham and Bursnall, 2006). The benefits of these protective individual and family processes are evident in both parent (Mazur, 2008) and youth (Pakenham and Bursnall, 2006) reports of the positive aspects of parental MS.

Another explanation is the recent developments in the treatment and management of MS, and in the services for children and families affected by MS. Findings support the view that with relevant resources and support, parental disability and/or illness in and of itself need not present a significant risk factor for youth (Blackford, 1999).

Although the focus of prior research has been on the adverse impact of parental MS on children, a theme of co-occurring positive impact has also emerged in many studies. Much of the positive impact appears to be associated with the rewards of taking on extra caregiving tasks and responsibilities, as mentioned above. Children of parents with MS have reported a wide range of benefits associated with supporting a parent with MS that are similar to those reported by adult MS caregivers (Pakenham and Bursnall, 2006). Commonly reported benefits include the skills and competencies that are developed through having to take on extra family responsibilities, and the sense of pride associated with undertaking these duties (Bogosian et al., 2011; Turpin et al., 2008). Caregiving is profoundly interpersonal, hence the relationship benefits of caregiving are frequently reported by youth. For example, strengthened family relationships and increased understanding of others with disability are frequently reported interpersonal benefits.

A FRAMEWORK FOR UNDERSTANDING THE EFFECTS OF PARENTAL MS ON CHILDREN

Much of the research on the effects of parental illness on children is descriptive and atheoretical and the parental MS field is no exception. The development of a framework that explains the effects of parental illness on children is essential, as it can identify the risk and protective processes that shape child adjustment, which will, in turn, directly inform the development of interventions and services that target them. There are several general theories that are relevant to understanding the effects of parental illness on children, including: parentification (mentioned above), stress and coping theory (Lazarus and Folkman, 1984), family systems theory (Rolland, 1999) and attachment theory (Bowlby, 1969). However, none of these theories have been comprehensively developed as frameworks that explain the mechanisms by which parental illness shapes child and family functioning and that can integrate the accumulated evidence in the field.

A framework that has been developed specifically to integrate findings in this field and to explain the effects of parental illness on children is the Family Ecology Framework (FEF; Pedersen and Revenson, 2005). This framework shows most promise and draws on some of the aforementioned theories relevant to this field, including general systems theory, human ecology, and stress and coping theory. The FEF describes a set of *mediating processes* and *buffering mechanisms* linking parental illness to youth and family functioning.

Regarding the *mediating processes*, the FEF proposes that parental illness affects youth and family functioning indirectly through four responses the child has to parental illness: an increase in caregiving duties undertaken by children as a result of redistribution of family roles due to parental illness; perceptions of stigma related to the parental illness; an increase in daily difficulties as routines are disrupted; and, most centrally, an increase in perceived stress. These four responses then affect youth and family functioning.

These pathways can also be affected by *buffering mechanisms*. Buffering mechanisms are hypothesised to ameliorate both the development of a youth stress response, and its negative effects on youth and family functioning. While some of the potential buffering mechanisms are not amenable to intervention, such as parent's gender, access to care, youth developmental stage and cultural norms, others are more malleable, such as children's coping strategies and social support.

Pakenham and Cox (2012b) found support for the application of the model in explaining youth adjustment and family functioning in families affected by parental MS over a 12-month interval. The study measured two aspects of MS-related disability: physical disability and depression. Depression was conceptualised as a potential dimension of parental MS-related disability because the lifetime prevalence rate for depression in MS is 50% (Siegert and Abernathy, 2005) and up to 59% of MS parents report depression (Steck et al., 2007). Furthermore, parental depression can exacerbate illness-related disability and interfere with parental functioning (Armistead et al., 1995), and there is evidence linking higher depression in parents with MS and poorer youth adjustment (De Judicibus and McCabe, 2004; Diareme et al., 2006; Steck et al., 2007). Parental disability was assessed at Time 1 and youth caregiving, youth stress, stigma, family functioning and youth well-being were assessed 12 months later, at Time 2 (Pakenham and Cox, 2012b). Results of structural equation modelling showed that, consistent with the model, youth caregiving, youth stress and stigma mediated the effects of parental MS physical disability on family functioning and youth well-being. However, parental depression was not mediated through the same processes; rather, parental depression directly affected family functioning, which, in turn, mediated the effects onto youth well-being. This research provides preliminary support for the utility of the FEF in explaining how parental MS affects youth and family functioning.

Youth coping strategies and social support are two important malleable potential buffering variables that were not examined in this study. However, several studies that have examined the relations between these variables and youth adjustment to parental illness suggest that better youth adjustment is associated with higher social support, less reliance on avoidant coping and greater reliance on problem-focused coping (e.g. Compas et al., 1996; Langrock et al., 2002; Pakenham and Bursnall, 2006). There is also a range of contextual variables that have been examined in other studies that have been shown to be associated with youth adjustment to parental MS and should be included in the FEF, including: choice in caregiving, parental illness unpredictability, single-parent family and multiple family members with illness (De Judicibus and McCabe, 2004; Pakenham and Bursnal, 2006; Pakenham and Cox, 2012a, 2012b). Future research testing the FEF should include a wider range of potential mediating and buffering variables, including social support, coping strategies and pertinent contextual variables.

INTERVENTIONS

Research on interventions to assist families, especially children, affected by MS is lacking. A review of interventions for children of a parent with MS identified two published interventions, but only one was evaluated (Horner, 2013). Coles, Pakenham and Leech (2007) developed an intervention for children of a parent with MS that employed primarily psycho-education about MS and cognitive and behaviour therapy strategies for targeting risk and protective factors identified within stress and coping theory: social support, appraisal and coping strategies. The manual-based intervention was called 'Fun in the Sun' and took the form of a six-day camp for children aged 9–14 years. Parents were provided with the same resources given to the children. Twenty children and their parents with MS participated. Children completed questionnaires at pre- and post-intervention and at a three-month follow-up, and parents completed questionnaires at pre-intervention and follow-up. Both quantitative and qualitative data were used to examine intervention efficacy.

The programme involved both recreational activities and eight half-hour group sessions providing education about MS, opportunities to share experiences within a supportive environment and training in coping strategies and life skills. The theme of each session is summarised as follows: Session 1 – getting to know each other; Session 2 – information on MS; Session 3 – enhancing awareness of feelings related to having a parent with MS; Session 4 – communication skills; Session 5 – cognitive restructuring; Session 6 – problem solving; Session 7 – coping with emotions; Session 8 – review and focus on personal strengths.

Results showed that after the intervention, children reported decreases in distress, stress appraisals and adverse caregiving experiences, and increases in social support and knowledge of MS. Parental data confirmed the significant increase in the children's knowledge of MS. Qualitative data showed that the intervention had indirect effects on some parents and families.

Providing information to children is important because without accurate and sufficient information they may develop inaccurate understandings of MS. For example, children have reported that they are in part responsible for their parent's MS and its progress. Some believe that their parent may die of MS (Cross and Rintell, 1999). Many MS symptoms are invisible and are very difficult for children to understand (e.g. fatigue and cognitive impairment). There is some evidence suggesting that children who are not adequately informed about their parent's MS are more at risk of developing problems (Paliokosta et al., 2009). However, there is a lack of data offering guidelines on 'how', 'what', 'how much' and 'when' to provide information. Mutch (2005) reported on the setting up of a series of information giving workshops for children of parents with MS aged 9–14 years; however, these were not evaluated.

IN PRACTICE

Best practice guiding principles for meeting the needs of children affected by parental MS should be enshrined in the clinical guidelines for managing MS. For example, in the UK the National Institute for Clinical Excellence guidelines for the management of MS includes guidance on meeting the needs of children who have a parent with MS. However, the extent to which such guidance is included in the national guidelines for managing MS varies across countries.

It should be noted that the majority of children of a parent with MS adjust relatively well. In most families, members pull together to meet the demands of parental MS. As documented above, there are many resources at the individual, family and community levels that can be accessed to empower family members to cope with the changing impact of parental MS. Providing assistance to families affected by MS should be guided by an empowerment framework; strengths and resources of families should be identified and built on and difficulties should be assessed and targeted where warranted. When intervention is necessary, it should be delivered in a way that respects the family and individual members and that draws on family resources.

Providing information is a fundamental first step in assisting families affected by MS. Healthcare professionals need to consider the information needs not only of the person with MS, but also of family members, including children. Age-appropriate information about MS and available support for children should be made available. However, giving information on MS can be confronting and frightening for children, so information should be delivered according to the needs of the child, the family context and the nature of the parent's MS. In this regard, information may best be delivered to children by parents, who can use their intimate knowledge of their child and the family to tailor the information giving. If the parent with MS has some cognitive impairment it may be preferable for the partner to deliver information on MS, or if it is a single-parent family, a healthcare professional and the parent who has MS may be better placed to provide the information together. Information giving is seldom a one-off event; parents need to be encouraged to provide information on MS consistent with the evolving developmental needs of the child and changes in the parent's MS. Provision of information by parents to children may be augmented by information from other sources (e.g. online information packages, booklets) via MS community organisations or other relevant services.

Healthcare professionals should routinely collect information regarding the parenting status of MS patients, so as to identify potential parenting, child and family needs. Parents with MS and their partners should be interviewed to screen for factors that may indicate the risk or presence of adjustment difficulties in the children. Risk factors that have been identified include: substantial youth caregiving responsibilities, less choice in opting to engage in caregiving, single-parent family, parental mental health problems (particularly depression) and the presence of multiple illnesses in the family.

Given the challenges confronting children in the context of parental MS, coping skills training interventions should be offered to children by MS community organisations or other relevant services. These interventions should provide information on MS and training in adaptive coping strategies, such as the one developed by Coles et al. (2006), which used cognitive and behaviour strategies to target key risk and protective factors.

Peer-support programmes such as support groups, camps, and mentoring and buddy systems can be helpful, particularly for those children who feel isolated and who are at risk. Audiovisual recordings of children talking about their experiences of coping with parental MS could be made available to other children facing similar difficulties. Children who have marked adjustment difficulties should be encouraged to seek counselling services. Other services that may assist children depending on individualised assessed needs include respite care and financial recognition and remuneration for caregiving. Some children may be eligible to receive 'young carer' services and support. Eligibility and availability of young carer services vary across countries. Children need to be represented and consulted about how the above-mentioned programmes and services are designed and delivered to ensure that they are responsive to children's needs.

For child-directed support and services to be optimised, they need to occur as part of a wider programme of support for the parent, and not in isolation. For example, flexible alternative care and support for parents with MS are necessary to lessen the load placed on children. For instance, regular home visits by nurses to assist the parent with MS with administering medication and personal hygiene will relieve the child from having to undertake such responsibilities. In general, there is growing recognition of the importance of a 'whole-family approach' in meeting the needs of children and the family member with care needs. A whole-family approach should underpin both service delivery and policy development to ensure the welfare of families affected by MS. Clinical management and community organisation protocols need to articulate clearly the engagement and involvement of the whole family.

RECOMMENDATIONS FOR FUTURE RESEARCH

In general, much of the research on children of a parent with MS is descriptive and atheoretical and many of the studies suffer from methodological weaknesses; hence the research agenda is broad. To further research and practice in this area, research developments are required with respect to theory testing, comparative research methodologies, measure development and intervention development and evaluation. Most of the research in this field is cross-sectional. Longitudinal research designs that track children and families over time are essential.

There is little data that reliably points to the most potent variables and processes that shape youth adjustment to parental MS over time. Developing and testing frameworks that explain the processes by which parental illness affects children is essential for the development of targeted interventions and services. As mentioned above, the FEF holds promise in this regard. Such a framework should be able to integrate the limited knowledge we have on the variables likely to shape youth adjustment and specify other, untested variables and processes.

In order to understand better the effects of parental MS on children, methodologically stronger studies (as specified above) that compare children of parents with MS to children of healthy parents and parents with other illnesses are required. For example, one study compared adolescent and adult children of a parent with MS to youth of a parent with Parkinson's disease and found that the two groups did not differ on the impact of parental illness (Morley et al., 2011). Similar studies are necessary to determine whether the effects of parental MS differ from those of other parental illnesses and the effects of parenting by healthy parents. Studies also need to investigate whether the effects of parental MS differ from the effects of having a non-parent family member with MS.

Given the dearth of intervention research in this area, studies that develop and test interventions for children of parents with MS are critical. The research agenda for intervention research in this area is wide. In view of the burgeoning literature on 'third-wave' cognitive and behaviour therapies, innovative interventions based on these more recent intervention trends need to be explored. Acceptance and Commitment therapy (ACT; Hayes et al., 2011) is one of the most widely researched 'third-wave' cognitive and behaviour therapies and has been shown to be effective in helping people cope with chronic illness (Hayes et al., 2006). ACT is based on mindfulness and acceptance processes which have been shown to be related to better adjustment outcomes for people with MS and their partners (Pakenham and Samios, 2013). ACT has also been effective in reducing mental health difficulties in youth (Livheim et al., 2015). At the core of ACT is fostering psychological flexibility. Put simply, this involves the acceptance of things that cannot be changed or controlled (e.g. parental illness and cognitive and emotional reaction to it), while at the same time modifying what can be changed (e.g. altering a homework routine), actively pursuing life values (e.g. engaging in a cherished hobby) and focusing on the present moment. Psychological flexibility is a cornerstone of mental health. ACT offers six evidence-based therapeutic processes for fostering psychological flexibility. Using ACT to enhance psychological flexibility in children coping with parental MS seems a promising research path.

The development of measures that are sensitive to the context of children coping with parental illness is necessary. Some progress has been made in this area with the development of measures of youth caregiving experiences, youth caregiving tasks, parental illness unpredictability and young carer benefit finding, all of which have been applied to children of a parent with MS (Cox and Pakenham, 2014; Morley et al., 2010; Pakenham and Bursnall, 2006; Pakenham and Cox, 2012b, 2014b). However, these measures have been only recently developed and require further testing and refinement. In addition, objective measures of child adjustment need to be developed.

Few studies have examined children at specific development stages. Given that biological, psychological and social issues differ across the developmental stages of childhood, research needs to explore whether the effects of parental MS varies across early, middle and late childhood phases.

Given that MS affects all family members, more research is required that includes data from multiple sources (parent with MS, healthy partner and children). Analytic approaches that can incorporate data from multiple sources will more effectively tap the family and interpersonal processes and context in which family members cope with MS.

Youth caregiving appears to play a central role in shaping youth adjustment to parental MS. However, it has emerged as a poorly conceptualised amorphous construct. A recent refinement of the conceptualisation of youth caregiving proposes that it is a tripartite construct comprising youth caregiving tasks, caregiving responsibilities and caregiving experiences (Pakenham and Cox, 2015). *Caregiving tasks* refer to the specific caregiving activities that youth undertake (e.g. shopping, cleaning). *Caregiving responsibilities* refers to the psychological sense of duty or responsibility related to roles involved in contributing to family functioning. A range of emotional, behavioural and social experiences emerge from taking on caregiving and are collectively labelled *caregiving experiences* (e.g. activity restrictions, isolation). To date the tripartite conceptualisation of youth caregiving has not been fully tested, nor included in a broader framework such as the FEF. Only individual subcomponents have been examined, with mixed samples and children of a parent with MS (e.g. Pakenham and Cox, 2012a, 2014a, 2014b). Future research needs to test this new conceptualisation of youth caregiving by examining both the individual and joint effects of each component within a broader framework (e.g. the FEF), and further refining the measures developed to assess these components.

CONCLUSION

Although parental MS poses many challenges to children, the process of coping with such difficulties should not be unduly pathologised. Life presents many unexpected and unwanted hardships that cannot be controlled; parental illness is one such life adversity. Most children demonstrate resilience and flexibility in adjusting to the difficulties associated with parental MS. Coping with parental MS involves dealing with many unpredictable and fluctuating challenges. It offers the potential to build skills, stimulate new perspectives and self-awareness, and foster resilience; facing challenges and taking risks can generate growth. Theory-testing research is required to identify the risk and protective factors and processes that shape youth adjustment to parental MS. Such research will help to identify the minority of children who are at risk for mental health problems, in addition to the processes and factors that should be targeted by interventions to help empower children to flourish in the face of adversity. Children who have a parent with MS are embedded in a family network, and research, services and interventions should be sensitive to the family context. Recognition of the needs of children who have parents with a serious health condition such as MS should be included in relevant government carer policies and in clinical practice guidelines.

REFERENCES

Armistead, L., Klein, K., Forehand, R. (1995). Parental physical illness and child functioning. *Clinical Psychology Review*, 15(5), 409–422.

Blackford, K.A. (1999). A child's growing up with a parent who has multiple sclerosis: Theories and experiences. *Disability and Society*, 14, 673–685.

Bogosian, A., Moss-Morris, R., Hadwin, J. (2010). Psychosocial adjustment in children and adolescents with a parent with multiple sclerosis: A systematic review. *Clinical Rehabilitation*, 24, 789–801.

Bogosian, A., Moss-Morris, R., Bishop, F.L., Hadwin, J. (2011). How do adolescents adjust to their parent's multiple sclerosis? An interview study. *British Journal of Health Psychology*, 16, 430–444.

Bowlby, J. (1969). *Attachment and loss, Vol. I: Attachment*. Middlesex: Penguin Books.

Braham, S., Houser, H.B., Cline, A., Posner, M. (1975). Evaluation of the social needs of non-hospitalized chronically ill persons: 1. Study of 47 patients with multiple sclerosis. *Journal of Chronic Diseases*, 28, 401–419.

Chase, N.D. (1999). *Burdened children: Theory, research, and treatment of parentification*. Thousand Oaks, CA: Sage.

Coles, A.R., Pakenham, K.I., Leech, C. (2007). Evaluation of an intensive psychosocial intervention for children of parents with multiple sclerosis. *Rehabilitation Psychology*, 52(2), 133–142.

Compas, B.E, Worsham, N.L., Ey, S., Howell, D.C. (1996). When Mom or Dad has cancer: II. Coping, cognitive appraisals, and psychological distress in children of cancer patients. *Health Psychology*, 15(3), 167–175.

Cox, S., Pakenham, K.I. (2014). Confirmatory factor analysis and invariance testing of the Young Carer of Parents Inventory (YCOPI). *Rehabilitation Psychology*, 59, 439–452.

Cross, T., Rintell, D. (1999). Children's perceptions of parental multiple sclerosis. *Psychology, Health and Medicine*, 4, 355–359.

De Judicibus, M.A., McCabe, M.P. (2004). The impact of parental multiple sclerosis on the adjustment of children and adolescents. *Adolescence*, 39, 551–569.

Deatrick, J.A., Brennan, D., Cameron, M.E. (1998). Mothers with multiple sclerosis and their children: Effects of fatigue and exacerbations on maternal support. *Nursing Research*, 47, 205–210.

Diareme, S., Tsiantis, J., Kolaitis, G., Ferentinos, S., Tsalamanios, E., Paliokosta, E., Anasontzi, S., Lympinaki, E., Anagnostopoulos, D., Voumvourakis, C., Romer, G. (2006). Emotional and behavioural difficulties in children of parents with multiple sclerosis: A controlled study in Greece. *European Child and Adolescent Psychiatry*, 15, 309–318.

Hayes, S.C., Luoma, J.B., Bond, F.W., Masuda, A., Lillis, J. (2006). Acceptance and commitment therapy: Model, processes and outcomes. *Behaviour Research and Therapy*, 44, 1–25.

Hayes, S.C., Strosahl, K.D., Wilson, K.G. (2012). Acceptance and commitment therapy: The process and practice of mindful change (2nd edn). New York: Guilford Press.

Horner, R. (2013). Interventions for children coping with parental multiple sclerosis: A systematic review. *Journal of the American Association of Nurse Practitioners*, 25, 309–313.

Ireland, M., Pakenham, K.I. (2010). The nature of young caregiving in families experiencing chronic illness/disability: Development of the Youth Activities of Caregiving Scale (YACS). *Psychology and Health*, 25, 713–731.

Kikuchi, J.F. (1987). The reported quality of life of children and adolescents of parents with multiple sclerosis. *Recent Advances in Nursing*, 16, 163–191.

Langrock, A.M., Compas, B.E, Keller, G., Merchant, M.J., Copeland, M.E. (2002). Coping with the stress of parental depression: Parent's reports of children's coping, emotional, and behavioral problems. *Journal of Clinical Child and Adolescent Psychology*, 31(3), 312–324.

Lazarus, R.S., Folkman, S. (1984). *Stress, appraisal, and coping*. New York: Springer.

Leary, S.M., Porter, B., Thompson, A.J. (2005). Multiple sclerosis: Diagnosis and the management of acute relapses. *Postgraduate Medical Journal*, 81, 302–308.

Livheim, F., Hayes, L., Ghaderi, A., Magnusdottir, T., Högfeldt, A., Rowse, J., Turner, S., Hayes, S.C., Tengström, A. (2015). The effectiveness of acceptance and commitment therapy for adolescent mental health: Swedish and Australian pilot outcomes. *Journal of Child and Family Studies*, 24(4), 1016–1030.

Mazur, E. (2008). Negative and positive disability-related events and adjustment of parents with acquired physical disabilities and their adolescent children. *Journal of Child and Family Studies*, 17, 517–537.

Morley, D., Selai, C., Schrag, A., Thompson, A.J., Jahanshahi, M. (2010). Refinement and validation of the Parental Illness Impact Scale, *Parkinsonism and Related Disorders*, 16, 181–185.

Morley, D., Selai, C., Schrag, A., Jahanshahi, M., Thompson, A.J. (2011). Adolescent and adult children of parents with Parkinson's disease: Incorporating their needs in clinical guidelines. *Parkinson's Disease*, 2011, 951874.

Mutch, K. (2005). Information for young people when multiple sclerosis enters the family. *British Journal of Nursing*, 14, 758–760.

Pakenham, K.I. (2005). The positive impact of multiple sclerosis (MS) on carers: Associations between carer benefit finding and positive and negative adjustment domains. *Disability and Rehabilitation*, 27(17), 985–997.

Pakenham, K.I. (2009). Children who care for their parents: The impact of disability on young lives. In C.A. Marshall, E. Kendall, M. Banks, R.M.S. Gover (Eds) *Disability: Insights from across fields and around the world, Vol. II* (pp. 39–60). Westport, CT: Praeger Press.

Pakenham, K.I. (2012). Multiple sclerosis. In P. Kennedy (Ed.), *The Oxford handbook of rehabilitation psychology* (pp. 211–234). New York: Oxford University Press.

Pakenham, K.I., Bursnall, S. (2006). Relations between social support, appraisal and coping and both positive and negative outcomes for children of a parent with multiple sclerosis and comparisons with children of healthy parents. *Clinical Rehabilitation*, 20, 709–723.

Pakenham, K.I., Cox, S. (2012a). The nature of caregiving in children of a parent with multiple sclerosis from multiple sources and the associations between caregiving activities and youth adjustment outcomes. *Psychology and Health*, 27(3), 324–346.

Pakenham, K.I., Cox, S. (2012b). Test of a model of the effects of parental illness on youth and family functioning. *Health Psychology*, 31(5), 580–590.

Pakenham, K.I., Cox, S. (2014a). The effects of parental illness and other ill family members on the adjustment of children. *Annals of Behavioral Medicine*, 48, 424–437.

Pakenham K.I., Cox, S. (2014b). Comparisons between youth of a parent with MS and a control group on adjustment, caregiving, attachment and family functioning. *Psychology and Health*, 29(1), 1–15.

Pakenham K.I., Cox, S. (2015). The effects of parental illness and other ill family members on youth caregiving experiences. *Psychology and Health*, 30(7), 857–878.

Pakenham, K.I., Samios, C. (2013). Couples coping with multiple sclerosis: A dyadic perspective on the roles of mindfulness and acceptance. *Journal of Behavioral Medicine*, 36, 389–400.

Pakenham, K.I., Stewart, C.A., Rogers, A. (1997). The role of coping in adjustment to multiple sclerosis-related adaptive demands. *Psychology, Health and Medicine*, 2, 197–211.

Pakenham, K.I., Bursnall, S., Chiu, J., Cannon, T., Okochi, M. (2006). The psychosocial impact of caregiving on young people who have a parent with an illness or disability: Comparisons between young caregivers and non-caregivers. *Rehabilitation Psychology*, 51, 113–126.

Pakenham, K.I., Chiu, J., Bursnall, S., Cannon, T. (2007). Relations between social support, appraisal and coping and both positive and negative outcomes in young carers. *Journal of Health Psychology*, 12, 89–102.

Pakenham, K.I., Tilling, J., Cretchley, J. (2012). Parenting difficulties and resources: The perspectives of parents with multiple sclerosis and their partners. *Rehabilitation Psychology*, 57(1), 52–60.

Paliokosta, E., Diareme, S., Kolaitis, G., Ferentinos, S., Lympinaki, E., Tsiantis, J., Romer, G., Karageorgiou C., Tsiantis A., Anasontzi S., Tsalamanios, E. (2009). Breaking bad news: Communication around parental multiple sclerosis. *Families, Systems and Health*, 27, 64–76.

Parker White, C., White, M.B., Fox, M.A. (2009). Maternal fatigue and its relationship to the caregiving environment. *Families, Systems and Health*, 27, 325–345.

Pedersen, S., Revenson, T.A. (2005). Parental illness, family functioning, and adolescent well-being: A family ecology framework to guide research. *Journal of Family Psychology*, 19(3), 404–409.

Power, P.W. (1985). Family coping behaviors in chronic illness: A rehabilitation approach. *Rehabilitation Literature*, 46, 78–83.

Rao, S.M., Huber S.J., Bornstein R.A. (1992). Emotional changes with multiple sclerosis and Parkinson's disease. *Journal of Consulting and Clinical Psychology*, 60, 369–378.

Razaz, N., Nourian, R., Marie R.A., Boyce W.T., Tremlett, H. (2014). Children and adolescents adjustment to parental multiple sclerosis: A systematic review. *BMC Neurology*, 14: 107.

Razaz, N., Tremlett, H., Boyce W.T., Guhn, M., Joseph, K.S., Marie, R.A. (2015). Impact of parental multiple sclerosis on childhood development: A retrospective cohort study. *Multiple Sclerosis Journal*, 21(9), 1172–1183.

Rolland, J.S. (1999). Parental illness and disability: A family systems framework. *Journal of Family Therapy*, 21, 242–266.

Siegert, R.J., Abernathy, D.A. (2005). Depression in multiple sclerosis: A review. *Journal of Neurology, Neurosurgery and Psychiatry*, 76, 469–475.

Sieh, D.S., Meijer, A.M., Oort, F.J., Visser-Meily, J.M.A., Van der Leij, D.A.V. (2010). Problem behavior in children of chronically ill parents: A meta-analysis. *Clinical Child and Family Psychology Review*, 13, 384–397.

Steck, B., Amsler, F., Kappos, L., Burgin, D. (2001). Gender-specific differences in the process of coping in families with a parent affected by a chronic somatic disease (e.g. multiple sclerosis). *Psychopathology*, 34, 236–244.

Steck, B., Grether, A., Amsler, F., Dillier, A.S., Schwald, A., Romer, G., Kappos L., Bürgin, D. (2007). Disease variables and depression affecting the process of coping in families with a somatically ill parent. *Psychopathology*, 40, 394–404.

Sturgess, N. (2012). Associations between disability and parenting outcomes and the moderating effects of marital adjustment in parents with multiple sclerosis and their partners. *Unpublished Doctoral Dissertation*, The University of Queensland, Brisbane, Australia.

Turpin, M., Leech, C., Hackenberg, L. (2008). Living with parental multiple sclerosis: Children's experience and clinical implications. *Canadian Journal of Occupational Therapy*, 75, 149–156.

Yahav, R., Vosburgh, J., Miller, A. (2005). Emotional responses of children and adolescents to parents with multiple sclerosis. *Multiple Sclerosis*, 11, 464–468.

CHAPTER 3

Parental Parkinson's disease

David Morley and Elaine Book

INTRODUCTION

This chapter details the emerging body of work focusing on the impact of parental Parkinson's disease (PD). PD is a chronic progressive condition characterised by tremor, bradykinesia and rigidity (Schapira, 1999). People with Parkinson's (PwP) are susceptible to psychiatric symptoms such as depression, hallucinations and confusion, as well as the likelihood of falls and freezing of gait as the condition progresses (Bloem et al., 2004). Although PD is commonly regarded as a disease of the elderly, a significant number are diagnosed before the age of 50 and in approximately 5–10% the condition is apparent prior to age 40 (Clarke and Moore, 2007). There is, therefore, the potential for children of a range of ages, from young to adult, to be affected in a variety of ways by their parent's condition.

The small evidence base to date will be reviewed and practical recommendations will be made regarding approaches to help children adjust to their parent's Parkinson's. As this is a relatively new field of investigation, the chapter will give significant space to highlighting future research requirements. Elements of the chapter have previously been discussed by Morley (2011) and Morley and Jenkinson (2013), discussions that are updated and further developed here.

LITERATURE REVIEW

Initial qualitative research

A study commissioned by the largest PD support charity in the United

Kingdom, the Parkinson's Disease Society (now Parkinson's UK), was conducted by Grimshaw in 1991. This was the first study to focus explicitly on children of parents with Parkinson's disease. As the first of its kind, the importance of this work should not be underestimated, particularly in light of its being a catalyst for later research. In his research Grimshaw took a qualitative approach and focused on the perspectives of pre-adolescent children aged 5–12, and young people aged 16–24. Data was collected through case studies of 10 families who participated in semi-structured interviews. The study aimed to gain a greater understanding of the processes through which parents and children react to change and then develop new ways of living. Importance was attached to concentrating not solely on the negative experiences of children, but also on displaying how their experiences and perceptions uncover a variety of issues that have been confronted – some successfully, others less so.

Grimshaw's final report highlighted a number of relevant issues for children confronted by parental Parkinson's. These included the changing roles of children within the family, both domestically and emotionally, as well as shifts in relationships with both the parent with Parkinson's and the healthy parent. Matters regarding children's social and emotional development and well-being, their level of independence, perceptions of disease and fears for the future were also brought to light. However, as Grimshaw himself acknowledged, the qualitative approach taken does not allow generalisations to be made regarding outcomes for a broader population. The qualitative nature of this research was therefore a major limitation, as was the selective nature of the sample and its size; 20 children and 20 adults participated.

Children's quality of life

A significant challenge for building on the work of Grimshaw was the development of a measure that would generate quantitative data and thereby enable greater generalisation of results. The Parental Illness Impact Scale (PIIS; Schrag et al., 2004a) and its revised version (PIIS-R; Morley et al., 2010a) were subsequently developed. The measure contains 51 items and was constructed broadly around a quality of life (QoL) model. A number of key demographic variables have subsequently been explored using this measure, with results suggesting three particular areas of concern for children's QoL; the age of the child, the duration of the parent's Parkinson's and the availability of sibling support.

Age of the child

The age of the child has been demonstrated as a significant indicator of adjustment to parental PD. In the first quantitative assessment of offspring of PwP,

Schrag et al. (2004b) reported significant associations between a child's age and a number of factors relating to QoL as measured by the PIIS. Results indicated that the younger the child, the greater the perceived burden of providing daily help, as well as greater difficulty with friends' reactions to their parent's Parkinson's. Conversely, the older the child, the greater the recognition of the effects of PD on both the affected and unaffected parent.

Schrag et al. also made comparisons between a group aged 12–24 and those aged 25 and above, with results largely supporting the associations reported above. The younger group reported a significantly heightened sense of burden in relation to their contribution to daily help in the parental home. As might be expected, they also reported far greater difficulty in dealing with friends' reactions. The older sample reported a significantly heightened impact on family functioning. Morley (2008) further assessed associations between age and QoL using the PIIS-R. Results confirmed those of Schrag et al. (2004b) in relation to perceived burden of daily help and relationships with friends. Findings also suggested that the perceived impact on a child's personal future increases as they get older. This is perhaps unsurprising since, with increasing age, children may become progressively more aware and realistic about their parent's condition. They are also better equipped educationally and emotionally to deal with the realistic prospects of their parent's condition (Lewandowski, 1992). What this data highlights is that children may require different types of support at different ages, and this needs to be considered in the management of their adjustment to parental Parkinson's.

Parental disease duration

The duration of the parent's Parkinson's has also been shown to be of significant importance. Schrag et al. (2004b) reported a reduction in children's overall QoL as parental disease duration increases. Such a pattern was also evident in three particular subscales of the PIIS. Longer disease duration was associated with worsening communication and understanding, reduced development and independence, and increased impact on family functioning. Morley (2008) reported similar findings, with longer disease duration again associated with inferior communication and understanding and deteriorating parent-child relationships. Such results reflect the progressive nature of PD and its impact on the child and highlight the need for ongoing support as the parental condition advances.

Number of siblings

Morley et al. (2010b) assessed the importance of sibling support within the family unit on adolescent and adult children's response to parental

Parkinson's, multiple sclerosis (MS) and stroke. Those children without siblings reported significantly greater emotional impact, elevated social impact, inferior communication and understanding with their affected parent, and heightened concerns for their personal future, as measured by the PIIS-R (Morley et al., 2010a). Total QoL scores were also significantly lower for children without the support of siblings. It is reasonable to speculate that these results reflect an inability to access support from siblings. This fits well with the Compensatory Siblings Hypothesis (Boer et al., 1992) where siblings use each other as a resource to make up for deficiencies in the parent-child relationship. This theory, however, is controversial and is contradicted by the Congruence Hypothesis (Sanders, 2004). Consistent with social learning theory the Congruence Hypothesis contends that it is positive interactions between children and their parents that foster positive interactions between the siblings themselves. However, a limitation of the Morley et al. (2010b) study is its sample size: although a sample of 168 adolescent and adult children participated, just 16 were an only child. Additionally, participants came from a range of parental neurological conditions and there are, therefore, limitations as to what can be concluded specifically in relation to parental PD. The results, however, stress the potential importance of recognising that children without the support of brothers or sisters may be at greater risk of responding negatively to their parent's condition, and this should be considered in the management of family adjustment to the parental condition.

Children's emotional well-being

Levels of depression in the offspring of PwP have been shown to be markedly higher than those in the general population. Incorporating the Birleson Depression Self Rating Scale (Birleson, 1981) for young people and the Beck Depression Inventory (Beck et al., 1961) for adult children, Schrag et al. (2004b) reported 17.2% of 12–24 year olds and 21.7% of participants aged 25 and above as mildly to moderately depressed. Further studies largely confirm these results, with 12.5% of 11–18 year olds and 17.7% of adult children experiencing mild to moderate depression (Morley 2008; Morley et al., 2011). Prevalence of depression in adults in the general population is estimated at 5–10% (Singleton et al., 2003) and in adolescents at 4–8% (Hazell, 2011; Son and Kirchner, 2000). Literature strongly indicates that the key to the effective treatment of depression remains its recognition and treatment in both adolescents and adults (Kessler et al., 1999; Rowe et al., 2004). It is therefore important that children confronted with parental PD, be they young or adult, are recognised as being at increased risk of mental health problems (Morley and Jenkinson, 2012).

Availability of information and support

The PIIS and PIIS-R incorporate a number of dichotomous questions focusing on the availability of support and information. Schrag et al. (2004b) reported that more than half of their sample (53.9%) felt they did not have enough information about PD, with an even greater proportion (67.4%) feeling they did not know enough about what would happen to their parent as their Parkinson's progressed. Nearly half of all participants (49.4%) felt that more information would lessen feelings of uncertainty and insecurity, with the same percentage relying solely on their parents as a source of information about PD. Morley (2011) reported similar results, with 37.5% feeling they did not have enough information about their parent's PD and over half (53.8%) not knowing enough about what would happen to their affected parent in the future. This study also found 61.1% relying solely on their parents as a source of information about PD. These results and those of previous studies with alternative parental conditions (i.e. Caton et al., 1998; Cross and Rintell, 1999; Mukherjee et al., 2002) emphasise the need to have appropriate and accessible information available for children of all ages when a parent has PD.

Regarding provision of support, Schrag et al. (2004b) reported 69.7% of participants wanting greater levels of help from local services and 48.3% feeling that it would be helpful if they had some influence over help provided. Of those families who participated in the study, 55.1% had outside help available to assist with care for the parent with PD. Only 40% of families had access to support from local services, whilst approximately 60% thought more support should be provided. Again, Morley (2011) largely mirrors these results, with 61% feeling greater levels of help should be provided by services and 40.5% suggesting it would help to be able to talk to relevant services about the care provided for their affected parent. Just 40.8% of families were receiving external help. Such results highlight the need for services first to be available where required, and second to engage with affected families regarding the level and nature of service provision.

IN PRACTICE

This section incorporates tentative guidance and recommendations for practitioners. This is based on the previously discussed research evidence and examples from clinical practice, alongside a recently undertaken series of interviews with children of PwP, a webinar focusing on Parkinson's and parenting and a roundtable session conducted for Parkinson's parents (Book, 2013, 2014a, 2014b, 2015). It is important to note that within the Parkinsonian family, adjustment issues for children may be related to a range of factors.

With regard to illness characteristics, some symptoms are potentially more challenging than others. For example, parental depression, anxiety and impulse control issues have the potential to have a significant negative impact. Additional factors might include the age and gender of the PwP and other family members, and the availability of informal or formal support (siblings, friends, grandparents, counsellors). The progressive nature of PD also means that new challenges may emerge as the illness progresses, with children continually being faced with a changing situation. Given this range of factors it is critical to pay attention to how well children are coping and address their needs as they arise. In order to do this, healthcare professionals need to better understand how PD might affect children, taking into account the broad range of feelings, experiences and occurrences that the children encounter.

Tables 3.1 and 3.2 provide summaries of a range of common feelings, experiences and occurrences highlighted by children of parents with PD. All of these clearly have the potential to impact upon social development and school achievement. Caregiving responsibilities, activity restrictions and feelings of isolation can lead to depression and anxiety and even somatisation. As previously mentioned in this chapter, it is therefore necessary to be sensitive and to recognise depression in children in order to treat it and improve their well-being. Healthcare professionals need to be proactive by screening PwP who might have children, assessing family functioning by directly asking about their children and how PD is affecting family life.

TABLE 3.1 Common feelings and experiences highlighted by children of parents with PD

Shame related to presentation of PD in parent, e.g. tremor, shuffling gait, speech problems
Concerns about socialising with peer group
Anxiety about stress in parental relationship
Fear and grief related to loss of shared experiences with affected parent
Loneliness, as healthy parent has to focus more on affected parent
Confusion and frustration with role changes and role reversal
Worry about developing PD themself
Concern that parents feel guilty about impact of PD on the family
Worry about financial impact of PD on the family
Concerns regarding aspirations and decisions for the future

TABLE 3.2 Common occurrences highlighted by children of parents with PD

Most do not know other children who have parents with PD
Most do not talk with friends about issues arising from their parent's PD
Many do not remember what life was like before PD entered the family
Majority of emotional support comes from within the family
Many indicate they would like to better understand PD in order to better understand the needs of the affected parent earlier on
Some express guilt related to asking for help from parents as their parents are dealing with the considerable burden of PD

Supporting PwP in their parenting role

Helping children to adjust to their parent's PD must include supporting the parents in this process. This support to the parents is particularly important because children rarely accompany their parent to the neurological appointment. Children are, in effect, supported by the education and support given to their parents. While parenting with PD presents additional challenges, it does not necessarily mean poor adjustment experiences for the children. With appropriately timed support and resources, the quality of life for each individual, as well as the family, can be addressed and optimised.

It is important to preserve the PwP parental role and to ensure that the healthy parent does not shield the affected parent from involvement with the children. As much as possible, it is important for children to continue to view the affected parent as having the same approaches to parenting, expectations, discipline and boundaries. Similarly, parents need to be mindful of the need to maintain family life activities and traditions, making adjustments over time as necessary. Parents may need to be reminded of the impact of age and developmental stage. It is important to remember that as children grow, they may experience social or emotional distress that may be much more related to their normal age and stage of development and that it can be completely unrelated to PD in the family. Similarly, it is important to remember that going through puberty, dealing with friendships and all things associated with growing up are realities in a child's life that can make it more challenging for them to then cope with PD in the family as well.

Counselling PwP to consider breaking the silence of the diagnosis with their children can decrease the anxiety children may have about a parent's health. Clinical practice suggests reminding parents with PD that children can be very intuitive and may sense an underlying cause for concern. They may also be concerned that something significantly worse than PD is apparent.

If 'the secret' goes public among teachers, friends or relatives before the parent has talked with the children, and the children hear of the diagnosis from someone else, this can damage trust between parent and child. Additionally, by sharing the diagnosis with children, it can be shared with those who are connected to them, such as teachers and coaches, people who can watch for signs of related stress and be a support to the child. It is also worthwhile suggesting that PwP provide the people within their network with accurate information about PD, as well as the philosophy and attitude they wish to be reinforced with the children. Sharing the PD diagnosis with children is therefore essential, as is providing age-appropriate information and communicating the best understanding of what might happen and how it will be dealt with as a family. The way the diagnosis is presented, the timing of the discussion, the tone of voice and the choice of words used can affect the way children cope from the start. Open communication is invaluable as time passes and the disease changes.

CASE EXAMPLE 1

A young girl, aged 10, was living with her father who has had PD for four years. Her father brought her to his annual neurologist visit because he had sensed a change in her recently. While she knew he had PD, she had become increasingly worried that he was going to die as a result of some physical changes he was now experiencing. By bringing her to his visit, her father created the opportunity to address her worries and fears and allowed for some accurate information to be shared with her. She acknowledged feeling relieved and comforted in knowing that she had someone to talk to if she needed to in the future.

Conversations with the children of PwP reveal that their coping may be related to the severity of symptoms and type of symptoms (motor and non-motor), but it may also be related to their parents' style of coping and attitude towards PD. Table 3.3 provides for a range of quotes from children that illustrates this. What these comments indicate is that the parents' attitude can be hugely significant, as children tend to model their own attitudes after those of their parents. Encouraging parents to foster and demonstrate good communication, honesty and even asking for help can set good examples for the children.

Positive outcomes for children of PwP

It is important to acknowledge the potential for positive outcomes for

TABLE 3.3 Quotes from children of PwP

'My mom has made it as normal as possible.'
'My mom's outlook has helped us manage well. Her attitude has been the most healing for all of us. She is inspiring.'
'It's not the end of the world. We are coping.'
'It's all a challenge but we have to live with it.'
'We can't do things the way we used to. We have to find new ways to spend time together.'

children. Clinical evidence and previous research detailing the impact of parental illness (e.g. Alexander et al., 2002; Blackford, 1992; Buck and Hohmann, 1981; Mukherjee et al., 2002) demonstrate that living life with challenging parental conditions can strengthen the family relationship, lead to improved coping skills for children and provide a sense of pride and maturity with a well-developed sense of empathy. If children are well supported, having PD in the family can actually enhance their quality of life and promote healthy personal growth and development.

CASE EXAMPLE 2

A teenage girl, aged 16, whose father has had PD since she was born. Her entire life has been impacted by his disease as it changes day to day and often hour to hour. With strong family support, avid interests and connections to faith, her experience with PD has contributed to her decision to pursue her education and a planned career in medicine.

RECOMMENDATIONS FOR FUTURE RESEARCH

This section identifies current limitations and key considerations for future research that should allow for a greater understanding of the needs of the offspring of PwP and the wider family unit.

Longitudinal research

Longitudinal studies should now become a priority as investigations into parental Parkinson's progress. There is a limit to what can be concluded from cross-sectional studies. Longitudinal research is required in order to assess families over time as the social, emotional, physical and practical demands of parental PD unfold. This is particularly important with chronic progressive conditions such as Parkinson's. The impact on the child and the challenges they might encounter, such as entering higher education or the decision to leave the parental home, may become more intense as the affected parent's Parkinson's advances. Longitudinal studies would also provide an avenue for the development of interventions, as well as identifying those families for whom the journey of Parkinson's is proving particularly challenging. Despite significant advances in understanding a range of parental conditions, few have been subject to longitudinal investigation, as is highlighted throughout this book. Longitudinal research should therefore remain an important priority for those investigating parental PD.

Comparative data

There is a limit to what can be concluded from current studies of parental PD in the absence of comparative data from adolescent and adult children with healthy parents. Few studies across a range of parental conditions have incorporated control groups to date, although there are some notable exceptions, such as those investigating children of parents with cancer (Harris and Zakowski, 2003) and multiple sclerosis (Pakenham and Cox, 2014, 2015; Yahav et al., 2005, 2007). Gaining such data for children of PwP should now become a significant priority. In the absence of control groups it is difficult to draw firm conclusions on a number of issues which are of importance when assessing the impact of parental illness.

Assessment of younger children

There is a further need to assess the impact of parental PD on younger children, and not solely on adolescent and adult children. Although the numbers of these children are likely to be small, the implications for children below the age of 11 are likely to be just as profound, if not more so, than for older children. Support groups and workshops, such as those provided for younger children of parents with cancer (Greening, 1999) and multiple sclerosis (Mutch, 2005), may well be valuable tools in helping younger children understand what is happening to their parent with Parkinson's. Resources such as this can allow children to meet with peers also experiencing parental illness and encourage them to discuss their fears and emotional concerns in a non-threatening, supportive environment. In addition, children can be provided with age-appropriate information to help them better understand the nature of their parent's condition.

Examination of further demographic variables

There remain further important demographic factors and groups that need to be addressed in a comprehensive examination of factors influencing the well-being of children of parents with Parkinson's. The need to examine different cultures is an important issue (Grimshaw, 1991). In doing so it is important to recognise that different cultures may require very different support. This is particularly so for those cultures where a far greater emphasis is placed on the social support network of the family. A further, and likely highly significant, group currently not assessed is single-parent families where the parent is chronically ill, this being of particular relevance to the caring role played by children (Becker et al., 1998). The importance of investigating this group is further highlighted by research indicating that the prevalence of mental health problems in children and young people from single-parent families is doubled when compared to those from two-parent families (Meltzer et al., 2003).

Implications on parenting for PwP

As indicated in the 'in practice' section of this chapter, the implications on parenting for PwP should not be underestimated. Formal lines of research are required to identify further what support is both needed and most effective. Detailed qualitative work with PwP of a range of ages and disease progression would be an appropriate starting point and should act as a catalyst for future quantitative assessment.

CONCLUSION

This chapter has presented current literature relating to children's responses to parental Parkinson's disease, along with a number of practical recommendations for those involved in this field. There is much research that remains to be conducted and there are significant gaps in our current understanding of children's needs, and it is vital that this research should become a priority if the needs of children and families touched by the effects of parental Parkinson's are to be met.

REFERENCES

Alexander, C.J., Hwang, K., Sipski, M.L. (2002). Mothers with spinal cord injury: Impact on marital, family, and children's adjustment. *Archives of Physical Medicine and Rehabilitation*, 83(1), 24–30.

Beck, A.T., Ward, C.H., Mendelson, M., Mock, J.E., Erbaugh, J.K. (1961). An inventory for measuring depression, *Archives of General Psychiatry*, 4(6), 561–571.

Becker, S., Aldridge, J., Dearden, C. (1998). *Young carers and their families*. Oxford: Blackwell Science.

Birleson, P. (1981). The validity of depressive disorder in childhood and the development of a self-rating scale: A Research Report. *Journal of Child Psychology and Psychiatry and Allied Disciplines*, 22(1), 73–88.

Blackford, K. (1992). Strategies for intervention and research with children or adolescents who have a parent with multiple sclerosis. *Axon*, 14, 50–54.

Bloem, B., Hausdorff, J., Visser, J., Giladi, N. (2004). Falls and freezing of gait in Parkinson's disease: A review of two interconnected, episodic phenomena. *Movement Disorders*, 19(8), 871–884.

Boer, F., Goedhart, A.W., Treffers, P.D.A. (1992). Siblings and their parents. In F. Boer, J. Dunn, J.F. Dunn (Eds) *Children's sibling relationships: Developmental and clinical issues* (pp. 41–54), Hillsdale, N.J: Lawrence Erlbaum Associates.

Book, E. (2013). Issues specific to Adolescents of Parents with Parkinson's disease. *Journal of Parkinson's Disease*, 3(S1), 42–43.

Book, E. (2014a). Interviews with children of people with Parkinson's disease. Unpublished data.

Book, E. (2014b). Parkinson's and Parenting: The Impact on Children and Young Adults. Available from http://event.netbriefings.com/event/pdeb/Archives/parenting/register.html (accessed 17 March 2015).

Book, E. (2015). Parkinson's and parenting: The impact on children, teens and young adults. *Movement Disorders*, 30(S1), S540.

Buck, F.M., Hohmann, G.W. (1981). Personality, behaviour, values, and family relations of children of fathers with spinal cord injury. *Archives of Physical Medicine and Rehabilitation*, 62(9), 432–438.

Caton, C.L.M., Cournos, F., Felix, A., Wyatt, R.J. (1998). Childhood experiences and current adjustment of offspring of indigent patients with Schizophrenia. *Psychiatric Services*, 49(1), 86–90.

Clarke, C.E., Moore, A.P. (2007). Parkinson's Disease. *American Family Physician*, 75(7), 1045–1048.

Cross, T., Rintell, D. (1999). Children's perceptions of parental MS. *Psychology Health and Medicine*, 4(4), 355–360.

Greening, K. (1999). Support groups for children of patients with cancer. *Cancer Practice*, 7(4), 208–211.

Grimshaw, R. (1991). Children of parents with Parkinson's disease. A research report for the Parkinson's Disease Society.

Harris, C.A., Zakowski, S.G. (2003). Comparisons of distress in adolescents of cancer patients and controls. *Psycho-Oncology*, 12(2), 173–182.

Hazell, P. (2011). Depression in children and adolescents. *BMJ Clinical Evidence*, Oct 21, pii, 1008.

Kessler, D., Lloyd, K., Lewis, G., Gray, D.P. (1999). Cross sectional study of symptom attribution and recognition of depression and anxiety in primary care. *British Medical Journal*, 318(7181), 436–440.

Lewandowski, L. (1992). Needs of children during the critical illness of a parent or sibling. *Critical Care Nursing Clinics of North America*, 4(4), 573–585.

Meltzer, H., Gatward, R., Goodman, R., Ford, T. (2003). Mental health of children and adolescents in Great Britain. *International Review of Psychiatry*, 15(1–2), 185–187.

Morley, D. (2008). The impact of parental neurological illness on adolescent and adult children: Quality of life, psychosocial factors, and relationship with parent well-being. PhD Thesis, University of London.

Morley, D. (2011). The psychosocial impact of Parkinson's disease on the wider family unit: A focus on the offspring of affected individuals. In A.Q. Rana (Ed.), *Symptoms of Parkinson's disease* (pp. 165–178). Rijeka: InTech Open Access.

Morley, D., Selai, C., Schrag, A., Thompson, A., Jahanshahi, M. (2010a). Refinement and validation of the Parental Illness Impact Scale. *Parkinsonism and Related Disorders*, 16(3), 181–185.

Morley, D., Selai, C., Thompson, A. (2010b). Sibling support and adjustment to parental neurological illness. *Quality of Life Research*, 19(S1), 143–144.

Morley, D., Selai, C., Schrag, A., Jahanshahi, M., Thompson, A. (2011). Adolescent and adult children of parents with Parkinson's disease: Incorporating their needs in clinical guidelines. *Parkinson's Disease*, 2011, 951874.

Morley, D., Jenkinson, C. (2012). The importance of recognising depression in adolescents affected by parental illness. *Psychology*, 3(9A), 756–757.

Morley, D., Jenkinson, C. (2013). Furthering our understanding of the needs of adolescent children of parents with Parkinson's disease. *Adolescent Health, Medicine and Therapeutics*, 4, 75–77.

Mukherjee, S., Sloper, P., Lewin, R. (2002). The meaning of parental illness to children: The case of inflammatory bowel disease. *Child: Care, Health and Development*, 28(6), 479–485.

Mutch, K. (2005). Information for young people when multiple sclerosis enters the family. *British Journal of Nursing*, 14(14), 758–767.

Pakenham, K.I., Cox, S. (2014). The effects of parental illness and other ill family members on the adjustment of children. *Annals of Behavioural Medicine*, 48(3), 424–437.

Pakenham K.I., Cox, S. (2015). The effects of parental illness and other ill family members on youth caregiving experiences. *Psychology and Health*, 30(7), 857–878.

Rowe, L., Tonge, B., Melvin, G. (2004). When should GPs prescribe SSRIs for adolescent depression? *Australian Family Physician*, 33(12), 1005–1008.

Sanders, R. (2004). The quality of sibling relationships. In R. Sanders (Ed.), *Sibling relationships: Theory and issues for practice* (pp. 82–108). New York: Palgrave.

Schapira, A. (1999). Parkinson's disease. *British Medical Journal*, 318, 311–314.

Schrag, A., Morley, D., Quinn, N., Jahanshahi, M. (2004a). Development of a measure of the impact of chronic parental illness on adolescent and adult children: The Parental Illness Impact Scale (Parkinson's disease). *Parkinsonism and Related Disorders*, 10(7), 399–405.

Schrag, A., Morley, D., Quinn, N., Jahanshahi, M. (2004b). Impact of Parkinson's disease on patients' adolescent and adult children. *Parkinsonism and Related Disorders*, 10(7), 391–397.

Singleton, N., Bumpstead, R., O'Brien, M., Lee, A., Meltzer, H. (2003). Psychiatric morbidity among adults living in private households, 2000. *International Review of Psychiatry*, 15(1–2) 65–73.

Son, S.E., Kirchner, J.T. (2000). Depression in children and adolescents. *American Family Physician*, 62(10), 2297–2308.

Yahav, R., Vosburgh, J., Miller, A. (2005). Emotional responses of children and adolescents to parents with multiple sclerosis. *Multiple Sclerosis*, 11(4), 464–468.

Yahav, R., Vosburgh, J., Miller, A. (2007). Separation-individuation processes of adolescent children of parents with multiple sclerosis. *Multiple Sclerosis*, 13(1), 87–94.

CHAPTER 4

Parental acquired brain injury

Rikke Kieffer-Kristensen

INTRODUCTION

The Brain Injury Association (2010) defines acquired brain injury (ABI) as 'damage to the brain, which occurs after birth and is not related to a congenital or a degenerative disease'. The most common types of ABI include stroke, traumatic brain injury (e.g. as a result of a traffic accident or sports injury), brain tumour, brain haemorrhage and viral infection (e.g. meningitis, encephalitis or septicaemia). The effects of ABI are impaired physical, cognitive, emotional and social functioning. These impairments impose a burden on the family system, as patients become dependent on their close relatives for an indefinite amount of time. Numerous studies on the consequences of a family member's brain injury on the family system have been conducted, finding that it results in a significant amount of stress for everyone involved.

Several factors have been found to contribute significantly to family stress after ABI. One the most distressing consequences of ABI for family members is the sudden changes in the brain-injured person's personality. In particular, changes in aggression, irritability, childishness and loss of empathy have been found to be important negative stressors (Ergh et al., 2002; Perlesz et al., 2000; Sander et al., 2003). In addition, such cognitive deficits as mental slowness, memory problems and fatigue are distressing for close relatives (Perlesz and O'Loughlan, 1998; Thomsen, 1984). Consequent stressors, such as a lack of social support, role changes and financial problems, have also been reported to influence the perceived stress in the family (Perlesz et al., 1999). Finally, family issues, such as having young children, less marital cohesion, more conflicts and sexual problems have been found to correlate with high levels of caregiver stress (Vaishnavi et al., 2009). For the most part, research has been aimed at studying the effect on spouses and parents of brain-injured persons. Studies of dependent children's adjustment to parental ABI have, in contrast, been very limited in the research, and are only sparsely described in the literature.

STUDIES OF ABI FAMILIES WITH DEPENDENT CHILDREN

Based on her clinical experience as a neuropsychologist, Lezak (1988: 121) noted:

> For most children, brain impairment in a parent or sibling typically brings a sharp reduction in parental attention, an equally sharp increase in responsibilities, an uncomprehended shame and guilt which ultimately is compounded by frustrations and anger of having a 'different' family, at being ashamed or unable to bring friends home, at not participating in school or community activities requiring a parent because the parent is occupied with the patient's care, and at the absence of parties or picnics and other kinds of good times the family had previously enjoyed.

One of the first empirical studies was that of Pessar et al. (1993) involving 24 families with a brain-injured parent. All children (n=56) between the ages of 2 and 20 were included. The healthy parents answered 11 questions about changes in the children's behaviour post-injury. Ninety per cent of the non-injured parents reported behavioural changes in their children, such as increased acting out, emotional or relationship problems. In 10 of the 24 families the children were reported as experiencing a significant breakdown in the relationship with the injured parent. The healthy parent described the children as being less loving towards the injured parent, not wanting to spend time with the injured parent and not bringing friends home. A limitation of this study was that there was not a control group. In addition, the authors did not collect data from the children themselves.

Uysal et al. (1998) published a study on the effect of parental traumatic brain injury (TBI) on parenting and child behaviour. In this study, 16 families with 18 children participated, and a matched control group was included. The children were between 8 and 18 years old. Four of the children were born post-injury. The mean number of years since injury was quite high, at nine years. The results showed that parents with TBI reported less active involvement, less cognitive competence, less conformity and less achievement on a parent behaviour rating scale, as compared to the control group. The children in the TBI families, however, did not confirm the above reported differences.

The only significant difference reported by children with a TBI parent as compared to children in the control group was that both parents in TBI families used a more lax form of control than parents in the control group used.

Butera-Prinzi and Perlesz (2004) conducted a pilot study based on a qualitative approach with a phenomenological frame of reference. The study consisted of in-depth semi-structured interviews of four children aged 7–12 years who had fathers with ABI. This small-scale study found that these children had many complex feelings after their fathers' injuries, and that their feelings of loss/grief were mainly due to their fathers' changed personalities. All children reacted emotionally, and were psychologically affected by the new family situation.

Visser-Meily et al. (2005) investigated 88 children aged 4–18 years from 55 families affected by parental strokes, at the start of an inpatient rehabilitation programme, two months after discharge and one year after the stroke. The results showed a significant improvement in the children's psychosocial functioning, as measured via Child Behavior Check List (Achenbach and Edelbrock, 1981) and the Child Depression Inventory (Kovacs, 1985) between admission and two months after discharge from the inpatient rehabilitation programme. However, no further improvement was found in the children's functioning between discharge and one year after the stroke.

A recent study from Finland investigated the long-term consequences for children with a parent with a TBI. In a retrospective population-based register study, all children (60 069) born in Finland in 1987 were followed up during a period of 21 years (1987–2008) through national health and social registers. Of these children, 1532 (2.6%) had a parent with TBI during this period. TBI was defined using the International Classification of Diseases (ICD) coding and divided into two groups: (i) severe TBI (skull fracture, brain contusion or other intracranial injuries as well as post-concussion syndrome or sequela of TBI) and (ii) mild TBI (concussions). The study found that almost one-quarter of these 1532 children (22.5%) were treated in a specialised psychiatric care unit as inpatients or as outpatients. Children with an injured mother were found to be more likely to use psychiatric services and interestingly so were children of a parent with mild TBI (Niemelä et al., 2014).

In summary, the lack of a control group, variability in injury severity, differences in rehabilitation services from country to country and small sample sizes serve as methodological challenges within this research field.

TABLE 4.1 Potential ABI-related disabilities that could lead to some degree of disrupted parenting

Physical disabilities:	Can affect the parent's efficiency and ability to play and be active with their children, and the children may need to help more around the house.
Cognitive disabilities:	Can make the parent less supportive with regards to schoolwork, intellectual stimulation and discipline.
Emotional problems:	Can make the parent more depressed, irritable, angry, and even aggressive. The stress tolerance can be low and the children must be aware of not annoying the parent ('walking on eggshells').

DISRUPTED PARENTING

An interesting concept regarding the effect of parental illness on children is that of 'disrupted parenting', introduced by Armistead et al. (1995). Disrupted parenting is defined as reduced parental support or less nurturing of the child. It may result directly or indirectly from parental physical illness because of altered family routines, fewer efforts at discipline, parental absence, depression, stress and marital conflicts between parents. Disrupted parenting can be viewed as a subtle or hidden interpersonal loss of one or perhaps both parents. It seems likely that the disabilities following ABI can result in some degree of disrupted parenting (see Table 4.1).

PARENTAL ABI: A STRESSOR FOR CHILDREN

Interpersonal loss is one of the most traumatising experiences a child can have. In cases of terminal illness, it is thus highly stressful for children to cope with the expected death of a loved one, and a high rate of symptoms associated with post-traumatic stress have been found in children and adolescents living with a parent diagnosed with cancer (Bruce, 2006; Huizinga et al., 2005; Osborn, 2007). Similarly, based on the onset, cause and associated disabilities of ABI, there seem to be a number of relational losses in cases of parental ABI for the children along with other illness-related stressors, many of which are ongoing (see Table 4.2).

To investigate the child-specific stressors of parental ABI as well as the possible post-traumatic stress symptoms in children, Kieffer-Kristensen et al. (2011) conducted a controlled study of 55 families. All families consisted of an ill parent, a healthy parent and a child between 7 and 14 years old. An important inclusion criterion was that the family members resided in the

TABLE 4.2 Potential ABI-related stressors

Acute Stress	Secondary Stress
Seeing the parent injured	Disrupted parenting
Hospitalisation	Relational changes/interpersonal loss
Fear of parent dying	Shifts in future perspectives
Parent's impaired physical, cognitive, emotional and social functioning	Declines in socio-economic status
Healthy parent's emotional reaction	Social stigmatisation

same household as they did prior to the illness or injury. The families were all visited at home by a trained child psychologist.

Results from this study demonstrated that children with a parent who has suffered a brain injury had significantly elevated post-traumatic stress symptoms as compared to a matched control group of children living with a parent with another chronic medical condition, hypothesised to be less traumatic (diabetes). On the screening questionnaire for child post-traumatic stress disorder (PTSD), the Children's Revised Impact of Events Scale (CRIES; Perrin et al., 2005), the brain injury group scored significantly and markedly higher than the diabetes group. Comparison of the two groups showed that almost half of the children (46%) in the brain injury group had post-traumatic stress symptoms above the clinical cut-off score (≥ 30), indicating a possible PTSD diagnosis, compared to 10% in the diabetes group. Findings indicated that the post-traumatic stress symptoms were so severe that referral to professional psychological counselling would have been recommended. Of course, a clinical diagnosis of PTSD in children must be based on a thorough clinical investigation and never on a single questionnaire.

PARENTAL ABI: A STRESSOR FOR THE PARENTS

Children who experience traumatic stress are very dependent on emotional support from their parents. Parents with ABI may be significantly less available to their children because of their cognitive and emotional impairments and disabilities. The healthy parent may also be preoccupied with the ill spouse and his or her own emotional reactions. This may lead the parents to respond less sensitively to the children in the family, who are similarly traumatised by the sudden illness/injury.

A recent study by Kieffer-Kristensen and Teasdale (2011) found that parents with ABI experience significantly more parental distress compared to parents with diabetes on the Parenting Stress Index (PSI; Abidin, 1983), indicating that brain-injured parents are more highly distressed by their lack of functioning in the parental role. This may be related to the reduced cognitive and emotional capacity of the ABI parents impacting on their parenting skills. On the other hand, the result may reflect a tendency of parents with ABI to be more critical of their own behaviour with regard to fulfilment of their parenting role. A significant difference was also observed on the Parent-Child Dysfunctional Interaction scale (a subscale of the PSI), indicating that ABI parents demonstrate problems redefining their relationships with their children. Similar results were found in a multiple family group study from Australia, where the most distressing experience for the parents with ABI was associated with the loss of, and fear of deterioration and breakdown of, their relationship and connectedness with their children (Charles et al., 2007).

The findings suggest that ABI can lead to relational problems between family members, and highlights the fact that the ABI parents themselves are aware of their difficulties in fulfilling the parenting role. We also examined whether parental and illness-related variables had an impact on the children's post-traumatic stress symptoms, and found only one significant relationship – namely that high levels of parental stress in the healthy parent seem to be related to high levels of post-traumatic stress symptoms in the children (Kieffer-Kristensen et al., 2013). This is an important finding that emphasises the need to understand the family dynamic after parental ABI. It may be that if the ill parent is unable to fulfil their parent role, the healthy parent is more vulnerable, as he or she must practically and emotionally support both the injured parent and the children, leading to an increased risk of stress that again has a negative effect on the children's well-being. In our study, an eight-year-old girl with a father with ABI explained:

> At home my mother also cried all the time, and my sister X, who lived at home at that point, she also cried, and I was still the only one who didn't react, so I had to comfort them every night and make sure that everything worked out at home and do the chores around the house because they were numb.

Children whose emotional needs are not met have a tendency to play a more adaptive role that makes it difficult for the parents and others in their surroundings to recognise that the child is reacting to the situation at home.

HIDDEN GRIEF

With parental ABI, the traumatic experience for the children may thus be related to significant changes in the parent-child relationship. Research has suggested that these losses may be complicated by the ambiguity of the loss, as the injured parent is physically present but psychologically absent (due to personality change, cognitive disabilities and emotional reactivity). This results in an ongoing loss that the children must deal with in their everyday life, putting a strain on their development (Boss and Couden, 2002).

To investigate this hypothesis Kieffer-Kristensen and Johansen (2013) conducted a qualitative study of 14 children with high levels of post-traumatic stress symptoms, in order to achieve an in-depth understanding of the possible trauma-related feelings and relational losses. Using a phenomenological child-friendly interview approach, some important themes were recognised, such as:

- *Traumatic experiences:* In most cases, the children had a vivid memory of witnessing the ABI or learning about it, but the memory of seeing the injured parent in the hospital was also vivid, and often they had felt very scared. The fear that the injured parent was going to die had been a strong emotional experience for most of the children in the acute stage following the ABI, even for the youngest subjects.
- *Relational changes/hidden loss:* We found that most children recognised that the ill parent had changed, but it was often painful for the children to think and talk about the changes, as it made them feel sad. Some thought frequently about what the ill parent could no longer do and whether the ill parent was emotionally affected by the ABI. Many spoke about how they missed having the old parent and remembered them as being more calm, fun, active and supportive.

Others found it hard to compare the mental state of their parent before and after the ABI, and said that they had become used to their parents as they are today and did not remember how it was before the brain injury. A 12-year-old boy with a severely aphasic mother said, 'She has always been the quiet type, and she hasn't changed a lot, because if I think she has changed, I get sad.' For others, the feeling of loss was clearer. As a 14-year-old girl said:

> For me, it is like he died, and I got a stepfather instead. This is a tough thought to have. It would have been 100% easier if he had died; then everybody would understand that he was gone. But I haven't felt that I could say this to him or anyone else.

Ambiguity was frequently present. One nine-year-old girl said, 'I really do like my mum as she is, but it is just that I sometimes really miss my old mum.'

Interestingly, the children also noticed changes in the healthy parents, whom, in contrast, they described as being stricter, more burdened, more stressed and less fun and spontaneous. Additionally, the healthy parent seemed to have the role of protecting the ill parent, asking the children not to bother them or otherwise put a strain on them. The children reported that they found this annoying and wished the healthy parents would be less protective of the ill parents and more supportive of the children's situation and needs.

The findings suggest that children affected by parental ABI experience several hidden losses as their relationship with both the injured and healthy parent is altered. The grief these changes cause is often suppressed or neglected, both by the child and the healthy parent, in order to protect the ill parent. The grief process is further complicated by the fact that those in their surroundings often do not verify the grief, as the cognitive disabilities and personality changes are difficult to observe, and the children therefore must cope with the feeling of relational loss and grief on their own.

INTERVENTIONS AND CLINICAL RECOMMENDATIONS

Patients with moderate to severe brain injury are often offered some form of specialised neuro-rehabilitation. Brain injury rehabilitation includes programmes with an interdisciplinary approach targeting the injury as well as the individual's life situation, with the goal of facilitating independency and life quality. Programmes can be in- or outpatient, and length varies from 2 to 12 months. Most rehabilitation programmes also include support for relatives, primarily spouses. Within the brain injury rehabilitation there is generally a limited focus on the well-being of dependent children in the family, and how the brain injury affects the brain-injured parent's ability to parent. Today, most children affected by parental ABI therefore receive no professional help. A national survey in England showed that few (19%) rehabilitation staff actively involved children in efforts to support the families of brain-injured people (Webster and Daisley, 2007). There were several explanations for this, and most of the professionals asked did not consider themselves skilled in working with children. Unfortunately, this often seems to be a barrier, not only within rehabilitation, but also in hospitals and elsewhere. It is, however, important to keep in mind that children do react emotionally when something dramatic and unexpected happens to their loved ones, as with ABI.

In the acute phase

In order to help the children, it is first necessary to identify them. Both in the hospital and in rehabilitation units, taking the patients' social history should include the question of whether there are children living at home. If this is the case, the functioning of the children should be discussed with the parents. An information dossier for parents with dependent children would be an improvement. Such a dossier should be available both in the hospital ward, and the in- and outpatient rehabilitation unit. It should contain information for both parents and children about brain injury, and information for the parents about children's reaction to parental illness and where to go if the children need professional help. Hospital staff should be trained in giving children age-appropriate information about the brain injury. At this stage it is also important to identify the adults in the extended family (such as a grandparent) who could support the child through this emotionally challenging time. The child will, for a temporary time, need to 'borrow' a grown-up for support, as both parents are unavailable at this point. For most children experiencing high levels of stress it is important to maintain structure and normality. This could be going to school and leisure activities, and keeping visits to the hospital to short daily visits. Family rooms and making the children feel comfortable in the ward is also of importance, as many children are quite uncomfortable being in a medical setting. In this phase there is often a lot of support and attention for the children from their extended family, friends and the community. However, as ABI is a chronic condition, many children may feel that the support stops – often when the injured parent is discharged from hospital and when, from the outside, it seems that family life is back to normal.

Sub-acute phase

Longitudinal studies have thus found the burden among family members to increase between three months post-injury and five years, without reducing after seven years (Oddy et al., 1985; Ponsford and Schonberger, 2010; Teasdale and Engberg, 2005). Recent research has found that teaching parents emotional coaching for children in distress seems to reduce the stress symptoms in children. This could be an important task for the rehabilitation team when the parent is discharged from hospital, and could be initiated by arranging a home visit with both parents and children attending. Rehabilitation staff should hereafter evaluate how the patient's emotional and cognitive deficits may influence their parenting skills and how these skills can be rehabilitated. First, parenting classes and family activities could be part of the rehabilitation programme in order to help the family to facilitate open communication about the brain injury and reconnect the bond between the parents and children. Second, education classes about the brain for the whole family could be good way to talk about the disabilities and changes in family life. Children like to be informed in an age-appropriate manner about the brain and for many it makes it easier to talk to peers about the injured parent when they have this information. Finally, health professionals must be aware not only of parenting limitations in the ill parent, but also of the potential stress and deterioration of parenting in the healthy parent, since the combination of both parents being unavailable would have a severe negative impact on their children's functioning. A psychosocial intervention to reduce the parental stress in both parents is therefore recommended. Arrangement for the children's well-being must be prioritised in these families until the parents again have the resources to take care of the children's needs – both practically and emotionally.

Chronic phase

The strain and burden can continue in ABI families for many years. It is therefore important to use the network in an appropriate manner, and not wear it out. Family network meetings can be arranged to keep up with how all family members are coping. Outsourcing some of the practical chores can be beneficial. This could be taking the children to football games on the weekend, helping with homework, or babysitting and giving the parents some time off. Family group meetings to meet other families can be a great way to share experiences and make new friends. Charles et al. (2007) conducted a pilot study exploring multifamily group work in families with a parent with an acquired brain injury. Six families met for a total of 12 sessions over a period of six months. Parents generally reported reduced levels of personal distress at follow-up but continuing high levels of marital and family dysfunction. Children were generally reported to be well functioning, although parents were particularly concerned about the impact of family disruption and violence on their children. Support groups for older children could also be beneficial and have been found to increase the quality of life for children faced with other interpersonal losses, such as death in the immediate family (Salloum and Overstreet, 2012). Individual psychological counselling for children with continuing psychological symptoms is in all cases, and in all phases, recommended.

RECOMMENDATIONS FOR FUTURE RESEARCH

The relationships between family processes and children's adjustment after parental ABI are complex, but it is evident that parental ABI can have an impact on the children and on family life. Much more research is, however, needed to confirm and explore these results. Larger prospective and longitudinal studies are recommended to explore fully the potentially traumatising/post-traumatic symptomatology of children affected by parental ABI. Special attention should be focused on the characteristics within the family system that may indirectly influence the children's adjustment to parental ABI, such as initial stress, communication, persistent parental conflict, disrupted parenting and loss of important relationships. It would be especially relevant to identify children at risk for developing psychopathology after parental ABI. The prior attachment patterns in the family may shed light on some of the dysfunctional relational processes that may occur after parental ABI.

To date, studies of parental illness have mainly focused on older children and adolescents, but future attention must also be directed towards younger children, as the relational aspects of ABI and adjustment may be most salient in infant and pre-school children because of their relatively greater dependence on caregivers. Trauma in young children can have long-term psychological effects and is often dismissed, as people expect that the child will be too young to grasp the changes and relational losses.

Future studies should pay attention to factors that have not yet been studied, such as previous and subsequent traumatic events, circumstances at the time of the parent's illness, the event of the illness, the secondary stressors, the consequences of the illness on family life, pre-existing emotional problems in the children, pre-existing family stressors, parenting styles, coping styles and support from peers and others. Finally, research on the effect of family-centred interventions which include the children in the treatment would be most interesting. Alternative programmes inspired by other serious illnesses would also be most welcomed.

CONCLUSION

Based on the recent research it seems that a major stressor for children, distinctive to parental ABI, may be the disrupted caretaking and lack of parental responsiveness (interpersonal loss) following the changes in the brain-injured parents' personality and cognitive capacity, which will usually stand in marked contrast to the parent's pre-injury personality.

Children living in families with a parent with an acquired brain injury seem at risk of developing post-traumatic stress symptoms. An understanding of the traumatic process and interpersonal losses experienced by children affected by parental ABI has implications for the provision of help. It is important to keep in mind when assessing these children that their symptoms may be related to the ABI. Internalisation (sadness, worry, anxiety) seems much more common than externalisation (acting out, aggression). As parents or teachers do not always report the children's symptoms, the assessment of children affected by parental ABI should therefore rely on the children's own self-report or clinical interview. Rehabilitation programmes should also be more aware of the role that the brain-injured person's disabilities and personality change has on their parenting role

This chapter points to a need for child-centred family support services to reduce the risk of children being traumatised by parental brain injury. Such interventions should focus on the (hidden) interpersonal losses experienced by the children and work towards re-establishing and reconnecting the relational bonds between children and their brain-injured parents.

REFERENCES

Abidin, R.R. (1983). *The parenting stress index*. Charlottesville, VA: Pediatric Psychology Press.

Achenbach, T.M., Edelbrock, C.S. (1981). Behavioral problems and competencies reported by parents of normal and disturbed children aged four through sixteen. *Monographs of the Society for Research in Child Development*, 46, 1–82.

Armistead, L., Klein, K., Forehand, R. (1995). Parental physical illness and child functioning. *Clinical Psychology Review*, 15, 409–422.

Boss, P., Couden, B.A. (2002). Ambiguous loss from chronic physical illness: Clinical interventions with individuals, couples, and families. *Journal of Clinical Psychology*, 58, 1351–1360.

Brain Injury Association. (2010). Definition of ABI. www.bcbraininjuryassociation.com.

Bruce, M. (2006). A systematic and conceptual review of posttraumatic stress in childhood cancer survivors and their parents. *Clinical Psychology Review*, 26, 233–256.

Butera-Prinzi, F., Perlesz., A. (2004). Through children's eyes: Children's experience of living with a parent with an acquired brain injury. *Brain Injury*, 18, 83–101.

Charles, N., Butera-Prinzi, F., Perlesz, A. (2007). Families living with acquired brain injury: A multiple family group experience. *NeuroRehabilitation*, 22, 61–76.

Ergh, T.C., Rapport, L.J., Coleman, R.D., Hanks, R.A. (2002). Predictors of caregiver and family functioning following traumatic brain injury: Social support moderates caregiver distress. *Journal of Head Trauma Rehabilitation*, 17, 155–174.

Huizinga, G.A., Visser, A., van der Graaf, W.T., Hoekstra, H.J., Klip, E.C., Pras, E., Hoekstra-Weebers, J.E. (2005). Stress response symptoms in adolescent and young adult children of parents diagnosed with cancer. *European Journal of Cancer*, 41, 288–295.

Kieffer-Kristensen, R., Teasdale, T.W. (2011). Parental stress and marital relationships among patients with brain injury and their spouses. *NeuroRehabilitation*, 28(4), 321–330.

Kieffer-Kristensen, R., Teasdale, T.W., Bilenberg, N. (2011). Post-traumatic stress symptoms and psychological functioning in children of parents with acquired brain injury. *Brain Injury*, 25(7–8), 752–760.

Kieffer-Kristensen, R., Siersma, V.D., Teasdale, T.W. (2013). Family matters: Parental-acquired brain injury and child functioning. *NeuroRehabilitation*, 32(1), 59–68.

Kieffer-Kristensen, R., Johansen, K.L.G. (2013). Hidden loss: A qualitative explorative study of children living with a parent with acquired brain injury. *Brain injury*, 27(13–14), 1562–1569.

Kovacs, M. (1985). The Children's Depression Inventory (CDI). *Psychopharmacology Bulletin*, 21, 995–998.

Lezak, M.D. (1988). Brain damage is a family affair. *Journal of Clinical and Experimental Neuropsychology*, 10, 111–123.

Niemelä, M., Kinnunen, L., Paananen, R., Hakko, H., Merikukka, M., Karttunen, V., Räsänen, S. (2014). Parents' traumatic brain injury increases their children's risk for use of psychiatric care: The 1987 Finnish Birth Cohort study. *General Hospital Psychiatry*, 36, 337–341.

Oddy, M., Coughlan, T., Tyerman, A., Jenkins, D. (1985). Social adjustment after closed head injury: A further follow-up seven years after injury. *Journal of Neurology, Neurosurgurgery and Psychiatry*, 48, 564–568.

Osborn, T. (2007). The psychosocial impact of parental cancer on children and adolescents: A systematic review. *Psychooncology*, 16, 101–126.

Perlesz, A., Kinsella, G., Crowe, S. (2000). Psychological distress and family satisfaction following traumatic brain injury: Injured individuals and their primary, secondary, and tertiary carers. *Journal of Head Trauma Rehabilitation*, 15, 909–929.

Perlesz, A., O'Loughlan, M. (1998). Changes in stress and burden in families seeking therapy following traumatic brain injury: A follow-up study. *International Journal of Rehabilitation Research*, 21, 339–354.

Perlesz, A., Kinsella, G., Crowe, S. (1999). Impact of traumatic brain injury on the family: A critical review. *Rehabilitation Psychology*, 44, 6–35.

Perrin, S., Meiser-Stedman, R., Smith, P. (2005). The children's revised impact of event scale (CRIES): Validity as a screening instrument for PTSD. *Behavioural and Cognitive Psychotherapy*, 33, 487–498.

Pessar, L.F., Coad, M.L., Linn, R.T., Willer, B.S. (1993). The effects of parental traumatic brain injury on the behaviour of parents and children. *Brain Injury*, 7, 231–240.

Ponsford, J., Schonberger, M. (2010). Family functioning and emotional state two and five years after traumatic brain injury. *Journal of the International Neuropsychology Society*, 16, 306–317.

Sander, A.M., Sherer, M., Malec, J.F., High, W.M., Jr., Thompson, R.N., Moessner, A.M., Josey, J. (2003). Preinjury emotional and family functioning in caregivers of persons with traumatic brain injury. *Archives of Physical Medicine and Rehabilitation*, 84, 197–203.

Salloum, S., Overstreet, S. (2012). Grief and trauma intervention for children after disaster: Exploring coping skills versus trauma narration, *Behaviour Research and Therapy*, 50, 169–179.

Teasdale, T.W., Engberg, A.W. (2005). Subjective well-being and quality of life following traumatic brain injury in adults: A long-term population-based follow-up. *Brain Injury*, 19, 1041–1048.

Thomsen, I.V. (1984). Late outcome of very severe blunt head trauma: A 10–15 year second follow-up. *Journal of Neurology, Neurosurgery and Psychiatry*, 47, 260–268.

Uysal, S., Hibbard, M.R., Robillard, D., Pappadopulos, E., Jaffe, M. (1998). The effect of parental traumatic brain injury on parenting and child behavior. *Journal of Head Trauma Rehabilitation*, 13, 57–71.

Vaishnavi, S., Rao, V., Fann, J.R. (2009). Neuropsychiatric problems after traumatic brain injury: Unraveling the silent epidemic. *Psychosomatics*, 50, 198–205.

Visser-Meily, A., Post, M., Meijer, A.M., Maas, C., Ketelaar, M., Lindeman, E. (2005). Children's adjustment to a parent's stroke: Determinants of health status and psychological problems, and the role of support from the rehabilitation team. *Journal of Rehabilitation Medicine*, 37, 236–241.

Webster, G., Daisley, A. (2007). Including children in family-focused acquired brain injury rehabilitation: A national survey of rehabilitation staff practice. *Clinical Rehabilitation*, 21, 1097–1108.

CHAPTER 5

Parental depression

Emily Crain and Tracy R.G. Gladstone

INTRODUCTION

One in five children in the United States is living with a depressed parent (National Research Council and Institute of Medicine, 2009). Research over the last several decades suggests that parental depression affects biological reactivity to stress, emotion regulation skills and attachment style early in life (Davé et al., 2005; McMahon et al., 2006; Volling et al., 2002;), and is associated with cognitive delays, academic difficulties and social and behavioural difficulties as children grow older (Barker et al., 2011; DeRose et al., 2014; Fihrer et al., 2009; Giallo et al., 2014, Murray et al., 2010). Being raised by a depressed parent also has been established as a risk factor for the onset of psychopathology, including both internalising (e.g. depression and anxiety) and externalising (e.g. conduct disorder, attention deficit disorder) disorders (Glasheen et al., 2010; Goodman and Rouse, 2010; Joorman et al., 2009; Kouros and Garber, 2010). Recently, interventions, preventative measures and psychotherapy practices have been developed and evaluated in order to address the increased risk of difficulties in children of depressed parents (Gladstone and Beardslee, 2002).

This chapter presents literature on the impact of parental depression on children throughout their lifespan, from infancy through to young adulthood, as parental depression affects children differentially at each developmental stage. In addition, literature is presented on interventions that address this increased risk in children of depressed parents at each stage of development. The chapter concludes with recommendations both for practice and for future research.

It should be noted that to date, much of the research on the intergenerational transmission of depression has focused on the relationship between depressed mothers and their children. Thus, throughout this review, when studies refer to fathers, or to both mothers and fathers, this is explicitly highlighted. In addition, in reviewing the literature for infants of depressed mothers, the focus is not on postpartum depression, but rather on maternal depression with a longer duration during the first few years of life. There is an extensive body of research on postpartum depression and on interventions targeting mothers during pregnancy, but this is not discussed in this chapter. Moreover, a range of definitions has been used to refer to depressive symptoms in parents. Specifically, some researchers label mothers as depressed if they endorse a standard number of symptoms on a self-report measure of depressive symptoms (e.g. Weissman et al., 2004); others define depression through structured diagnostic interviews (e.g. Garber et al., 2009). These diagnostic distinctions are clarified throughout this review. Finally, it should be noted that some child outcomes are also contingent on the vulnerability status of the family (e.g. socio-economic status, minority status); where relevant, these additional risk factors will be highlighted.

LITERATURE REVIEW

Infants

Infancy, defined as birth until 12 months, is a critical time for healthy emotional, behavioural, cognitive and language development in children (Davies, 2011). Healthy infants are alert, active and socially aware from the first days of life. From birth, infants have the ability to respond to parental, particularly maternal, stimuli (Chase-Brand, 2008). Infants are also born with goals of maintaining homeostasis and regulating their emotions (Tronick, 2007); both goals are contingent on the quality of the parent-infant dyad. Research suggests that caretaking can significantly impact behavioural, emotional and cognitive outcomes, and parental depression or depressive symptoms can have a negative impact on parenting abilities and the familial environment (Bernard-Bonnin, 2004).

Behavioural and emotional development

During the first six to nine months of an infant's life, the mother-child relationship significantly grows and develops. However, even the first four months of life are crucial for healthy attachment development (Chase-Brand, 2008; Moheler et al., 2006). Even from the first moments of birth, infants and mothers engage in reciprocal behaviour, and depressed mothers often are unable to maintain the 'developmental duet' (Chase-Brand, 2008). Depressed mothers are less likely to smile, speak to and make eye contact with their babies. They also have different vocal patterns when communicating with their children, relative to mothers who are not depressed (Reissland et al., 2003). Researchers explain that depressed mothers have often inconsistent emotional responses around their children (Field, 2010), making it difficult for children to regulate their own emotions (Tronick, 2007). Depressed mothers are often more distracted and preoccupied during interactions with their infants, and may exhibit either intrusive or withdrawn patterns of behaviour, contributing to the difficulty of matching emotional states (Field, 2010; Hoffman et al., 2006).

Research suggests that infants will mirror this lack of engagement displayed by their mothers. These infants are often observed avoiding gazes and displaying less positive affect, and are less likely to engage in 'turn-taking' speech with their caregivers than babies of mothers who are not depressed (Ferber et al., 2008; Reck et al., 2004; Righetti-Veltema et al., 2003). Relative to infants of mothers who are not depressed, infants of depressed mothers show evidence of more sleep problems and crying (Dennis and Ross, 2005; Hiscock and Wake, 2001) and have been described as more tense, less content, fussier and less physically active (Field, 2010).

Research suggests that mothers suffering from depression, in comparison to mothers who are not depressed, less frequently touch their children in an affectionate manner (Ferber et al., 2008). As a result, the child may become passive, withdrawn and may engage in maladaptive self-regulatory behaviour, such as looking away or sucking their thumb (Bernard-Bonnin, 2004). Multiple research groups have discovered that infants of depressed mothers spend more time touching their own skin (Herrera et al., 2004), a behaviour that may develop as a consequence of the lack of touch they receive from their mothers in these critical months of life. Finally, children of depressed mothers have been observed to engage in less play, suggesting that this is a consequence of the poor engagement and attachment with their child (Righetti-Veltema et al., 2003). Ultimately, with repeated negative interaction experiences, infants develop representations of themselves as ineffective; when infants' efforts to achieve their goals are thwarted by insensitive or inconsistent maternal response, negative affective responses may result.

It is important to note that not only maternal depression has had negative outcomes on infants. A study by Davé, Nazareth, Sherr and Senior explored the relation between paternal depression/mood and the temperament (i.e. fussiness) of their infants and found a significant association between fathers' self-reported depressive symptoms and infants' negative temperament (Davé et al., 2005).

Cognitive development

During the early months of life, infants are also developing skills in cognition, attention regulation and arousal. Research suggests that even during infancy, children of depressed mothers demonstrate reduced cognitive functioning (Cicchetti et al., 2000; Galler et al., 2000; Sutter-Dalley et al., 2010). As mentioned earlier, relative to mothers who are not depressed, depressed mothers are less likely to provide sufficient stimulation and display positive affect with their infants (Ferber et al., 2008). Studies also show that depressed parents engage less in enrichment activities with their infants, such as reading, singing and playing (Paulson et al., 2006). Research has suggested that this lack of stimulation/attention and positive affect impedes infants' ability to process information and learn (Bernard-Bonnin, 2004).

There may be some gender differences in the relation between cognitive development and parental depression. Azak found that in homes with a depressed parent, female infants' cognitive scores tended to increase over time, but this effect was not seen among male infants (Azak, 2012). Milgrom, Westley and Gemmill (2004) followed depressed and non-depressed mother-infant dyads from birth until 42 months of age. They found that at six months, the interactions between depressed mothers and their children were dysfunctional, and by 42 months the children showed cognitive deficits measured by IQ. However, interestingly, male infants of depressed mothers were disproportionately vulnerable to impaired cognitive abilities, relative to female infants of depressed mothers (Milgrom et al., 2004).

Toddlers

During toddlerhood, ages 1–3, children develop an abundance of skills (e.g. language skills, motor skills, developing empathy and gaining independence) that help them navigate the world around them (Albers and Grieve, 2007; Davies, 2011). Achieving these milestones is important in the trajectory of the child's healthy behavioural, socio-emotional and cognitive functioning. Research suggests that growing up with a depressed parent may interfere with a toddler's development in these areas (Petterson and Albers, 2001).

Behavioural and emotional development

According to Bowlby (1969, 1973, 1980), a primary task in the early years of life is the formation of an attachment relationship with a primary caregiver. Through repeated positive interactions with the primary caregiver, toddlers form secure internal working models of this relationship, which enable them to tolerate brief separations. Ultimately, toddlers are able to use this secure relationship as a base for the development of healthy relationships throughout life. However, Bowlby (1969, 1973, 1980) argued that children with parents who are unavailable, either physically or psychologically, might develop an insecure primary attachment that may ultimately impede their social and emotional growth.

The relationship between maternal depression and toddler attachment-autonomy behaviour has been established with some consistency. Specifically, research suggests that attachment relationships between depressed mothers and toddlers are more insecure, relative to those of non-depressed mother-toddler dyads (Coyl et al., 2002; Gravener et al., 2012). Insecure and disorganised attachment is significantly correlated with negative behavioural and emotional outcomes in children (Fearon et al., 2010; McCartney et al., 2004). Thus, it is not surprising that children with depressed parents are more likely to develop internalising and externalising behaviour issues than their counterparts with parents who are not depressed (Civic and Holt, 2000; Fihrer et al., 2009; Fisher et al., 2015; Halligan et al., 2007; Trapolini et al., 2007;). Despite the consistency of findings related to depressed parents and attachment, it is important to remember that not all children of depressed parents are insecurely attached. Attachment is most contingent on parenting, yet not all depressed parents have poor parenting styles and behaviour (Toth et al., 2009).

Research indicates that both maternal and paternal depression can increase a toddler's risk of developing behavioural and emotional problems (Fisher et al., 2015; Giles et al., 2011; Velders et al., 2011). As children are acquiring basic behavioural and emotional skills, their parents often serve as their role models for appropriate behaviour. Depressed parents often can be poor models for negative mood regulation and problem-solving behaviour (Maughan et al., 2007). Consequently, efforts to connect parental depression and socio-emotional competence have revealed that toddlers with depressed caregivers exhibit deficits in their socio-emotional development and competency (Luoma et. al., 2001). In a study by Langrock et al., in comparison to children of parents who are not depressed, young children with depressed parents experienced higher rates of anxiety, depressive and aggressive symptoms (Langrock et al., 2002). Importantly, recurrent parental depression, as opposed to single isolated episodes during young childhood, is significantly correlated with child impairments (Giles et al., 2011).

Cognitive development

Parental depression also has been found to negatively impact toddlers' cognitive development. Experts suggest that having a depressed parent may hinder the activation of a child's exploration system that contributes to cognition (Speranza et al., 2006). Specifically, cognitive-linguistic functioning also can be negatively affected by parental depression (Chapin and Altenhofen, 2010). Language development, like emotional development, is contingent upon social interactions between the child and caregiver (Chapin and Altenhofen, 2010; Paulson et al., 2009). For example, parent-to-child reading supports early expressive language, school readiness, academic achievement and literacy in children (Roberts et al., 2005; Westerlund and Lagerberg, 2008); research shows that, in homes with a depressed parent, less parent-to-child reading occurs, and when it does the quality is poorer (Bigatti et al., 2001; McLennan and Kotelchuck, 2000; Paulson et al., 2009; Reissland et al., 2003). Research also reveals that prenatal maternal depression is associated with more abnormal speech errors in children by the age of two (Wong et al., 2013). Furthermore, across early child development, maternal depressive symptoms have been found to have the strongest negative effect on children's cognitive development, intelligence, and social engagement from ages 2–5 (Feldman and Eidelman, 2009).

It is important to note that parents experiencing depression can still facilitate healthy cognitive functioning in their toddlers. A study by Milgrom et al. (2004) suggests that, within households with a depressed parent, parental responsiveness may mediate the relation between poor language development and psychopathology (Milgrom et al., 2004). Also worthy of mention, Paulson et al. found that there was a stronger association between *paternal* depression and limited expressive language in children, in comparison to *maternal* depression and language development (Paulson et al., 2009).

School-age children

Consistent with other research, parental depression is a risk factor for the healthy development of school-aged children. During school years, children with depressed parents are at risk of experiencing more complex internalising and externalising problems that affect both their family and peer relationships. They are also vulnerable to the onset of cognitive difficulties, such as attention deficit/hyperactivity disorder (ADHD), which compromises their academic achievement moving into adolescence (Lesesne et al., 2003).

Behavioural and emotional development

School-age children of depressed parents display deficits in adaptive functioning (i.e. how well one deals with common life demands), leading to internalising and externalising problems (Goodman et al., 2011). Researchers suggest that the relation between parental depression and child behaviour is a transactional process (Bagner, 2013), whereby parenting behaviour (e.g. hostility, criticism) results in behavioural issues for children (Goodman and Tully,

2008), and children's externalising behaviour problems, hostile interactions and negative affective displays are associated with more parental depression (Goodman et. al., 2011). A study in the UK found that depressed mothers were more likely to engage in harsh disciplinary practices, which were significantly associated with conduct problems among their children (Kiernan and Huerta, 2008). There is also evidence to suggest that there is an association between ADHD in children and maternal mental health, even when adjusted for the child's age, sex, race, household income and type of family structure (Lesene, Visser and White, 2003).

Children of depressed parents are at higher risk of developing internalising psychopathology (Sanger et al., 2015) as well. In Sweden, Agnafors et al. (2013) conducted a longitudinal study following infant-mother dyads up to 12 years of age. They found that concurrent maternal depression (i.e. depression experienced beyond the postpartum period) was the strongest predictor of the child's risk of developing internalising problems by age 12. Their work also suggested that there was a correlation between reports of children's depressed-withdrawn symptoms and maternal postnatal depression. Mothers who experienced both postnatal and concurrent depression were more likely to have children who reported elevated depressive symptoms (Agnafors et al., 2013). Specifically, young girls of depressed mothers exhibit more passive styles of emotional regulation, which in fact might increase their risk for developing psychopathology (Silk et al., 2005).

Additional research in the field has examined different familial or depressive factors that can moderate child outcomes. Interestingly, studies suggest that chronic, concurrent parental depressive symptoms have a stronger effect on child psychopathology outcomes than brief postnatal depressive episodes (Goodman et al., 2010). The severity of parental psychopathology also seems to moderate child behaviour (Barker et al., 2011). Also, a study by Barker et al. concluded that in comparison to maternal anxiety, maternal depression had a larger impact on child maladjustment and externalising disorders. Finally, it is important to note that there is inconsistent literature regarding behavioural differences among boys and girls with depressed parents during their school years (Cummings et al., 2005). It is also likely that genetic susceptibility influences children's development. As a result, it can often be difficult to delineate children's behaviour as a product of maternal depression or other environmental factors.

Cognitive development

Although not adequately researched, there are a few studies that assess the cognitive development of school-age children with depressed parents. More research is needed to examine the cognitive development of these children more comprehensively. Hay et al. (2001) conducted a longitudinal study to assess attention difficulties of 11-year-old boys and girls. Children whose mothers were depressed at three months postpartum were found to have lower IQ scores, increased attentional problems, increased difficulties in mathematical reasoning and increased special educational needs (Hay et al., 2001). Interestingly, male children appeared to be more affected by maternal depression than female children, most significantly on performance IQ. These academic difficulties were not mediated by socio-demographic variables, parental IQ or concurrent maternal depression (Hay et al., 2001).

Adolescents and young adults

Adolescence is defined broadly as the developmental transition between youth and adulthood (Spear, 2000). Across the population, adolescents are particularly vulnerable to the onset of significant psychiatric disorders such as major affective illness, substance abuse and psychosis (Paus et al., 2008). Research has noted that the onset of such disorders can be mediated by family relationships and interactions (National Research Council and Institute of Medicine, 2009). Thus it is not surprising that adolescents of depressed parents are more likely than their peers with non-depressed parents to develop psychopathology (e.g. depression, ADHD) and to exhibit elevated levels of internalising and externalising behaviour (Halligan et al., 2007; Pawlby et al., 2009; Sanger et al., 2015).

Behavioural and emotional development

Similar to the behavioural and emotional findings for toddlers and school-age children, adolescents of depressed parents often experience an increasing number of behavioural and emotional difficulties (Sanger et al., 2015). Fear et al. (2009) examined parental conflict and internalising and externalising behaviour among adolescents with depressed parents and found that a higher level of depression among parents was correlated with higher levels of interparental conflict. Of significance, these higher levels of interparental conflict were positively associated with internalising and externalising behaviour among teens (Fear et al., 2009). Brennan et al. (2002) sampled 522 Australian families and examined the relationship between both paternal psychopathology and maternal depression, and adolescent outcomes (Brennan et al., 2002). Specifically, these researchers were interested in exploring youth depression, non-depressive externalising disorders (i.e. ADHD, conduct disorder, oppositional-defiant disorder or substance-use disorder) and non-depressive internalising disorders (i.e. anxiety disorders, eating disorders). Results revealed that there was a significant correlation between maternal and paternal depression and externalising disorders in youth (Brennan et al., 2002).

As mentioned above, adolescents with depressed parents are at a higher risk for the onset of their own psychiatric disorders (Halligan et al., 2007; Pawlby et al., 2009). Pawlby and her team followed 152 mother-child dyads from pregnancy to age 16 of the child. During the lifetime of their child, two-thirds of the mothers in the study reported a depressive episode, most of them reporting more than one episode. Of the children in the study, 14% were diagnosed with a depressive disorder by age 16, and all of these adolescents were exposed to maternal depression during their lifetime. Strikingly, teens exposed to maternal depression were 4.7 times more likely to develop depression themselves, relative to teens whose mothers were never depressed (Pawlby et al., 2009). Other research supports these findings as well. Research suggests that experiencing stressful life events during adolescence puts teens at a higher risk of developing depressive problems (Goodyer et al., 2000). Bouma et al. examined reactions to stressful life events among adolescents with and without a depressed parent. Their findings concluded that when teens of depressed parents experience stressful life events, they are more sensitive to the depressogenic effect than teens of parents who are not depressed (Bouma et al., 2006).

Some research suggests that socio-emotional impairments among children with depressed parents may vary based on gender. Korhonen et al. (2012) found that adolescent boys with depressed mothers exhibited more deficits on measures of social competency than their female counterparts. At age 13, however, teenage girls with depressed parents experienced elevated levels of emotional sensitivity and insecure attachment (Murray et al., 2006).

Cognitive development

Some studies have examined the effect of parental depression on academic achievement among adolescents. A series of studies, conducted by Murray et al. in the UK, suggest that boys with depressed mothers score significantly lower on standardised tests, relative to girls with depressed mothers, and in comparison to teens with mothers who are not depressed (Murray et al., 2010). Ensminger and his research team revealed that teen boys with depressed mothers more than doubled their risk of high school dropout. However, girls seemed to be unaffected (Ensminger et al., 2003). More research regarding adolescent cognitive function and the impact of parental depression is needed to develop a comprehensive understanding of teens' outcomes and experiences.

INTERVENTIONS

New information about the effects of parental depression on children highlights the need for intervention and prevention efforts to address the risk in this population. The Institute of Medicine (2009) summarised six models of preventative interventions for adverse outcomes in children of depressed parents, including: (i) treatment of depression in parents, (ii) early childhood interventions, (iii) cognitive behavioural intervention to address children's risk factors, (iv) teaching parenting skills, (v) family cognitive behavioural interventions to teach both parenting skills to depressed parents and coping skills for their children, and (vi) interventions to strengthen family functioning (National Research Council and Institute of Medicine, 2009). Below, we review intervention programmes for children of depressed parents across the lifespan.

Infants

Research on the prevention of negative outcomes in children of depressed mothers has gained popularity over the last several decades. In a review by Dennis and Creedy (2004) that looked at preventions for postpartum depression, the most successful interventions appeared to be ones that focused on the postnatal, rather than the prenatal, experience of the mothers (Dennis and Creedy, 2004; Field, 2010). The studies described below focus on alleviating maternal depressive symptoms and improving the postnatal relationship and interactions between infants and their mothers.

Home visit intervention programme

Van Doesum et al. (2005) developed a transactional, early-intervention programme aimed at improving the interactions between the depressed mother-infant dyad and preventing developmental problems among these children. This intervention programme, known as the Dutch KOPP, was inspired by other infant-depressed mother interventions from previous generations (e.g. Field, 1998). This intervention included components previously found to be effective, such as interaction coaching for the mother, massaging and increasing touch for the infant, and facilitating increased support from the partner who is not depressed (Van Doesum et al., 2005). The intervention was implemented through six to eight home visits by mental health clinicians over the course of three to four months. Three months after the termination of the invention, one follow-up visit occurred. Depressed mothers were randomly assigned to the intervention condition or the control condition (i.e. parenting support by telephone). Results indicate that the intervention did have a positive effect on the quality of mother-infant interactions.

Dyads in the intervention condition experienced higher scores on attachment security as measured by the Attachment Q Sort (Waters, 1995) and socio-emotional competency as assessed via the Infant Toddler Social and Emotional Assessment (Carter et al., 2003), relative to dyads in the control group (Van Doesum et al., 2008).

Psychotherapy interventions

Forman et al. studied an interpersonal psychotherapy intervention for mothers experiencing postpartum depression. The goal of the intervention was to help mothers interact more effectively with their children. Researchers compared child outcomes of both depressed mothers and mothers who were not depressed. Depressed mothers were either assigned to the control (wait list) condition or the psychotherapy condition, and mothers who were not depressed comprised the control group. Results at 18 months post-treatment suggest that depressed mothers who received the interpersonal psychotherapy significantly decreased their levels of parenting stress, but there were not similar findings among the mothers who were not depressed. Unfortunately, based on reports given by mothers, children of depressed mothers still showed lower attachment security, more internalising and externalising problems, and higher negative temperament than children of mothers who were not depressed (as assessed via the Attachment Q Sort; Waters, 1995; Child Behavior Checklist; Achenbach, 1992; and Child Behavior Questionnaire; Rothbart et al., 2001). Even children whose mothers recovered from depression as a result of the intervention did not show any more benefit from the programme than children with mothers who did not recover from depression (Forman et al., 2007).

In 2006, Howard, Battle, Pearlstein and Rosene-Montella developed a Day Hospital programme for depressed mothers and their infants. The Day Hospital programme included group psychotherapy, individual psychotherapy, and family psychoeducation and counselling. In addition, the programme provided observation and support of the mother-infant dyad, and pharmacological treatments if appropriate. The theoretical approach to this intervention was mainly cognitive behavioural therapy and interpersonal psychotherapy. No randomised controlled trial has been conducted, but preliminary results (Battle et al., 2006) suggest that this programme is associated with a significant reduction in depressive symptoms (i.e. 53.2% of women had 'recovered' at the end of the programme, and 96% of participants endorsed the programme as helpful; Howard et al., 2006).

Intervention for adolescent mothers

Field et al. (2000) conducted an intervention for depressed mothers who were 'at risk' for unremitting depression (Field et al., 2000). In anticipation of the intervention, Field et al. identified a number of factors that may be predictive of maternal depression past six months postnatal. These variables included: right frontal EEG activation, elevated levels of norepinephrine, serotonin and cortisol, poor vagal tone and fewer positive interactions with their infant (Field et al., 2000). Selected from the criteria mentioned above, participants in this study were primarily low-income, adolescent mothers and their infants. Women were randomised into the no-treatment control group or the intervention group. The intervention aimed to decrease mothers' depressive symptoms and increase positive interactions with their infants. In addition, the intervention included a component to enhance the mother's general education/vocational skills. Twice a week mothers in the intervention group received progressive muscle relaxation, massage therapy, music therapy and visual imagery. Their infants also received massages twice a week. Finally, the mother-infant dyad also participated in interaction coaching with the goal of increasing maternal sensitivity and infant responsiveness. The intervention for mother and child lasted a total of four weeks. Results of this intervention revealed that mothers' depressive symptoms (as assessed by the Beck Depression Inventory; Beck et al., 1961 and Diagnostic Interview Schedule for Children; Costello et al., 1985) significantly decreased, and the infants' cognitive (assessed by Bayley's Scale of Infant Development; Bayley, 1969) and social (assessed by the Early Social Communications Scale; Seibert and Hogan, 1982) functioning improved significantly as well.

Toddlers

Interventions for toddlers have targeted toddlers' formation and maintenance of secure attachments, and have encouraged the development of prosocial behaviour and social competence, in order to encourage healthy peer relationships in middle childhood. Several researchers have focused on attachment during this developmental stage, and have emphasised the importance of healthy parenting practices among depressed mothers.

Toddler-parent psychotherapy

The study reviewed in this section was designed to explore the utility of applying toddler-parent psychotherapy (TPP; Lieberman, 1992) as a preventive intervention for families with maternal depressive disorder. TPP uses joint mother-toddler sessions and concepts drawn from attachment theory to alter the relationship between the mother and the child. Drawing on research connecting attachment insecurity to maternal depression, Cicchetti et al. (2000) hypothesised that depressed mother-toddler dyads who participated in TPP would show evidence of more secure attachment relationships at the conclusion of the intervention than would depressed mother-toddler dyads in the control group. It was further expected that the percentage of secure attachments in the group of depressed mother-toddler dyads participating in the intervention would mimic findings for a non-depressed control group. Results indicated that, at baseline, more toddlers of depressed mothers were classified as insecurely attached, relative to toddlers in the non-depressed control group (Cicchetti et al., 2000). At follow-up, as predicted, fewer toddlers of depressed mothers in the TPP group were classified as insecurely attached (26%), relative to toddlers with depressed mothers assigned to the control group (47%). Moreover, as hypothesised, the frequency of toddlers classified as insecurely attached in the depressed TPP group was statistically comparable to the frequency of toddlers classified as insecurely attached in the non-depressed control group. Cicchetti and his colleagues suggested that these results support an understanding of attachment security as malleable, and provide support for an attachment theory model of intervention in protecting children of depressed mothers from a host of social and emotional difficulties.

Group cognitive behavioural therapy

Verduyn et al. (2003) developed a group cognitive behavioural therapy (GCBT) targeting depressed mothers and their two-and-a-half- to four-year-old children. The intervention aimed to reduce maternal depressive symptoms and reduce child behavioural problems through play therapy for the children, and cognitive therapy, psychoeducation and parenting for the mothers. At 6- and 12-month follow-ups, there were no group differences in maternal depressive symptoms or child behavioural problems for mothers in the GCBT group, relative to mothers in a support group control condition and to mothers in a no-treatment condition; however, within the GCBT condition, there did seem to be significant improvements in the child behavioural difficulties at 6- and 12-month follow-ups, and a significant decrease in maternal depressive symptoms. Although the results of this study were somewhat disappointing, the inclusion of psychoeducation regarding the child's development was a great strength of this study, as endorsed by the Institute of Medicine (2009).

School-age children

To date, two research groups have developed family-based interventions for school-age children of depressed parents, and several other researchers have focused their interventions on the functioning and behaviour of the parents, excluding the children from participation.

Family-based intervention programmes

In 2009, Compas et al. conducted a randomised clinical trial examining the efficacy of a family-based cognitive behavioural intervention to prevent adverse effects of parental depression on children aged 9–16 (Compas et al., 2009), relative to a control condition (i.e. written materials only). The active intervention provided coping-skills training for children and parenting-skills training for depressed adults and spouses who were not depressed. They found that, at 18 months post-intervention, children who received the cognitive behavioural intervention reported significantly lower levels of anxiety, depression, internalising, and externalising symptoms, relative to controls, and externalising symptoms and rates of depression seemed to continue to decrease at 24 months. Parents who participated in the intervention group also displayed a significant decrease in depressive symptoms, using a self-report measure (Beck Depression Inventory – II; Beck et al., 1996) at the 2-, 6- and 12-month follow-up (Compas et al., 2009).

Sanders and McFarland also developed a cognitive behavioural family intervention (CBFI) focused on treating child externalising behaviour and parental depression. Participants in this study included depressed mothers (diagnosed major depressive disorder), their spouses (all fathers in this study) and their young children who were diagnosed with oppositional defiant disorder or conduct disorder. Similar to other studies, the goals of this intervention were twofold: to improve parents' depressed moods and also to improve the relationship between parent and child. To achieve these goals, Sanders and McFarland created a 12-session intervention, involving two components: the behavioural family intervention (BFI) and cognitive behavioural treatment (CBT). The BFI involved parenting skills training that promoted positive parenting behaviours and effective management of poor child behaviour (Sanders and McFarland; 2000). The second component, CBT, engaged the parents to identify and interrupt dysfunctional cognitions related to their children during family activities, and used relaxation techniques and coping skills to deal with these negative feelings and emotions. Both the CBFI and BFI conditions were associated with reduced maternal depressive symptoms and automatic thoughts (i.e. internalised perceptions involuntarily triggered by a situation or event). At a six-month post-intervention follow-up, mothers' perceptions of social support and parenting competency showed an elevated rate from baseline. The spouses also displayed a reduction of depressive symptoms and increased parenting competency post-intervention within both conditions. Interestingly enough, however, these changes were not maintained at the six-month follow-up, as they were with mothers. Regarding child behaviour outcomes, both observational measures and mothers' reports indicated a reduction in behavioural issues in both the CBFI and BFI intervention conditions. These child outcome results also were sustained at a six-month follow-up. As described, both the CBFI and BFI interventions had similar effects, so that it is not clear whether the CBFI intervention was in fact more beneficial than BFI alone (Boyd and Gillham, 2009).

Targeting a slightly different population, Sandler et al. (2003) developed the Family Bereavement Program (FBP), which aimed to prevent mental health problems in children (ages 8–16) who have experienced parental loss. With the understanding that bereaved parents may also be experiencing depressive symptoms, the FBP also aimed to promote resilient outcomes among all family members and children. During the interventions, families participated in pre-test, post-test and 11-month follow-up assessments. Findings from this study suggest that the FBP was indeed effective. Families in the FBP group experienced improvements in parenting, coping and caregiver mental health immediately following the intervention. The FBP condition was also significantly correlated with reductions in stressful events experienced at the post-test measure. Unfortunately, the FBP was less strongly associated with a change in children's mental health problems post-intervention. At the 11-month follow up, FBP only led to a reduction in internalising and externalising behaviour problems for girls, and for children who had originally reported elevated problem scores at baseline (Sandler et al., 2003). Six years after this study, Sandler et al. followed up again with youth in their study and found that there were main effects for youths' self-esteem and externalising behaviour (Sandler et al., 2003).

Parent-only group interventions

In 2005, Ha and Oh developed a cognitive behavioural group therapy for depressed mothers with children aged 5–12. To be eligible for this study, the mothers' children also had to be demonstrating significant behavioural problems. Thirty-four mothers were recruited from child psychiatric clinics and enrolled in the study; half the mothers were placed in the cognitive-behavioural therapy group, and the other half in the Wait List control group (this included receiving referrals for parent education). The cognitive-behavioural group therapy aimed to: improve the relationship between mother and child and the mother's feelings of control over their child(ren)'s behaviour; reduce maternal stress, negative automatic thoughts and depressive symptoms; and reduce child behaviour issues (Ha and Oh, 2005). Results demonstrated that mothers in the CBT group reported less stress and fewer maternal depressive symptoms, negative thoughts, parent-child problems, punishing-parenting behaviour, and fewer behavioural problems and less externalising behaviour among their children, in comparison to the Wait List condition post-intervention. At three-month follow-up, adverse child behaviour and maternal symptoms continued to decrease compared to the pre-intervention assessments, and mothers even reported higher social competency among their children (Ha and Oh, 2005).

In a similar group format, Sanford and his research team developed a parent education group for families with young children (ages 6–13) and a parent with depression (Sanford et al., 2003). The parent education programme comprised psychoeducation and parental training to increase knowledge about depression and its impact on the family, spousal support, positive family communication and positive parenting strategies (Sanford et al., 2003). Depressed parents who were enrolled in the treatment group reported improved levels of family functioning and parenting competency, and a lower incidence of family and parent conflict than parents in the control group. Interestingly, however, there were no differences found in depression knowledge between the groups or in child outcomes of depressive symptoms, peer relationships or school problems. One of the major limitations of this study was a poor retention rate: 27% of participants did not complete the post-intervention assessment and 43% did not complete the eight-week post-intervention follow-up. Participants with more severe depression dropped out at a higher rate than participants with less severe major depressive disorder. Researchers hypothesise that this could have been a result of heightened stress and competing treatment and social service needs (Sanford et al., 2003).

Adolescents and young adults

Several research groups have studied directly the treatment or prevention of dysfunction in adolescents of depressed parents (Beardslee et al., 1993; Clarke et al., 2001). These interventions address the onset of adolescent depression, given the developmental risk for depression onset during this life stage.

Family-based intervention programme

Beardslee et al. (1993) have focused their work on families with parental affective disorder, with the goal of preventing the onset of the disorder in non-symptomatic early adolescents aged 8–15 years. Eighty dual- and single-parent families were included in the study, all of which had at least one parent who had experienced an episode of affective disorder in the past 18 months, and at least one child who had never been treated for an episode of affective disorder. Families were assigned to either a six- to ten-session clinician-facilitated condition or to a two-session lecture control condition. Results indicated that both approaches were associated with positive changes in parenting, improved family functioning and decreased internalising symptoms in youth; participants in the clinician-facilitated condition reported significantly greater levels of parenting change and child understanding of parental illness than did participants in the lecture condition (Beardslee et al., 2003, 2007).

Several research groups have adapted the general principles of the Beardslee clinician-facilitated intervention to other populations around the globe (reviewed by Boyd and Gillham, 2009). Podorefsky et al. (2001) evaluated the effectiveness of an adapted version of the clinician-facilitated approach in a low-income, urban population and D'Angelo et al. investigated this approach in a version adapted specifically for Latino mothers. Both studies found that families who participated in the intervention exhibited positive changes in family functioning, including better communication, understanding and focus on children (D'Angelo et al., 2009; Podorefsky et al., 2001). Solantaus et al. (2010) adapted the Beardslee intervention for countrywide use in Finland, targeting children with parents suffering from mental illness. Multiple interventions were implemented, and the clinician-facilitated component was proven to be successful and beneficial for children and families (Solantaus et al., 2010).

Adolescent group intervention programmes

Based on the social learning model of depression, Clarke and Lewinsohn (1995) developed the Coping with Stress (CWS) course, a manual-based psychoeducational group programme that targets adolescents who are at risk for the development of significant depressive disorders. CWS aims to assist vulnerable adolescents in gaining control over negative moods, resolving conflicts that arise at home and with peers, and altering maladaptive thought patterns. Participants included symptomatic adolescents with depressed parents, who were enrolled in a programme maintained by a health maintenance organisation. On measures of self-report (assessed by the Center for Epidemiologic Studies Depression Scale; Radloff, 1977) of depressive symptoms and on interview diagnostic assessments (assessed by the Kiddie-SADS-Epidemiological Version; Orvaschel et al., 1986; and the Hamilton Rating Scale for Depression; Endicott et al., 1981), adolescents assigned to the experimental condition generally reported lower rates of depression than did adolescents assigned to the usual care condition. Moreover, participants in the experimental group were less likely than those in the control group to develop an episode of diagnosable depression both immediately following group participation and throughout the two-year follow-up interval (Clarke et al., 2001). Clarke and his colleagues have concluded that participation in their group intervention programme brought the rate of depressive illness in demoralised (adolescents who presented with sub-diagnostic levels of depressive symptoms or an elevated score on a self-report measure of depressive symptoms) offspring of depressed parents to a level consistent with the general rate of depression in community samples (i.e. in samples with no particular risk for illness).

Using the CWS programme, Garber et al. (2009) conducted a multi-site randomised controlled trial called the Prevention of Depression in At-Risk Adolescents (Garber et al., 2009) study. In this programme, Garber et al. modified Clarke's CWS programme and randomly assigned at-risk teens with a depressed parent to either the group cognitive behavioural condition or to usual care. According to clinician-rated diagnostic clinical interviews, adolescents in the group cognitive behavioural prevention condition were less likely to experience an episode of major depressive disorder than were adolescents assigned to usual care at nine-month follow-up. Current parental depression moderated the intervention effects, such that, when adolescents' parents were not experiencing a depressive episode at baseline, the group cognitive behavioural condition was more effective than the usual care condition in preventing the incidence of depression among teens (Garber et al., 2009); however, this group difference disappeared among adolescents whose parents were currently depressed (Garber et al., 2009). Longer-term data suggest that these findings persist over time (Beardslee et al., 2013; Brent et al., 2015).

IMPLICATIONS FOR PRACTICE

Given the wide-ranging effects of parental depression on children throughout the lifespan, it is important to outline directions for work in clinical settings to address the needs of children with depressed parents.

1. Efforts to prevent negative outcomes in children of depressed parents should not replace efforts to treat parental depression itself. Depression remains one of the most treatable of all mental illnesses, and there are several evidence-based treatments for adult depression, including cognitive behavioural therapy, interpersonal psychotherapy, and psychopharmacological interventions. Depressed parents can engage in healthy parenting practices and foster healthy attachment with their children despite their affective disorder.
2. Interventions for children with depressed parents need to be

developmentally focused, and should include parents in some way. For younger children, it is important to include parents to work on parent interactions, parenting strategies, and parent communication skills. But parental involvement is appropriate with adolescents as well. Parents can play a significant role in how well teens respond to interventions (Garber et al., 2009), and parents can support their children's healthy development and resilience (Beardslee and Podorefsky, 1988).

3. Family-based interventions clearly hold promise. Strong family-based approaches need to support boundaries between parents and their children and should not be initiated during times of severe illness in parents (e.g. during stays in hospital). Family-based interventions should consider including:
   a. Education for all family members about depression, including information about depression as an illness, and reviewing common symptoms of depression and treatments for this disorder. In addition, as part of a discussion of depression, family members can be encouraged to discuss ways that this illness affects them personally.
   b. Information about resilience, including information about how parents can support resilience in themselves and in their children. Research suggests that, although children of depressed parents are at increased risk for negative outcomes, many of these children are resilient (Beardslee and Podorefsky, 1988). Factors associated with resilience in children of depressed parents include being involved in activities outside the home, maintaining meaningful relationships, and understanding that they are separate from their parent's depressive disorder. Families should receive more support in identifying resources for their children in order to foster resiliency and optimal health.
   c. Maintain a strength-based focus, promoting the family's strengths, and also the individual strengths of people within the family. Taking a strength-based approach helps to eliminate stigma and potentially support positive outcomes for both parents and children.

RECOMMENDATIONS FOR FUTURE RESEARCH

We suggest several directions for future research on children of depressed parents.

1. Boyd and Gillham (2009) note a number of limitations associated with the intervention research on children of depressed parents, including the use of non-randomised designs, small sample sizes, non-representative

samples, and short follow-up intervals. Future research in this area must: (i) examine the effects of both maternal and paternal depression on children across the life span; (ii) study both short- and long-term effects of interventions targeting children of depressed parents; (iii) explore effects of the severity of parental depression on children; (iv) examine the effects of interventions for parents and children from marginalised populations; and (v) consider bi-directional influences (i.e. the effects of parental depression on youth, and the effects of youth behaviour on parents' symptoms).

2. Recent evidence suggests that parental depression may be associated with a child's ability to respond to treatment and preventive interventions targeting internalising disorders. For example, in an effectiveness study of a cognitive behavioural prevention intervention targeting adolescents at risk for depression (adolescents of parents with a current and/or past diagnosis of depression), Garber et al. (2009) found that the intervention was successful in preventing episodes of depression in teens without a currently depressed parent, but no intervention effect emerged for teens with a parent who was currently depressed. Similar findings regarding the effect of parental mental illness on children's intervention responses have been reported in studies of parents with general psychopathology (Bodden et al., 2008; Cooper et al., 2008; Creswell et al., 2008; Phillips et al., 2000; Rishel et al., 2006a, 2006b) and for children's response to interventions targeting a range of youth behaviour and disorders (e.g. Kazdin 1989, 1995; Owens et al., 2003). Thus, when studying interventions for children of depressed parents, it is important to investigate the effects of parental depression on children's responses to interventions targeting youth symptoms.
3. An important direction for future research involves exploring new avenues for encouraging depressed parents to seek treatment, and also new approaches to helping depressed parents get the treatment they need. Motivational interviewing strategies (Miller and Rollnick, 2003) have been used to help people move through the stages of behaviour change and may hold promise in encouraging parents to seek treatment for their own symptoms. Motivational interviewing is a person-centred, directive method of communication that aims to enhance one's intrinsic motivation to change by exploring and resolving ambivalence. It may be that motivational interviewing strategies, such as asking open-ended questions, using active/reflective listening, eliciting self-motivational statements and supporting parents in balancing the positives and negatives of seeking treatment, could help parents begin to accept the need to address

their own depressive illness. Likewise, patient navigator models, which were initially developed for patients with cancer or other chronic medical problems, have been found to play an important role in helping adults to access timely care. Specifically, the use of patient navigators among adults with cancer, HIV and chronic disease is associated with greater adherence to treatment recommendations, decreased anxiety and increased patient satisfaction (e.g. Bradford et al., 2007; Esperat et al., 2012; Robinson-White et al., 2010). It is possible that patient navigators can similarly assist depressed parents in accessing appropriate treatment resources.

4. Research is required on new approaches that may help at-risk youth to access interventions to prevent negative outcomes, particularly when many youths from disadvantaged backgrounds may have difficulty accessing services within traditional specialty mental health settings. For example, technology-based depression prevention approaches hold promise (Van Voorhees et al., 2011) and provide an area in need of further exploration.

CONCLUSION

Children of depressed parents have been identified as a population at high risk for a variety of emotional problems, including depression and other forms of psychopathology. Parental depression affects children differentially at each developmental stage. During infancy, maternal depression has been found to interfere with children's internal and social goals and with the regulation of emotion and attention. During toddlerhood, maternal depression has been associated with insecure attachment and with deficits in socio-emotional development. Throughout the school years, children of depressed parents exhibit more externalising and internalising symptoms and cognitive limitations, which have an impact on their social and school functioning. During adolescence, maternal depression has been associated with negative self-concept and with the use of poor interpersonal strategies. In this chapter, treatment and intervention research addressing these issues has been reviewed, and suggestions for practice and research have been offered. Ultimately, we argue for the development of primary prevention programmes targeting the children of depressed parents as they negotiate developmental tasks from infancy through young adulthood (Gladstone and Beardslee, 2002).

REFERENCES

Achenbach, T.M. (1992). *Manual for the Child Behavior Checklist/2–3 and 1992 profile.* Burlington, VT: University of Vermont.

Agnafors, S., Comasco, E., Bladh, M., Sydsjö, G., DeKeyser, L., Oreland, L., Svedin, C.G. (2013). Effect of gene, environment and maternal depressive symptoms on pre-adolescence behavior problems. A longitudinal study. *Child and Adolescent Psychiatry and Mental Health*, 7(1), 10.

Albers, C.A., Grieve, A.J. (2007). Review of Bayley Scales of infant and toddler development (3rd edn). *Journal of Psychoeducational Assessment*, 25(2), 180–190.

Azak, Schale. 2012. Maternal depression and sex differences shape the infants' trajectories of cognitive development. *Infant Behavior and Development*, 35(4), 803–814.

Bagner, D.M., Pettit, J.W., Lewinsohn, P.M., Seeley, J.R., Jaccard, J. (2013). Disentangling the temporal relationship between parental depressive symptoms and early child behavior problems: A transactional framework. *Journal of Clinical Child and Adolescent Psychology*, 42(1), 78–90.

Barker, E.D., Jaffee, S.R., Uher, R., Maughan, B. (2011). The contribution of prenatal and postnatal maternal anxiety and depression to child maladjustment. *Depression and Anxiety*, 28(8), 696–702. doi:10.1002/da.20856.

Battle, C.L., Zlotnick, C., Miller, I.W., Pearlstein, T., Howard, M. (2006). Clinical characteristics of perinatal psychiatric patients: A chart review study. *Journal of Nervous and Mental Disease*, 194(5), 369–377.

Bayley, N. (1969). *Bayley scales of infant development.* New York: The Psychological Corporation.

Beardslee, W.R., Podorefsky, D. (1988). Resilient adolescents whose parents have serious affective and other psychiatric disorders: Importance of self-understanding and relationships. *The American Journal of Psychiatry*, 145(1), 63–69.

Beardslee, W.R., Keller, M.B., Lavori, P.W., Staley, J.E., Sacks, N. (1993). The impact of parental affective disorder on depression in offspring: A longitudinal follow-up in a nonreferred sample. *Journal of the American Academy of Child and Adolescent Psychiatry*, 32(4), 723–730.

Beardslee, W.R., Gladstone, T.R., Wright, E.J., Cooper, A.B. (2003). A family-based approach to the prevention of depressive symptoms in children at risk: Evidence of parental and child change. *Pediatrics*, 112(2), e119–e131.

Beardslee, W.R., Wright, E.J., Gladstone, T.G., Forbes, P. (2007). Long-term effects from a randomized trial of two public health preventive interventions for parental depression. *Journal of Family Psychology*, 21(4), 703–713.

Beardslee, W.R., Brent, D.A., Weersing, V.R., Clarke, G.N., Porta, G., Hollon, S.D., Gladstone, T.R., Gallop, R., Lynch, F.L., Iyengar, S., DeBar, L., Garber, J. (2013). Prevention of depression in at-risk adolescents: Longer-term effects. *JAMA Psychiatry*, 70(11), 1161–1170.

Beck, A.T., Ward, C.H., Mendelson, M., Mock, J., Erbaugh, J. (1961). An inventory for measuring depression. *Archives of General Psychiatry*, 4561–4571.

Beck, A.T., Steer, R.A., Ball, R., Ranieri, W.F. (1996). Comparison of Beck Depression

Inventories IA and II in psychiatric outpatients. *Journal of Personality Assessment*, 67, 588–597.

Bernard-Bonnin, A. (2004). Maternal depression and child development. *Paediatrics and Child Health*, 9(8), 575–583.

Bigatti, S.M., Cronan, T.A., Anaya, A. (2001). The effects of maternal depression on the efficacy of a literacy intervention program. *Child Psychiatry and Human Development*, 32(2), 147–162.

Bodden, D.H.M., Bogels, S.M., Nauta, M.H., De Haan, E., Ringrose, J., Appelboom, C. et al. (2008). Child versus family cognitive-behavioral therapy in clinically anxious youth: An efficacy and partial effectiveness study. *Journal of the American Academy of Child and Adolescent Psychiatry*, 47(12), 1384–1394.

Bouma, E.C., Ormel, J., Verhulst, F.C., Oldehinkel, A.J. (2008). Stressful life events and depressive problems in early adolescent boys and girls: The influence of parental depression, temperament and family environment. *Journal of Affective Disorders*, 105(1–3), 185–193.

Bowlby, J. (1969). *Attachment and loss: Vol. 1.* New York: Basic Books.

Bowlby, J. (1973). *Attachment and loss: Vol. 2. Separation.* New York: Basic Books.

Bowlby, J. (1980). *Attachment and loss: Vol. 3. Loss, sadness, and depression.* New York: Basic Books.

Boyd, R.C., Gillham, J.E. (2009). Review of interventions for parental depression from toddlerhood to adolescence. *Current Psychiatry Reviews*, 5(4), 226–235.

Bradford, J.B., Coleman, S., Cunningham, W. (2007). HIV system navigation: An emerging model to improve HIV care access. *AIDS Patient Care and STDs*, 21(Suppl1), S49–S58.

Brennan, P.A., Hammen, C., Katz, A.R., Le Brocque, R.M. (2002). Maternal depression, paternal psychopathology, and adolescent diagnostic outcomes. *Journal of Consulting and Clinical Psychology*, 70(5), 1075–1085.

Brent, D., Brunwasser, S., Hollon, S., Weersing, V., Clarke, G., Dickerson, J., Beardslee, W., Gladstone, T., Porta, G., Lynch, F., Iyengar, S., Garber, J. (2015). Prevention of depression in at-risk adolescents: Impact of a cognitive behavioral prevention program on depressive episodes, depression-free days, and developmental competence 6 years after the intervention. *JAMA Psychiatry*, 72(11), 1110–1118.

Carter, A.S., Briggs-Gowan, M., Jones, S.M., Little, T.O. (2003). The Infant-Toddler Social and Emotional Assessment (ITSEA): Factor structure, reliability, and validity. *Journal of Abnormal Child Psychology*, 31, 495–514.

Chapin, L.A., Altenhofen, S. (2010). Neurocognitive perspectives in language outcomes of Early Head Start: Language and cognitive stimulation and maternal depression. *Infant Mental Health Journal*, 31(5), 486–498.

Chase-Brand, J. (2008). Effects of maternal postpartum depression on the infant and older siblings. In S. Dowd Stone, A.E. Menken (Eds) *Perinatal and postpartum mood disorders: Perspectives and treatment guide for the health care practitioner* (pp. 41–64). New York: Springer.

Cicchetti, D., Rogosch, F.A., Toth, S.L. (2000). The efficacy of toddler-parent psychotherapy for fostering cognitive development in offspring. *Journal of Abnormal Child Psychology*, 28(2), 135–148.

Civic, D., Holt, V.L. (2000). Maternal depressive symptoms and child behavior problems in a nationally representative normal birthweight sample. *Maternal and Child Health Journal*, 4(4), 215–221.

Clarke, G.N., Lewinsohn, P.M. (1995). Instructor's manual for the Adolescent Coping with Stress Course. Unpublished work.

Clarke, G.N., Hornbrook, M., Lynch, F., Polen, M., Gale, J., Beardslee, W., O'Connor, E., Seeley, J. (2001). A randomized trial of a group cognitive intervention for preventing depression in adolescent offspring of depressed parents. *Archives of General Psychiatry*, 58(12), 1127–1134.

Compas, B.E., Forehand, R., Keller, G., Champion, J.E., Rakow, A., Reeslund, K.L., McKee, L., Fear, J.M., Colletti, C.J., Hardcastle, E., Merchant, M.J., Roberts, L., Potts, J., Garai, E., Coffelt, N., Roland, E., Sterba, S.K., Cole., D.A. (2009). Randomized controlled trial of a family cognitive-behavioral preventive intervention for children of depressed parents. *Journal of Consulting and Clinical Psychology*, 77(6), 1007–1020.

Cooper, P.J., Gallop, C., Willets, L., Creswell, C. (2008). Treatment response in child anxiety is differentially related to the form of maternal anxiety disorder. *Behavioural and Cognitive Psychotherapy*, 36, 44–48.

Costello, E.J., Edelbrock, C.S., Costello, A.J. (1985). Validity of the NIMH Diagnostic Interview Schedule for Children: A comparison between psychiatric and pediatric referrals. *Journal of Abnormal Child Psychology*, 13(4), 579–595.

Coyl, D.D., Roggman, L.A., Newland, L.A. (2002). Stress, maternal depression, and negative mother-infant interactions in relation to infant attachment. *Infant Mental Health Journal*, 23(1–2), 145–163.

Creswell, C., Willets, L., Murray, L., Singhal, M., Cooper, P. (2008). Treatment of child anxiety: An exploratory study of the role of maternal anxiety and behaviors in treatment outcome. *Clinical Psychology and Psychotherapy*, 15, 38–44.

Cummings, E.M., Keller, P.S., Davies, P.T. (2005). Towards a family process model of maternal and paternal depressive symptoms: Exploring multiple relations with child and family functioning. *Journal of Child Psychology and Psychiatry*, 46(5), 479–489.

D'Angelo, E.J., Llerena-Quinn, R., Shapiro, R., Colon, F., Rodriguez, P., Gallagher, K., Beardslee, W.R. (2009). Adaptation of the preventive intervention program for depression for use with predominantly low-income Latino families. *Family Process*, 48(2), 269–291.

Davé, S., Nazareth, I., Sherr, L., Senior, R. (2005). The association of paternal mood and infant temperament: A pilot study. *British Journal of Developmental Psychology*, 23(4), 609–621.

Davies, D. (2011). *Child development: A practitioner's guide* (3rd edn). New York: Guilford Press.

Dennis, C.L., Creedy, D. (2004). Psychosocial and psychological interventions for preventing postpartum depression [review]. *The Cochrane Database of Systematic Reviews*, (4).

Dennis, C., Ross, L. (2005). Relationships among infant sleep patterns, maternal fatigue, and development of depressive symptomatology. *Birth: Issues in Perinatal Care*, 32(3), 187–193.

DeRose, L.M., Shiyko, M., Levey, S., Helm, J., Hastings, P.D. (2014). Early maternal depression and social skills in adolescence: A marginal structural modeling approach. *Social Development*, 23(4), 753–769.

Endicott, J., Cohen, J., Nee, J., Fleiss, J., Sarantakos, S. (1981). Hamilton Depression Rating Scale: Extracted from regular and change versions of the schedule for affective disorders and schizophrenia. *Archives of General Psychiatry*, 38(1), 98–103.

Ensminger, M.E., Hanson, S.G., Riley, A.W., Juon, H. (2003). Maternal psychological distress: Adult sons' and daughters' mental health and educational attainment. *Journal of the American Academy of Child and Adolescent Psychiatry*, 42(9), 1108–1115.

Esperat, M.C., Flores, D., McMurry, L., Feng, D., Song, H., Billings, L., Masten, Y. (2012) Transformacion para salud: A patient navigation model for chronic disease self-management. *OJIN: The Online Journal of Issues in Nursing*, 17(2).

Fear, J.M., Champion, J.E., Reeslund, K.L., Forehand, R., Colletti, C., Roberts, L., Compas, B.E. (2009). Parental depression and interparental conflict: Children and adolescents' self-blame and coping responses. *Journal of Family Psychology*, 23(5), 762–766.

Fearon, R.P., Bakermans-Kranenburg, M.J., van IJzendoorn, M.H., Lapsley, A., Roisman, G.I. (2010). The significance of insecure attachment and disorganization in the development of children's externalizing behavior: A meta-analytic study. *Child Development*, 81(2), 435–456.

Feldman, R., Eidelman, A.I. (2009). Biological and environmental initial conditions shape the trajectories of cognitive and social-emotional development across the first years of life. *Developmental Science*, 12(1), 194–200.

Ferber, S.G., Feldman, R., Makhoul, I.R. (2008). The development of maternal touch across the first year of life. *Early Human Development*, 84(6), 363–370.

Field, T. (1998). Maternal depression effects on infants and early interventions. *Preventive Medicine: An International Journal Devoted to Practice and Theory*, 27(2), 200–203.

Field, T. (2010). Postpartum depression effects on early interactions, parenting, and safety practices: A review. *Infant Behavior and Development*, 33(1), 1–6.

Field, T., Pickens, J., Prodromidis, M., Malphurs, J., Fox, N., Bendell, D., Yando, R., Schanberg, S., Kuhn, C. (2000). Targeting adolescent mothers with depressive symptoms for early intervention. *Adolescence*, 35(138), 381–414.

Fihrer, I., McMahon, C.A., Taylor, A.J. (2009). The impact of postnatal and concurrent maternal depression on child behaviour during the early school years. *Journal of Affective Disorders*, 119(1–3), 116–123.

Fisher, S.D., Brock, R.L., O'Hara, M.W., Kopelman, R., Stuart, S. (2015). Longitudinal contribution of maternal and paternal depression to toddler behaviors: Interparental conflict and later depression as mediators. *Couple and Family Psychology: Research and Practice*, 4(2), 61–73.

Forman, D.R., O'Hara, M.W., Stuart, S., Gorman, L.L., Larsen, K.E., Coy, K.C. (2007).

Effective treatment for postpartum depression is not sufficient to improve the developing mother–child relationship. *Development and Psychopathology*, 19(02), 585–602.

Galler, J.R., Harrison, R.H., Ramsey, F., Forde, V., Butler, S.C. (2000). Maternal depressive symptoms affect infant cognitive development in Barbados. *Journal of Child Psychology and Psychiatry*, 41(6), 747–757.

Garber, J., Clarke, G.N., Weersing, V.R., Beardslee, W.R., Brent, D.A., Gladstone, T.G., DeBar, L.L., Lynch, F.L., D'Angelo, E., Hollon, S.D., Shamseddeen, W., Iyengar, S. (2009). Prevention of depression in at-risk adolescents: A randomized controlled trial. *JAMA: Journal of the American Medical Association*, 301(21), 2215–2224.

Giallo, R., Cooklin, A., Wade, C., D'Esposito, F., Nicholson, J.M. (2014). Maternal postnatal mental health and later emotional–behavioural development of children: The mediating role of parenting behaviour. *Child: Care, Health and Development*, 40(3), 327–336.

Giles, L.C., Davies, M.J., Whitrow, M.J., Warin, M.J., Moore, V. (2011). Maternal depressive symptoms and child care during toddlerhood relate to child behavior at age 5 years. *Pediatrics*, 128(1), e78–e84.

Gladstone, T.G., Beardslee, W.R. (2002). Treatment, intervention, and prevention with children of depressed parents: A developmental perspective. In S.H. Goodman, I.H. Gotlib, S.H. Goodman, I.H. Gotlib (Eds) *Children of depressed parents: Mechanisms of risk and implications for treatment* (pp. 277–305). Washington, DC, US: American Psychological Association.

Glasheen, C., Richardson, G.A., Fabio, A. (2010). A systematic review of the effects of postnatal maternal anxiety on children. *Archives of Women's Mental Health*, 13(1), 61–74.

Goodman, S.H., Rouse, M.H. (2010). Perinatal depression and children: A developmental perspective. In R.E. Tremblay, R.G. Barr, Peters, R. De V., M. Boivin (Eds) *Encyclopedia on early childhood development* (pp. 1–7). Montreal, Quebec: Centre of Excellence for Early Childhood Development.

Goodman, S.H., Tully, E. (2008). *Children of depressed mothers: Implications for the etiology, treatment, and prevention of depression in children and adolescents*. New York: Guilford Press.

Goodman, S.H., Rouse, M.H., Connell, A.M., Broth, M.R., Hall, C.M., Heyward, D. (2011). Maternal depression and child psychopathology: A meta-analytic review. *Clinical Child and Family Psychology Review*, 14(1), 1–27.

Goodyer, I.M., Herbert, J., Tamplin, A., Altham, P.E. (2000). First-episode major depression in adolescents: Affective, cognitive and endocrine characteristics of risk status and predictors of onset. *The British Journal of Psychiatry*, 176(2), 142–149.

Gravener, J.A., Rogosch, F.A., Oshri, A., Narayan, A.J., Cicchetti, D., Toth, S.L. (2012). The relations among maternal depressive disorder, maternal expressed emotion, and toddler behavior problems and attachment. *Journal of Abnormal Child Psychology*, 40(5), 803–813.

Ha, E.H., Oh, K.J. (2006). Effects of cognitive-behavioral group therapy for depressive mothers of children with behavior problems. *Child and Family Behavior Therapy*, 28(2), 1–13.

Halligan, S.L., Herbert, J., Goodyer, I., Murray, L. (2007). Disturbances in morning cortisol secretion in association with maternal postnatal depression predict subsequent depressive symptomatology in adolescents. *Biological Psychiatry*, 62(1), 40–46.

Hay, D.F., Pawlby, S., Sharp, D., Asten, P., Mills, A., Kumar, R. (2001). Intellectual problems shown by 11-year-old children whose mothers had postnatal depression. *Journal of Child Psychology and Psychiatry*, 42(7), 871–889.

Herrera, E., Reissland, N., Shepherd, J. (2004). Maternal touch and maternal child-directed speech: Effects of depressed mood in the postnatal period. *Journal of Affective Disorders*, 81(1), 29–39.

Hiscock, H, Wake, M. (2001). Infant sleep problems and postnatal depression: A community-based study. *Pediatrics*, 107, 1317–1322.

Hoffman, C., Crnic, K.A., Baker, J.K. (2006). Maternal depression and parenting: Implications for children's emergent emotion regulation and behavioral functioning. *Parenting: Science and Practice*, 6(4), 271–295.

Howard, M., Battle, C.L., Pearlstein, T., Rosene-Montella, K. (2006). A psychiatric mother-baby day hospital for pregnant and postpartum women. *Archives of Women's Mental Health*, 9(4), 213–218.

Joormann, J., Eugene, F., Gotlib, I.H. (2009). Parental depression: Impact on offspring and mechanisms underlying transmission of risk. In S. Nolen-Hoeksema, L.M. Hilt, S. Nolen-Hoeksema, L.M. Hilt (Eds) *Handbook of depression in adolescents* (pp. 441–472). New York: Routledge/Taylor and Francis Group.

Kazdin, A.E. (1989). Hospitalization of antisocial children: Clinical course, follow-up status, and predictors of outcome. *Advances in Behavior Research and Therapy*, 11(1), 1–67.

Kazdin, A.E. (1995). Child, parent, and family dysfunction as predictors of outcome in cognitive-behavioral treatment of antisocial children. *Behavior and Research Therapy*, 33(3), 271–281.

Kiernan, K.E., Huerta, M.C. (2008). Economic deprivation, maternal depression, parenting and children's cognitive and emotional development in early childhood. *British Journal of Sociology*, 59(4), 783–806.

Korhonen, M., Luoma, I., Salmelin, R., Tamminen, T. (2012). A longitudinal study of maternal prenatal, postnatal and concurrent depressive symptoms and adolescent well-being. *Journal of Affective Disorders*, 136(3), 680–692.

Kouros, C.D., Garber, J. (2010). Dynamic associations between maternal depressive symptoms and adolescents' depressive and externalizing symptoms. *Journal of Abnormal Child Psychology*, 38(8), 1069–1081.

Langrock, A.M., Compas, B.E., Keller, G., Merchant, M.J., Copeland, M.E. (2002). Coping with the stress of parental depression: Parents' reports of children's coping, emotional, and behavioral problems. *Journal of Clinical Child and Adolescent Psychology*, 31(3), 312–324.

Lesesne, C.A., Visser, S.N. White, C.P. (2003). Attention-deficit/hyperactivity disorder in school-aged children: Association with maternal mental health and use of health care resources. *Pediatrics*, 111, 1232–1327.

Lieberman, A.F. (1992). Infant-parent psychotherapy with toddlers. *Development and Psychopathology*, 4, 559–574.

Luoma, I., Tamminen, T., Kaukonen, P., Laippala, P., Puura, K., Salmelin, R., Almqvist, F. (2001). Longitudinal study of maternal depressive symptoms and child well-being. *Journal of the American Academy of Child and Adolescent Psychiatry*, 40(12), 1367–1374.

Maughan, A., Cicchetti, D., Toth, S.L., Rogosch, F.A. (2007). Early-occurring maternal depression and maternal negativity in predicting young children's emotion regulation and socioemotional difficulties. *Journal of Abnormal Child Psychology*, 35(5), 685–703.

McCartney, K., Owen, M.T., Booth, C.L., Clarke-Stewart, A., Vandell, D.L. (2004). Testing a maternal attachment model of behavior problems in early childhood. *Journal of Child Psychology and Psychiatry*, 45(4), 765–778.

McLennan, J.D., Kotelchuck, M. (2000). Parental prevention practices for young children in the context of maternal depression. *Pediatrics*, 105(5), 1090–1095.

McMahon, C.A., Barnett, B., Kowalenko, N.M., Tennant, C.C. (2006). Maternal attachment state of mind moderates the impact of postnatal depression on infant attachment. *Journal of Child Psychology and Psychiatry*, 47(7), 660–669.

Milgrom, J., Westley, D.T., Gemmill, A.W. (2004). The mediating role of maternal responsiveness in some longer term effects of postnatal depression on infant development. *Infant Behavior and Development*, 27(4), 443–454.

Miller, W., Rollnick, S. (2003). Motivational interviewing: Preparing people for change. *Journal for Healthcare Quality*, 25(3), 46.

Moehler, E., Brunner, R., Wiebel, A., Reck, C., Resch, F. (2006). Maternal depressive symptoms in the postnatal period are associated with long-term impairment of mother-child bonding. *Archives of Women's Mental Health*, 9(5), 273–278.

Murray, L., Arteche, A., Fearon, P., Halligan, S., Croudace, T., Cooper, P. (2010). The effects of maternal postnatal depression and child sex on academic performance at age 16 years: A developmental approach. *Journal of Child Psychology and Psychiatry*, 51(10), 1150–1159.

Murray, L., Halligan, S.L., Adams, G., Patterson, P., Goodyer, I.M. (2006). Socioemotional development in adolescents at risk for depression: The role of maternal depression and attachment style. *Development and Psychopathology*, 18(2), 489–516.

National Research Council and Institute of Medicine. (2009). Depression in parents, parenting, and children: Opportunities to improve identification, treatment, and prevention. Washington, DC: National Academies Press.

Orvaschel, H., Puig-Anticj, J., Chambers, W., Tabrizi, M., Johnson, R. (1982). Retrospective assessment of prepubertal major depression with the Kiddie-SADS-E. *Journal of the American Academy of Child Psychiatry*, 21(4), 392–397.

Owens, E.B., Hinshaw, S.P., Kraemer, H.C., Arnold, L.E., Abikoff, H.B., Cantwell, D.P. et al. (2003). Which treatment for whom for ADHD? Moderators of treatment response in the MTA. *Journal of Consulting and Clinical Psychology*, 71(3), 540–552.

Paulson, J.F., Dauber, S., Leiferman, J.A. (2006). Individual and combined effects of postpartum depression in mothers and fathers on parenting behavior. *Pediatrics*, 118(2), 659–668.

Paulson, J.F., Keefe, H.A., Leiferman, J.A. (2009). Early parental depression and child language development. *Journal of Child Psychology and Psychiatry*, 50(3), 254–262.

Paus, T., Keshavan, M., Giedd, J.N. (2008). Why do many psychiatric disorders emerge during adolescence? *Nature Reviews Neuroscience*, 9(12), 947–957.

Pawlby, S., Hay, D.F., Sharp, D., Waters, C.S., O'Keane, V. (2009). Antenatal depression predicts depression in adolescent offspring: Prospective longitudinal community-based study. *Journal of Affective Disorders*, 113(3), 236–243.

Petterson, S.M., Albers, A.B. (2001). Effects of poverty and maternal depression on early child development. *Child Development*, 72(6), 1794–1813.

Phillips, S.D., Hargis, M.B., Kramer, T.L., Lensing, S.Y., Taylor, J.L., Burns, B.J., Robbins, J.M. (2000). Toward a level playing field: Predictive factors for the outcomes of mental health treatment for adolescents. *Journal of the American Academy of Child and Adolescent Psychiatry*, 39(11).

Podorefsky, D.L., McDonald-Dowdell, M., Beardslee, W.R. (2001). Adaptation of preventive interventions for a low-income, culturally diverse community. *Journal of the American Academy of Child and Adolescent Psychiatry*, 40(8), 879–886.

Radloff, L.S. (1977). The CES-D Scale: A self-report depression scale for research in the general population. *Applied Psychological Measurement*, 1(3), 385–401.

Reck, C., Hunt, A., Fuchs, T., Weiss, R., Noon, A., Moehler, E., Downing, G., Tronick, E.Z., Mundt, C. (2004). Interactive regulation of affect in postpartum depressed mothers and their infants: An overview. *Psychopathology*, 37(6), 272–280.

Reissland, N., Shepherd, J., Herrera, E. (2003). The pitch of maternal voice: A comparison of mothers suffering from depressed mood and non-depressed mothers reading books to their infants. *Journal of Child Psychology and Psychiatry*, 44(2), 255–261.

Righetti-Veltema, M., Bousquet, A., Manzano, J. (2003). Impact of postpartum depressive symptoms on mother and her 18-month-old infant. *European Child and Adolescent Psychiatry*, 12(2), 75–83.

Rishel, C.W., Greeno, C.G., Marcus, S.C., Anderson, C. (2006a). Effect of maternal mental health problems on child treatment response in community-based services. *Psychiatric Services*, 57(5), 716–719.

Rishel, C.W., Greeno, C.G., Marcus, S.C., Sales, E., Shear, M.K., Swartz, H.A., Anderson, C. (2006b). Impact of maternal mental health status on child mental health treatment outcome. *Community Mental Health Journal*, 42(1).

Roberts, J., Jurgens, J., Burchinal, M. (2005). The role of home literacy practices in preschool children's language and emergent literacy skills. *Journal of Speech, Language, and Hearing Research*, 48(2), 345–359.

Robinson-White, S., Conroy, B., Slavish, K.H., Rosenzweig, M. (2010). Patient navigation in breast cancer: A systematic review. *Cancer Nursing*, 33(2), 127–140.

Rothbart, M.K., Ahadi, S.A., Hershey, K.L., Fisher, P. (2001). Investigations of temperament at three to seven years: The Children's Behavior Questionnaire. *Child Development*, 72, 1394–1408.

Sanders, M.R., McFarland, M. (2000). Treatment of depressed mothers with disruptive children: A controlled evaluation of cognitive behavioral family intervention. *Behavior Therapy*, 31(1), 89–112.

Sandler, I.N., Ayers, T.S., Wolchik, S.A., Tein, J., Kwok, O., Haine, R.A., Twohey-Jacobs, J., Suter, J., Lin, K., Padgett-Jones, S., Weyer, J.L., Cole, E., Kriege, G., Griffin, W.A. (2003). The Family Bereavement Program: Efficacy evaluation of a theory-based prevention program for parentally bereaved children and adolescents. *Journal of Consulting and Clinical Psychology*, 71(3), 587–600.

Sanford, M., Byrne, C., Williams, S., Atley, S., Ridley, T., Miller, J., Allin, H. (2003). A pilot study of a parent-education group for families affected by depression. *The Canadian Journal of Psychiatry/La Revue Canadienne de Psychiatrie*, 48(2), 78–86.

Sanger, C., Iles, J.E., Andrew, C.S., Ramchandani, P.G. (2015). Associations between postnatal maternal depression and psychological outcomes in adolescent offspring: A systematic review. *Archives of Women's Mental Health*, 18(2), 147–162.

Seibert, J., Hogan, A. (1982). Procedures manual for early social communication scales. Unpublished manuscript, University of Miami.

Silk, J.S., Shaw, D.S., Skuban, E.M., Oland, A.A., Kovacs, M. (2006). Emotion regulation strategies in offspring of childhood-onset depressed mothers. *Journal of Child Psychology and Psychiatry*, 47(1), 69–78.

Solantaus, T., Paavonen, E.J., Toikka, S., Punamäki, R. (2010). Preventive interventions in families with parental depression: Children's psychosocial symptoms and prosocial behaviour. *European Child and Adolescent Psychiatry*, 19(12), 883–892.

Spear, L.P. (2000). The adolescent brain and age-related behavioral manifestations. *Neuroscience and Biobehavioral Reviews*, 24(4), 417–463.

Speranza, A.M., Ammaniti, M., Trentini, C. (2006). An overview of maternal depression, infant reactions and intervention programmes. *Clinical Neuropsychiatry: Journal of Treatment Evaluation*, 3(1), 57–68.

Sutter-Dallay, A., Murray, L., Dequae-Merchadou, L., Glatigny-Dallay, E., Bourgeois, M., Verdoux, H. (2011). A prospective longitudinal study of the impact of early postnatal vs. chronic maternal depressive symptoms on child development. *European Psychiatry*, 26(8), 484–489.

Toth, S.L., Rogosch, F.A., Sturge-Apple, M., Cicchetti, D. (2009). Maternal depression, children's attachment security, and representational development: An organizational perspective. *Child Development*, 80(1), 192–208.

Trapolini, T., McMahon, C.A., Ungerer, J.A. (2007). The effect of maternal depression and marital adjustment on young children's internalizing and externalizing behaviour problems. *Child: Care, Health and Development*, 33(6), 794–803.

Tronick, E. (2007). *The neurobehavioral and social-emotional development of infants and children*. WW Norton and Company.

Van Doesum, K.M., Hosman, C.H., Riksen-Walraven, J.M. (2005). A model-based intervention for depressed mothers and their infants. *Infant Mental Health Journal*, 26(2), 157–176.

Van Doesum, K.M., Riksen-Walraven, J.M., Hosman, C.H., Hoefnagels, C. (2008). A randomized controlled trial of a home-visiting intervention aimed at preventing relationship problems in depressed mothers and their infants. *Child Development*, 79(3), 547–561.

Van Voorhees, B.W., Mahoney, N., Mazo, R., Barrera, A.Z., Siemer, C.P., Gladstone, T.R.G., Munoz, R.F. (2011). Internet-based depression prevention over the life course: A call for behavioral vaccines. *Psychiatric Clinics of North America*, 34, 167–183.

Velders, F.P., Dieleman, G., Henrichs, J., Jaddoe, V.V., Hofman, A., Verhulst, F.C., Hudziak, J.J., Tiemeier, H. (2011). Prenatal and postnatal psychological symptoms of parents and family functioning: The impact on child emotional and behavioural problems. *European Child and Adolescent Psychiatry*, 20(7), 341–350.

Verduyn, C., Barrowclough, C., Roberts, J., Tarrier, N., Harrington, R. (2003). Maternal depression and child behaviour problems: Randomised placebo-controlled trial of a cognitive-behavioural group intervention. *The British Journal of Psychiatry*, 183(4), 342–348.

Volling, B.L., McElwain, N.L., Notaro, P.C., Herrera, C. (2002). Parents' emotional availability and infant emotional competence: Predictors of parent-infant attachment and emerging self-regulation. *Journal of Family Psychology*, 16(4), 447–465.

Waters, E. (1995). The attachment Q-set. In E. Waters, B.E. Vaughn, G. Posada, K. Kondo-Ikemura (Eds) Caregiving, cultural and cognitive perspectives on secure base behavior and working models. *Monographs of the Society for Research in Child Development*, 60 (Serial No. 244), 234–246.

Weissman, M.M., Feder, A., Pilowsky, D.J., Olfson, M., Fuentes, M., Blanco, C., Lantigua, R., Gameroff, M.J., Shea, S. (2004). Depressed mothers coming to primary care: Maternal reports of problems with their children. *Journal of Affective Disorders*, 78(2), 93–100.

Westerlund, M., Lagerberg, D. (2008). Expressive vocabulary in 18-month-old children in relation to demographic factors, mother and child characteristics, communication style and shared reading. *Child: Care, Health and Development*, 34(2), 257–266.

Wong, G.Y., To, C.S., Lee, A.M., Chan, C., Lam, G.L. (2013). Effect of prenatal maternal depression on early speech sound acquisition: A preliminary study. *Speech, Language and Hearing*, 16(4), 215–220.

CHAPTER 6

Parental alcoholism

Peggy S. Keller, Lauren R. Gilbert, Eric A. Haak and Shuang Bi

INTRODUCTION

Any discussion of the impact of parental alcoholism on children must first consider varying definitions of alcoholism and related conditions. The DSM-IV included two alcohol use disorders: alcohol dependence (commonly referred to as alcoholism) and alcohol abuse (American Psychiatric Association, 2000). Alcohol dependence was diagnosed when at least three of the following were present: (i) tolerance to alcohol, (ii) withdrawal symptoms or using alcohol to recover from withdrawal, (iii) using alcohol in greater quantities than was intended, (iv) a desire or unsuccessful attempts to cut down on drinking, (v) spending large amounts of time drinking alcohol or recovering from the effects of alcohol, (vi) reducing other activities to spend more time drinking and (vii) continued drinking despite the problems it causes. Alcohol abuse was diagnosed only when criteria for alcohol dependence were not met and alcohol use resulted in at least one of the following: (i) problems at work or school, (ii) blackouts, (iii) recurrent legal problems, (iv) injury to self, (v) injury to another person, (vi) alcohol use in risky situations, such as while driving, (vii) others expressing concern about alcohol use and (viii) continued drinking despite the problems it causes.

DSM-V combined alcohol dependence and alcohol abuse into a single diagnosis called alcohol use disorder but removed the criterion for persistent legal problems and added a new criterion of craving for alcohol (American Psychiatric Association, 2013). A distinction was also made between mild (two to three criteria present), moderate (four to five criteria present) and severe (six or more criteria present) alcohol use disorder. The National Institute of Alcohol Abuse and Alcoholism (NIAAA) also has a classification for binge drinking (consuming enough alcohol in a two-hour period to reach a blood alcohol concentration of .08 g/dL) (NIAAA, n.d.). Definitions of heavy drinking differ slightly, with the Centers for Disease Control (CDC) defining heavy drinking as 15 or more drinks per week for men or eight or more drinks per week for women (CDC, 2014) and the Substance Abuse and Mental Health Services Administration (SAMHSA) defining heavy drinking as five or more drinks on the same occasion at least five times in the past 30 days (SAMHSA, 2014). Both binge drinking and heavy drinking are considered hazardous (CDC, 2014). However, problem drinking falls along a continuum, and subclinical levels of problem drinking can have an impact on functioning and affect children (Keller et al., 2005). We use the term *problem drinking* as an umbrella term to encompass the variety of alcohol use diagnoses and classifications, including subclinical levels of alcohol dependence, alcohol abuse or alcohol use disorder, and use the more specific terms only when appropriate (i.e. when diagnostic or classification criteria have been met).

Alcohol is the most commonly used drug, and alcohol use disorders are some of the most common mental disorders in the US and around the world. According to the World Health Organization (WHO), rates of alcohol use disorders among men are highest (> 6.3% prevalence) in England, Eastern Europe, Norway, the Philippines, Russia, South America and parts of South Asia, and among women are highest (> 1.6% prevalence) in the US, Canada, England, Norway, Sweden, Eastern Europe, Columbia, Argentina, Russia, Australia and New Zealand (WHO, 2010). Rates of problem drinking are consistently higher among men than women. In the US, nearly 25% of adults engage in binge drinking in a given month, 7.1% engage in heavy drinking in a given month and 7.2% have an alcohol use disorder in a given year (SAMHSA, 2012a). Among women of child-bearing age in the US, 15.0% of non-pregnant and 1.4% of pregnant women engaged in binge drinking in the past 30 days, with both groups averaging three binge episodes per month and six drinks per binge episode (CDC, 2012). The result is that over 10% of US children (more than 7 million) are living with a parent meeting criteria for an alcohol use disorder (SAMHSA, 2012b).

LITERATURE REVIEW

Thousands of studies on children of alcoholics (CoAs) have been published. This review cannot cover such a large volume of research, but consistent themes and recent and notable studies will be highlighted. We begin with an overview of conditions across the lifespan associated with CoA status. We next consider the role of parent and child gender in associations between CoA status and adverse outcomes. Finally, we consider the various explanatory mechanisms through which CoA status confers risk for dysfunction.

RISKS ASSOCIATED WITH COA STATUS

There is a multifinality of outcomes associated with CoA status. The most commonly studied outcome is problem drinking and alcoholism. CoAs are at a significantly increased risk for developing drinking problems of their own (e.g. Anda et al., 2002; Kendler et al., 2013; Murphy and Kelley, 2015). A recent meta-analysis on the subject indicated that a positive family history of alcoholism has a small to moderate relation to negative drinking consequences and symptoms of alcohol use disorder (Elliott et al., 2012). Hussong et al. (2012) suggest that the development of alcohol problems in CoAs is greater where exposure to parental alcoholism occurs during early childhood as opposed to later childhood or adolescence. This may reflect genetic processes. Although molecular genetic research is still ongoing, the genes encoding alcohol dehydrogenase and aldehyde dehydrogenase, which oxidise alcohol to acetaldehyde and acetaldehyde to acetate, respectively, are the most well-established genetic mechanisms of alcoholism (Wang et al., 2012). Further, CoAs do seem to have neurological abnormalities and altered physiological responses to alcohol that predate their initial alcohol consumption. For example, CoAs in middle childhood exhibit blunted activity in the neural circuitry involved in inhibitory control (Hardee et al., 2014). At the same time, alcohol appears to impact behavioural inhibition less among CoAs than among non-CoAs, consistent with a theory that CoAs inherit a genetic profile that makes them less sensitive to the effects of alcohol and therefore at increased risk of drinking hazardously (Kereken et al., 2013). CoAs may also have alcohol expectancies that differ from those of non-CoAs, likely due to witnessing the effects of alcohol on their parents. For example, CoAs have significantly greater social and relaxation alcohol expectancies compared to non-CoAs beginning around age 9–11 years; such expectancies are tied to earlier onset of binge drinking (Jester et al., 2015).

Drinking problems are just one of many types of problems observed in CoAs. CoA status is associated with risk for more general drug abuse and dependence (Elliott et al., 2012; Schuckit et al., 2000). CoAs are also more likely to exhibit externalising problems. Toddlers of alcoholic fathers exhibit greater externalising symptoms than toddlers of non-alcoholic fathers

(Edwards et al., 2006). Father alcoholism during the toddler years also predicts increased externalising symptoms in kindergarten (Eiden et al., 2007). Adolescent CoAs are at two to three times the risk for meeting criteria for attention deficit/hyperactivity disorder (ADHD), oppositional defiant disorder, conduct disorder and antisocial behaviour (Marmorstein et al., 2009). An especially interesting longitudinal study found long-term prospective effects of parental problem drinking on externalising problems from age 2–17 years, and in addition the manifestation of these symptoms temporally coincides with parental symptoms of problem drinking (Hussong et al., 2010). This study is especially important because some evidence has raised questions about the role of parental alcoholism in child externalising symptoms. For example, conduct disorders, oppositional defiant disorders and ADHD are no more likely to occur among CoAs than among non-CoAs once familial antisocial disorders and family socio-economic status (SES) are controlled (Schuckit et al., 2000). Similar results have been reported for associations between maternal postnatal heavy drinking and toddler behaviour problems in Norway (Knudsen et al., 2015). It is also important to note that externalising problems in children may causally contribute to parental drinking problems, as parents may turn to alcohol to cope with their difficult children (Kashdan et al., 2013).

Internalising symptoms have also been observed at higher rates among CoAs than in the general population. CoAs are at increased risk for general internalising problems, even after controlling for parental antisocial behaviour and depression (Hussong et al., 2008a). There are long-term effects of mother and father problem drinking in childhood on adolescent internalising, and also short-term effects of mother problem drinking on adolescent internalising (Hussong et al., 2008b). Specific internalising problems associated with CoA status include low self-esteem (Rangarajan, 2008), loneliness (Martin, 1995), behavioural inhibition (Hill et al., 1999), feelings of shame and guilt (Haverfield and Theiss, 2014), post-traumatic stress disorder (Hanson et al., 2006), numerous other anxiety disorders such as panic disorder, social phobia, simple phobias and generalised anxiety (Morgan et al., 2010), depression (Chen and Weitzman, 2005) and suicidality (Arendt et al., 2007). Depression in particular has been frequently observed in CoAs. Parental alcoholism is linked to offspring depression even after controlling for numerous other negative life events (physical and sexual abuse, domestic violence, parental mental illness, parental drug abuse and parental antisocial behaviour) (Anda et al., 2002). Compared to depressed non-CoAs, depressed CoAs make more suicide attempts and have greater intention to succeed in suicide (Sher et al., 2005).

A popular framework for understanding the problems of CoAs is codependency. This term is defined in various ways, but generally encompasses focusing on the needs and wants of others instead of the self, sacrificing one's needs in favour of the needs of others, belief in one's ability to fix the problems and mental health conditions of others and emotional suppression (Dear et al., 2004). Codependency is a common component of the self-help literature for CoAs, and is frequently utilised by non-academic clinicians (Beattie 2013a, 2013b; Wegscheide-Cruse and Cruse, 2012). However, scientific evidence for the construct validity of codependency is weak. First, there are important questions about whether codependency is better explained by validated mental health conditions such as borderline or dependent personality disorders (Hoenigmann-Lion and Whitehead, 2007). Second, the most validated measure of codependency does not directly coincide with most common definitions of the term (Dear and Roberts, 2005). Third, some studies have found no differences in codependency between CoAs and non-CoAs (Jones et al., 2007). Nevertheless, use of the codependency construct persists in the CoA treatment field.

Research on the personality features of CoAs continues in other directions as well. For example, a large sample of doctoral-level mental health professionals provided Q-sort personality ratings of randomly chosen adolescent and adult CoAs under their care (Hinrichs et al., 2011). Results identified four consistent personality subtypes of CoAs: (i) *externalising*, characterised by feelings of anger, defiance towards authority, eagerness to disagree with others, manipulative behaviour towards others, being highly critical of others, little empathy for others and impulsivity, (ii) *inhibited*, characterised by shyness, poor social skills, few friendships or social supports, difficulties dealing with frustration or challenge, lower self-esteem and passiveness, (iii) *emotionally dysregulated*, characterised by tendencies toward extreme emotions, rapid changes in emotions, extreme reactions to perceived criticism, inability to soothe or comfort oneself, immature coping strategies and neediness, (iv) *high-functioning*, characterised by conscientiousness, a good sense of humour, empathy for others, focus on moral standards, being well liked by others, ability to have meaningful and intimate relationships, but also high levels of depression and anxiety. Notably, none of these categories conforms to the concept of codependency. In terms of validated personality disorders, CoAs are at increased risk for all DSM-IV Axis II conditions (paranoid, schizoid, antisocial, histrionic, avoidant, dependent and obsessive-compulsive personality disorders) (Morgan et al., 2010).

It is notable that these findings are consistent across cultures, even those that are traditionally more accepting of heavy alcohol use than the US. For example, a study of Spanish CoAs found they suffer from increased risk for ADHD, depression, phobias, enuresis and tic disorders (Diaz et al., 2008). Slovenian CoAs aged 12–18 years report significantly lower school performance, more sedentary lifestyles, greater use of alcohol, tobacco and other drugs, greater externalising problems and increased suicidality, all even after controlling for family SES (Serec et al., 2012). Slovenian CoAs aged 12–24 years showed more arousal-focused implicit alcohol expectancies than non-CoAs, although no differences on explicit expectances were observed (Belles et al., 2011). Australian CoAs are at increased risk for internalising and externalising symptoms compared to Australian non-CoAs (Waldron et al., 2009). Research has also investigated the consequences of CoA status in cultures that traditionally disapprove of heavy alcohol use or have lower rates of problem drinking. A study of adolescent CoAs in Mangalore, India found that 21.7% experienced mild symptoms, 61.7% experienced moderate symptoms and 16.6% experienced severe symptoms of psychosocial problems resulting from father alcoholism (Shaji, 2012). Korean fourth graders who are CoAs exhibited higher levels of depression, lower levels of self-esteem and greater bullying of other children (Kim et al., 2011). Korean fifth graders whose parents engage in problem drinking have greater difficulties expressing emotions and lower social competence than children of parents who do not have drinking problems (Lee and Kweon, 2014). In college, Korean CoAs are still exhibiting higher levels of depression but are also engaged in greater problem drinking than their non-CoA counterparts (Lee and Bong, 2014).

RESILIENCE IN CHILDREN OF ALCOHOLICS

Despite the wide range of problems that CoAs tend to experience, there is also the possibility of resilience. In fact, associations between CoA status and mental health conditions are only small to moderate in most cases. As noted above, a relatively high-functioning subtype of CoAs has been identified in personality research on mental health patients (who are likely seeking treatment for anxiety or depression) (Hinrichs et al., 2012). Therefore, a key goal for research is to identify factors that contribute to CoA resilience. One of the more commonly studied protective factors is social support and positive relationships with parents. Korean adult CoAs reporting greater social support were less likely to exhibit psychological disturbances otherwise associated with CoA status (Kim and Lee, 2011). Similarly, a sense of belonging provided protection against psychosocial problems among Korean adult CoAs (Lee and Williams, 2013). When support comes from healthy fathers, the relation between mother alcoholism and child externalising problems is ameliorated

(McKelvey et al., 2012). Better parent-child communication serves as a protective factor against depression otherwise observed in adolescent CoAs (Ohannessian, 2013). Support from extended family may be important for promoting resilience in African American CoAs (Hall 2007). A less frequently studied protective factor is religiosity (Kim and Lee, 2011), although this may simply be a marker for higher family functioning (Harden, 2010).

It is also possible that there are biological differences between vulnerable and resilient CoAs. Higher vagal tone in children (suggesting greater biological support for emotion regulation) reduces associations between parental problem drinking and child internalising and externalising problems (El-Sheikh, 2005). Resilient CoAs (defined as those not exhibiting alcohol problems of their own) exhibit greater activation of the orbital frontal gyrus, ventral striatum and extended amygdala, and less activation of the dorsomedial prefrontal cortex in response to emotional stimuli than vulnerable CoAs exhibit (Heitzeg et al., 2008). Whether these biological differences are genetically based or driven by exposure to different levels of environmental stress is unclear.

An interesting qualitative study of children of substance-abusing parents questioned children about factors they believed would allow them to become happy and healthy adults (Moe et al., 2007). Children reported that resilience may be achieved if parents stop using substances and seek treatment, they themselves avoid alcohol and drugs, they can avoid blaming themselves for their parents' substance use, they have someone they trust to whom they can express their feelings and they foster an optimistic outlook about their future. Unfortunately, there has been little to no quantitative research examining these factors as contributing to resilience in CoAs.

GENDER DIFFERENCES IN EFFECTS

Does it matter which parent suffers from alcoholism? This is a difficult question to answer, as investigation of the impact of mother alcoholism may be confounded with the teratogenic effects of prenatal exposure to alcohol. For example, mother alcohol consumption during pregnancy predicts child externalising problems above and beyond her postnatal alcohol consumption or problem drinking (Kendler et al., 2013). On the other hand, it may also be more difficult to observe effects of mother alcoholism compared to father alcoholism because the former is far less common than the latter. However, several researchers have examined the potential impact of mother vs father problem drinking. In most cases, risks for mental health conditions are significantly higher for CoAs than for non-CoAs, regardless of whether the alcoholic parent is the mother or father (e.g. Keller et al., 2011; Kendler et al., 2013). There are some exceptions. In one study, father problem drinking was found to predict adolescent alcohol use, while mother problem drinking was found to predict adolescent depression (Ohannessian, 2013). There is also some research suggesting that having more than one parent with an alcohol problem conveys the highest level of risk for children, including risk for externalising problems (Hussong et al., 2007).

Gender-specific effects may only become apparent when child gender is taken into account. Female CoAs may be more likely to choose romantic partners with drinking problems than are male CoAs (Kelley et al., 2014). For drinking motives, there is greater similarity between fathers and sons than between fathers and daughters, and greater similarity between mothers and daughters than between mothers and sons (Windle and Windle, 2012). Similarly, female college students have the greatest levels of problem drinking when only their mothers are alcoholics, while male college students have the greatest level of problem drinking when both their mothers and fathers are alcoholics (Pearson et al., 2012). Another study found that both mother and father problem drinking were related to female CoA depression, while only father problem drinking was related to male CoA depression (Chen and Weitzman, 2005). At the same time, an examination of a broad range of DSM-IV diagnoses revealed a very complex gender-related pattern in which the father alcoholic-daughter pairing was related to greater risk for alcohol abuse than the father alcoholic-son pairing, but the opposite was found for mania. The mother alcoholic-daughter pairing was associated with greater risk for mania, nicotine dependence, alcohol abuse and schizoid personality disorder than the mother alcoholic-son pairing, but the opposite was found for panic disorder (Diaz et al., 2008). Thus, while there is evidence that same gender parent-child relationships carry the greatest risk for children, and that having two parents with alcohol problems is riskiest, questions still remain about the role of gender in the effects of parental problem drinking on children.

MECHANISMS OF RISK

Several potential mechanisms through which parental alcoholism conveys risk to offspring have been identified. We divide these into two groups: environmental and internal mechanisms. In terms of environmental mechanisms, parental problem drinking is related to problems with parenting and the marital relationship. Persons struggling with addiction have difficulties functioning in a parental role, possibly because of the effects of intoxication, time spent obtaining alcohol and drinking, legal problems related to alcohol use and typical features of alcoholism including denial of problems, placing blame on others, selfishness and manipulative behaviour (Dare and Derigne, 2010; Morjaria-Keval and Orford, 2002). It is therefore not surprising that mother alcoholism is associated with adult children perceiving greater alienation, less communication, less trust and more negative attitudes about the mother, while father alcoholism is associated with similar perceptions about the father-child relationship (Keller et al., 2011). Even alcohol problems limited to early adulthood predict poor parenting skills years later, likely due to increases in negative emotions (Bailey et al., 2013). In addition, father problem drinking is related to problems in the mother-child relationship, suggesting that having a spouse with an alcohol problem may undermine parenting as well. For example, father problem drinking was associated with poor mother-child communication, which partially accounted for poorer social skills and greater self-blame in adolescents (Peleg-Oren et al., 2013). Similarly, insecure attachment to mothers mediates the relation between father problem drinking and behaviour problems in toddlers (Edwards et al., 2006). The stress mothers experience because of their male partners' drinking problems may prevent them from fully engaging with their children, make them more likely to lash out at children and cause them to suffer problems such as anxiety and depression (Dawson et al., 2007).

Another important environmental mechanism of risk may be exposure to marital conflict. There are well-established associations between alcohol and aggression (Giancola et al., 2012; Kachadourian et al., 2012), and alcohol and marital conflict (Floyd et al., 2006; Keller et al., 2009; Leonard and Eiden, 2007), including domestic violence (Drapkin et al., 2005; Foran and O'Leary, 2008). Prior to fathers' alcohol treatment, CoAs were exposed to significantly greater levels of interparental conflict than non-CoAs were; levels of interparental conflict significantly decreased following treatment and at the six-month follow-up conflict was no different from that in control families (although conflict was significantly higher again at the 12-month follow-up) (Rounsaville et al., 2014). Exposure to marital conflict can be very detrimental to children; children report that it is one of the most stressful events they experience (Lewis et al., 1984). Decades of research have documented the link between marital conflict and children's development (Cummings and Davies, 2011). Research testing marital conflict as a mediator of associations between parental problem drinking and child adjustment consistently support it as a mechanism of risk. For example, marital conflict mediates associations between father problem drinking and children's internalising and externalising problems from kindergarten to second grade (Keller et al., 2008). Marital aggression also mediates the association between father problem drinking and child anxiety across early childhood (Eiden et al., 2009). Emotional security theory (which proposes that children have a fundamental need to feel secure in their family and that insecurity is manifested in terms of emotional, behavioural and cognitive reactions to family conflict) is a prominent theory explaining the effects of marital conflict on children (Cummings and Davies, 2011). Research suggests that parental problem drinking undermines children's sense of emotional security. For example, from kindergarten through the second grade, higher levels of parental problem drinking are related to stronger emotional reactions, caretaking behaviour and negative expectations for the future of the family (Keller et al., 2007; Keller et al., 2011).

Some mental health professionals conceptualise CoAs as falling into one of a variety of family roles, the most widely adopted being those identified by Wegscheider-Cruse (1989) based on clinical experience (enabler, hero, scapegoat, lost child and mascot). These family roles are purported to protect children from the effects of parental problem drinking, but also allow the problem drinker to continue their pattern of behaviour, and are manifested in terms of psychological and interpersonal features. Enablers are most commonly spouses of alcoholics rather than the children; their role is to protect the alcoholic from any negative consequences, for example by taking on responsibilities that the alcoholic cannot fulfil, and as a result they neglect their own needs and experience feelings of stress, anxiety and depression. The family hero, typically the oldest child in the family, also takes on additional responsibilities on behalf of the alcoholic, and focuses on achievement in arenas that are highly valued by the family (such as school or work). Heroes may leave the family at a young age but will return to the family any time they feel needed. Lost children are children who are emotionally neglected and frequently overlooked as the rest of the family attempts to cope with the alcoholic; they are withdrawn within the family and develop their own world outside it. Lost children may feel lonely and depressed, and have difficulties forming relationships with others. The family mascot is typically the youngest child, and takes the role of enhancing positive effect in the family by being cute or funny, leading to difficulties confronting and solving problems throughout life. Finally, the scapegoat also attempts to distract the family from the problems caused by the alcoholic, but these attempts involve causing problems themselves, such as by getting into trouble at school or engaging in delinquent behaviour.

Despite the popularity of family-role typology among self-help authors and some clinicians, there is little empirical support for their construct validity or clinical utility (Vernig, 2011). CoAs do not fit neatly into these categories, and like codependency, in some cases these so-called family roles appear to be tapping into more valid constructs (including the general family dynamics described above). However, there is some research to support parentification in families characterised by alcohol problems. Parentification is the process when children take on the role of parents, attempting to take care of them physically and emotionally, and fulfilling the responsibilities of parents when they cannot do so. Adult CoAs report higher levels of parentification, including instrumental and emotional caregiving, and feelings of past unfairness in their family, than adult non-CoAs report (Kelley et al., 2007). Parentification is reported by adult CoAs with regard to their experiences growing up and their current family relationships (Pasternak and Schier, 2012). Parentification is associated with adverse outcomes for children, as parental roles likely get in the way of more appropriate and critical developmental goals, and children's success at parental roles tends not to be very high, leading to feelings of guilt, anxiety and depression (Khafi et al., 2014).

Some of the most commonly studied internal mechanisms of risk include self-regulatory abilities, such as emotion regulation, coping skills and impulsivity. These difficulties may arise because families are important for teaching children and promoting the development of these abilities. CoA status is associated with alexithymia, a condition in which a person has difficulty identifying and describing emotions (Lyvers et al., 2012). Temperamental emotionality mediates the association between parental alcoholism and adolescent substance use (Chassin et al., 1993). Low self-regulation also mediates associations between father problem drinking and child externalising behaviour in early childhood (Eiden et al., 2007). The risk for problem drinking among adult CoAs is ameliorated in the context of strong self-regulation (Pearson et al., 2012). Parental problem drinking also predicts problems with offspring coping. Adult CoAs report greater maladaptive coping strategies than adult non-CoAs report, such as behavioural disengagement, focus on and venting of emotions, and denial, all of which are related to higher levels of depressive symptoms (Klostermann et al., 2011).

Another widely studied internal mechanism of risk is impulsivity. Children and adolescents with problem drinking fathers exhibit higher levels of novelty seeking than other children and adolescents, especially if they have short alleles of the DRD4 gene (Lahti et al., 2010). Parent substance-use disorders are linked to a lack of planning behaviour in adolescents (Handley et al., 2011). These tendencies toward impulsive behaviour can be observed at the neurological level (DeVito et al., 2013), including activation of neural circuitry involved in behavioural inhibition (Kareken et al., 2013), responsivity to reward (Yarosh et al., 2014) and error processing (Hardee et al., 2015).

RELEVANT INTERVENTIONS

In considering interventions for CoAs, there is the obvious choice of treating the parental alcohol problem. A comparison of behavioural couples therapy (BCT), individual-based treatment for addiction (IBT) and a control group receiving couple-related psychoeducation indicated that BCT was associated with the greatest improvements in functioning for children with alcoholic fathers (Kelley and Fals-Stewart, 2002). A later study compared BCT to IBT and BCT with an additional component focusing on parent skills; results supported the modified version of BCT as the most effective in promoting adjustment in children (Lam et al., 2008). These findings are consistent with numerous studies supporting the joint involvement of family members in treatment of alcoholic relatives (Copello et al., 2005) and also with marital conflict and family dysfunction serving as mechanisms of risk in the context of parental problem drinking (Keller et al., 2008).

Behavioural couples therapy has been modified for use with alcoholics; this modification is known as Alcohol-Focused Behavioural Couples Therapy (ABCT). There are four major components of ABCT, all of which make use of cognitive behavioural principles: (i) strategies to improve coping and stop drinking in the alcoholic, (ii) strategies to improve coping in the non-alcoholic partner and to help the partner support abstinence in the other, (iii) strategies to improve the quality of the relationship, and (iv) creation of behavioural contracts among the partners to ensure compliance with medication regimes (Roberts and McCrady, 2003). There are also 'pressure to change' treatments for adult family members of alcoholics, in which the family member is counselled on strategies for preparing and pressuring the alcoholic to enter treatment (Barber and Crisp, 1995). One of the most widely studied of these is Community Reinforcement and Family Training, which focuses on teaching adult family members of alcoholics how to use a reinforcement training programme to encourage treatment seeking and abstinence in alcoholics (Meyers et al., 1999; Meyers and Miller, 2001).

There are fewer interventions available for addressing the problems experienced by COAs. One approach has been to provide some attention to adult family members of alcoholics by listening to them, providing them with information and encouraging them to find sources of social support and to seek treatment for their psychological problems (Copello et al., 2000). Another approach is to teach family members that alcoholism is a 'family disease' (i.e. they are part of the problem by enabling the alcoholic) and discourage enabling behaviour that also undermines the psychological health of the family member (Dittrich, 1993). Unfortunately, there is little evidence that these approaches are effective (Halford et al., 2001). However, the most widely used support programme for family members impacted by alcoholism is Al-Anon, which has been in existence since 1951 (www.al-anon.org). In Al-Anon, family members of alcoholics attend group meetings in which they are able to share stories and experiences about their lives and listen to the stories and experiences of others; key goals are to help group members feel less alone and take their own lessons from what others say rather than learning specific strategies to improve their mental health (see Roth and Tan, 2008). In that sense, Al-Anon contrasts with most empirically validated treatments for mental illness. There are few methodologically sound empirical investigations of Al-Anon, but those studies that are available suggest that Al-Anon participation may improve coping and decrease depression, anger, and family conflict (Humphreys, 2004; Timko et al., 2012).

Like most other therapies, Al-Anon is designed for use with adults. Alateen is the companion programme to Al-Anon for use with teens affected by alcoholism in family or friends (www.al-anon.org/for-alateen). Alateen groups are similar to Al-Anon groups, although somewhat greater emphasis is placed on developing coping strategies, and reducing feelings of self-blame or responsibility for the behaviour of the alcoholic. Other than Alateen, there are few intervention programmes for young children of alcoholics. Most are school-based programmes, and are focused on providing social support, helping children to cope with the emotional and other problems associated with parental alcoholism and providing information about alcoholism. Unfortunately, there is little evidence supporting the effectiveness of these interventions (Copello et al., 2005).

IN PRACTICE

Based on the research we have reviewed, some recommendations for clinical practice with CoAs can be made. Our major recommendation is to avoid the use of the concepts known as codependency and family roles such as mascot, lost child, etc. There are two important reasons for this recommendation. First, these concepts are not empirically validated. To the extent that practitioners rely on them, they spend less time considering and treating empirically validated mental health conditions (such as depression) with evidence-based treatments that are known to be effective (such as cognitive-behaviour therapy). Therefore, codependency and family roles are distractions from effective treatment. Second, these concepts have strong undercurrents of blaming the victims. Their proponents adhere to the idea that alcoholism is a 'family disease', made possible by the behaviour of family members. The family members 'allow' the alcoholic to drink and to hurt them. Work with family members therefore focuses, sometimes exclusively, on making them understand how they have encouraged the alcoholic and must change to help the alcoholic. In reality, alcoholics are responsible for their own behaviour. They have a tendency to blame others for their problems, and when clinicians support this belief, it not only prevents alcoholics from taking full responsibility for themselves and the pain they have caused, it represents additional victimisation of the family members.

An additional recommendation is to use behavioural couples therapy (BCT), and alcohol-focused behavioural couples therapy (ABCT), with families in which one or both of the parents is/are an alcoholic. These are evidence-based treatments that have been shown to reduce drinking, improve family functioning and benefit children. When CoAs are adults or teens, we also recommend encouraging them to participate in Alateen or Al-Anon, as these group therapies appear to be helpful for some people. However, all CoAs, regardless of their age, should be evaluated for a range of clinical and subclinical mental disorders and appropriate evidence-based treatments for them should be implemented. A final recommendation is to consider the possibility of violence in homes with an alcoholic parent. Practitioners should be prepared to contact the appropriate authorities when abuse or neglect of minors is suspected.

RECOMMENDATIONS FOR FUTURE RESEARCH

Despite the large volume of scientific research available on CoAs, there are a number of gaps requiring additional research. First, alcoholism is frequently comorbid with a number of other conditions, including major depression (Hasin et al., 2005), bipolar disorder (Frye and Salloum, 2006), post-traumatic stress disorder (Ullman et al., 2006), attention deficit/hyperactivity disorder (Ohlmeier et al., 2008) and personality disorders, especially obsessive-compulsive personality disorder (Echeburua et al., 2007). However, very few studies have examined the role of parental alcoholism in the context of other parental mental health problems. This role may be important. As an example, when alcohol abuse or dependence co-occurs with bipolar disorder, the bipolar presentation is more likely to be characterised by mixed or dysphoric mania, rapid cycling, greater impairment, suicidal ideation, impulsivity and aggression (Frye and Salloum 2006). Alcoholics with comorbid anxiety are more likely to relapse after treatment (Kushner et al., 2005). Thus, when alcoholism is comorbid with other mental health conditions, it may be especially detrimental to children.

Second, additional research is needed on resilience in CoAs. Resilience is a complex process and difficult to define. CoAs may exhibit resilience in some domains (e.g. alcohol or other substance use) but manifest risk in others (e.g. depression or anxiety). They may exhibit resilience at one point in development only to manifest maladaptation later. Research on resilience in CoAs has rarely considered these issues. Furthermore, the range of possible factors contributing to resilience that have been investigated is very limited and there are few studies available on those that have been investigated. Social support, particularly from the other parent, is most widely studied, but additional research on support would be beneficial. Alternative protective factors that have rarely if ever been examined include religiosity, intelligence and socio-economic status.

Third, there are few biopsychosocial models of risk associated with CoA status. There are prominent theoretical models of biological stress response that have been applied to other forms of family stress, such as parental depression, marital conflict and child maltreatment, but these models have rarely been applied to parental alcoholism. For example, the autonomic balance model (Berntson et al., 2008) proposes that the branches of the sympathetic and parasympathetic nervous system interact to predict adaptation and maladaptation. The theories of biological sensitivity to context (Boyce and Ellis, 2005) and differential susceptibility to the environment (Belsky and Pluess, 2009) are similar in that they propose that certain patterns of biological stress response will increase vulnerability in stressful contexts but result in advanced adaptation in stable and enriched environments, while other patterns of stress response lead to acceptable levels of adaptation in any context. There is some evidence to support parasympathetic nervous system activity as a moderator of relations between parental problem drinking and child adjustment problems (El-Sheikh 2001, 2005), but few such studies have been conducted. Although these models consider biological stress response as a moderator of associations, it may also be possible that biological stress response serves as a mediator. According to allostatic load theory, exposure to a stressful environment can cause wear and tear on biological systems, reducing their effectiveness and leading to physical and mental health problems (McEwen, 1998). In support of parental problem drinking as a contributor to allostatic load, mother problem drinking was found to predict increased reactivity of the hypothalamic-pituitary-adrenal axis in children, even after controlling for family functioning and father problem drinking (Keller et al., 2014). Additional research is needed to further explicate the role of biological stress response in the context of parental alcoholism.

However, the greatest need for additional research is in the area of interventions for CoAs. There are, of course, numerous evidence-based treatments available for the conditions associated with CoA status, including depression, anxiety and conduct problems. However, even the most well-established programmes do not work equally well for everyone. An important goal for clinical research is to identify moderators of treatment outcomes, and CoA status may be one such moderator. In other words, it is not clear whether various evidence-based programmes are as effective for CoAs as they are for other populations. There is also a need for the development of interventions that address the specific needs of CoAs, interventions that are based on theory and translational research, and that have demonstrated effectiveness in randomised clinical trials. Programmes that are currently available, including Al-Anon and Alateen, would also benefit from additional evaluation (Timko et al., 2012).

REFERENCES

American Psychiatric Association. (2000). *Diagnostic and statistical manual of mental disorders* (4th edn, text revision). Arlington, VA: American Psychiatric Publishing.

American Psychiatric Association. (2013). *Diagnostic and statistical manual of mental disorders* (5th edn). Arlington, VA: American Psychiatric Publishing.

Anda, R.F., Whitfield, C.L., Felitti, V.J., Chapman, D., Edwards, V.J., Dube, S.R., Williamson, D.F. (2002). Adverse childhood experiences, alcoholic parents, and later risk of alcoholism and depression. *Psychiatric Services*, 53, 1001–1009.

Arendt, M., Sher, L., Fjordback, L., Brandholdt, J., Munk-Jorgensen, P. (2007). Parental alcoholism predicts suicidal behavior in adolescents and young adults with cannabis dependence. *International Journal of Adolescent Medicine and Health*, 19(1), 67–77.

Bailey, J.A., Hill, K.G., Guttmannova, K., Oesterle, S., Hawkins, J.D., Catalano, R.F., McMahon, R.J. (2013). The association between parent early adult drug use disorder and later observed parenting practices and child behavior problems: Testing alternative models. *Developmental Psychology*, 49(5), 887–899.

Barber, J.G., Crisp, B.R. (1995). The 'pressures to change' approach to working with the partners of heavy drinkers. *Addiction*, 90, 269–276.

Beattie, M. (2013a). *Codependent no more: How to stop controlling others and start caring for yourself.* Center City, MN: Hazelden Publishing.

Beattie, M. (2013b). *Beyond codependency: And getting better all the time*. Center City, MN: Hazelden Publishing.

Belles, S., Budde, A., Moesgen, D., Klein, M. (2011). Parental problem drinking predicts implicit alcohol expectancy in adolescents and young adults. *Addictive Behaviors*, 36(11), 1091–1094.

Belsky, J., Pluess, M. (2009). Beyond diathesis stress: Differential susceptibility to environmental influences. *Psychological Bulletin*, 135(6), 885–908.

Berntson, G.G., Norman, G.J., Hawkley, L.C., Cacioppo, J.T. (2008). Cardiac autonomic balance vs. cardiac regulatory capacity. *Psychophysiology*, 45(4), 643–652.

Boyce, W.T., Ellis, B.J. (2005). Biological sensitivity to context: I. an evolutionary-developmental theory of the origins and functions of stress reactivity. *Development and Psychopathology*, 17, 271–301.

Centers for Disease Control and Prevention. (2012). Alcohol use and binge drinking among women of childbearing age – United States, 2006–2010. *Morbidity and Mortality Weekly Reports*, 61(28), 534–538.

Centers for Disease Control and Prevention. (2014). Frequently asked questions. Available from www.cdc.gov/alcohol/faqs.htm#heavyDrinking (accessed 21 February 2015).

Chassin, L., Pillow, D.R., Curran, P.J., Molina, B.S.G., Barrera, M. (1993). Relation of parental alcoholism to early adolescent substance use: A test of three mediating mechanisms. *Journal of Abnormal Psychology*, 102(1), 3–19.

Chen, Y.Y., Weitzman, E.R. (2005). Depressive symptoms, DSM-IV alcohol abuse and their comorbidity among children of problem drinkers in a national survey: effects of parent and child gender and parent recovery status. *Journal of Studies on Alcohol*, 66(1), 66–73.

Copello, A.G., Templeton, L.J., Krishnan, M., Orford, J., Velleman, R.D.B. (2000) A treatment package to improve primary care services for the relatives of people with alcohol and drug problems. *Addiction Research*, 8, 471–484.

Copello, A.G., Velleman, R.D.B., Templeton, L.J. (2005). Family interventions in the treatment of alcohol and drug problems. *Drug and Alcohol Review*, 24, 369–385.

Cummings, E.M., Davies, P.T. (2011). *Marital conflict and children: An emotional security perspective*. New York: Guilford Press.

Dare, P.A.S., DeRigne, L. (2010). Denial in alcohol and other drug use disorders: A critique of theory. *Social Work Faculty Publications*. Paper 19.

Dawson, D.A., Grant, B.F., Chou, S.P., Stinson, F.S. (2007). The impact of partner alcohol problems on women's physical and mental health. *Journal of Studies on Alcohol and Drugs*, 68(1), 66–75.

Dear, G.E. (2004). Test-retest reliability of the Holyoake codependency index with Australian students 1. *Psychological reports*, 94(2), 482–484.

Dear, G.E., Roberts, C.M. (2005). Validation of the Holyoake codependency index. *The Journal of psychology*, 139(4), 293–314

DeVito, E.E., Meda, S.A., Jiantonio, R., Potenza, M.C., Krystal, J.I., Pearlson, G.D. (2013). Neural correlates of impulsivity in health males and females with family histories of alcoholism. *Neuropsychopharmacology*, 38, 1854–1863.

Díaz, R., Gual, A., García, M., Arnau, J., Pascual, F., Cañuelo, B., Rubio, G., de Dios, Y., Fernández-Eire, M.C., Valdés, R., Garbayo, I. (2008). Children of alcoholics in Spain: From risk to pathology. Results from the ALFIL program. *Social Psychiatry and Psychiatric Epidemiology*, 43(1), 1–10.

Dittrich, J. (1993). Group programs for wives of alcoholics. In T.J. O'Farrell (Ed.), *Treating alcohol problems: Marital and family interventions* (pp 78–114). New York: Guilford Press.

Drapkin, M.L., McCrady, B.S., Swingle, J.M., Epstein, E.E. (2005). Exploring bidirectional couple violence in a clinical sample of female alcoholics. *Journal of Studies on Alcohol and Drugs*, 66(2), 213–219.

Echeburua, E., De Medina, R.B., Aizpiri, J. (2007). Comorbidity of alcohol dependence and personality disorders: A comparative study. *Alcohol and Alcoholism*, 42(6), 618–622.

Edwards, E.P., Eiden, R.D., Leonard, K.E. (2006). Behavior problems in 18- to 36-month-old children of alcoholic fathers: Secure mother infant attachment as a protective factor. *Development and Psychopathology*, 18(2), 395–407.

Eiden, R.D., Edwards, E.P., Leonard, K.E. (2007). A conceptual model for the development of externalizing behavior problems among kindergarten children of alcoholic families: Role of parenting and children's self-regulation. *Developmental Psychology*, 43(5), 1187–1201.

Eiden, R.D., Molnar, D.S., Colder, C., Edwards, E.P., Leonard, K.E. (2009). A conceptual model predicting internalizing problems in middle childhood among children of alcoholic and nonalcoholic fathers: The role of marital aggression. *Journal of Studies on Alcohol and Drugs*, 70(5), 741–750.

El-Sheikh, M. (2001). Parental drinking problems and children's adjustment: Vagal regulation and emotional reactivity as pathways and moderators of risk. *Journal of Abnormal Psychology*, 110(4), 499–515.

El-Sheikh, M. (2005). Does poor vagal tone exacerbate child maladjustment in the context of parental problem drinking? A longitudinal examination. *Journal of Abnormal Psychology*, 114(4), 735–741.

Elliott, J.C., Carey, K.B., Bonafide, K.E. (2012). Does a family history of alcohol problems influence college and university drinking or substance use? A meta-analytical review. *Addiction*, 107(10), 1774–1785.

Floyd, F.J., Cranford, J.A., Daugherty, M.K., Fitzgerald, H.E., Zucker, R.A. (2006). Marital interaction in alcoholic and nonalcoholic couples: Alcoholic subtype variations and wives' alcoholism status. *Journal of Abnormal Psychology*, 115(1), 121–130.

Foran, H.M., O'Leary, K.D. (2008). Problem drinking, jealousy, and anger control: Variables predicting physical aggression against power. *Journal of Family Violence*, 23(3), 141–148.

Frye, M.A., Salloum, I.M., 2006, Bipolar disorder and comorbid alcoholism: Prevalence rate and treatment considerations. *Bipolar Disorders*, 8(6), 677–685.

Giancola, P.R., Godlaski, A.J., Roth, R.M. (2012). Identifying component processes of executive functioning that serve as risk factors for the alcohol-aggression relation. *Psychology of Addictive Behaviors*, 26(2), 201–211.

Halford, W., Price, J., Kelly, A., Bouma, R., Young, R. (2001). Helping the female partners of men abusing alcohol: A comparison of three treatments. *Addiction*, 96, 1497–1508.

Hall, J.C. (2007). Kinship ties: Attachment relationships that promote resilience in African American adult children of alcoholics. *Advances in Social Work*, 8(1), 130–140.

Handley, E.D., Chassin, L., Haller, M.M., Bountress, K.E., Dandreaux, D., Beltran, I. (2011). Do executive and reactive disinhibition mediate the effects of familial substance use disorders on adolescent externalising outcomes? *Journal of Abnormal Psychology*, 120(3), 528–542.

Hanson, R.F., Self-Brown, S., Fricker-Elhai, A., Kilpatrick, D.G., Saunders, B.E., Resnick, H. (2006). Relations among parental substance use, violence exposure and mental health: the national survey of adolescents. *Addictive behaviors*, 31(11), 1988–2001.

Hardee, J.E., Weiland, B.J., Nichols, T.E., Welsh, R.C., Soules, M.E., Steinberg, D.B., Zubieta, J.K., Zucker, R.A., Heitzeg, M.M. (2014). Development of impulse control circuitry in children of alcoholics. *Biological Psychiatry*, 76(9), 708–716.

Hardee, J.E., Zucker, R.A., Heitzeg, M.M. (2015). Development of error processing in children of alcoholics. *Drug and Alcohol Dependence*, 146, e136.

Harden, K.P. (2010). Does religious involvement protect against early drinking? A behavior genetic approach. *Journal of Child Psychology and Psychiatry*, 51(7), 763–771.

Hasin, D.S., Goodwin, R.D., Stinson, F.S., Grant, B.F. (2005). Epidemiology of major depressive disorder: Results from the National Epidemiologic Survey on Alcoholism and Related Conditions. *Archives of General Psychiatry*, 62(10), 1097–1106.

Haverfield, M.C., Theiss, J.A. (2014). A theme analysis of experiences reported by adult children of alcoholics in online support forums. *Journal of Family Studies*, 20(2), 166–184.

Heitzeg, M.M., Nigg, J.T., Yau, W.Y.W., Zubieta, J.K., Zucker, R.A. (2008). Affective circuitry and risk for alcoholism in late adolescence: Differences in frontostriatal responses between vulnerable and resilient children of alcoholic parents. *Alcoholism: Clinical and Experimental Research*, 32(3), 414–426.

Hill, S.Y., Lowers, L., Locke, J., Snidman, N., Kagan, J. (1999). Behavioral inhibition in children from families at high risk for developing alcoholism. *Journal of the American Academy of Child & Adolescent Psychiatry*, 38(4), 410–417.

Hinrichs, J., DeFife, J., Westen, D. (2012). Personality subtypes in adolescent and adult children of alcoholics: A two part study. *Journal of Nervous and Mental Disorders*, 199(7), 487–498.

Hoenigmann-Lion, N.M., Whitehead, G.I. (2007). The relationship between codependency and borderline and dependent personality traits. *Alcoholism Treatment Quarterly*, 24(4), 55–77.

Humphries, K. (2004). *Circles of recovery: Self-help organisations for addictions.* Cambridge University Press, Cambridge.

Hussong, A.M., Wirth, R.J., Edwards, M.C., Curran, P.J., Chassin, L.A., Zucker, R.A. (2007). Externalizing symptoms among children of alcoholic parents: Entry points for an antisocial pathway to alcoholism. *Journal of Abnormal Psychology*, 116(3), 529–542.

Hussong, A.M., Flora, D.B., Curran, P.J., Chassin, L.A., Zucker, R.A. (2008a). Defining risk homogeneity for internalizing symptoms among children of alcoholic parents. *Development and Psychopathology*, 20(1), 165–193.

Hussong, A.M., Cai, L., Curran, P.J., Flora, D.B., Chassin, L.A., Zucker, R.A. (2008b). Disaggregating the distal, proximal, and time-varying effects of parent alcoholism on children's internalizing symptoms. *Journal of Abnormal Child Psychology*, 36(3), 335–346.

Hussong, A.M., Huang, W., Curran, P.J., Chassin, L., Zucker, R.A. (2010). Parent alcoholism impacts the severity and timing of children's externalizing symptoms. *Journal of abnormal child psychology*, 38(3), 367–380.

Hussong, A.M., Huang, W., Serrano, D., Curran, P.J., Chassin, L. (2012). Testing whether and when parent alcoholism uniquely affects various forms of adolescent substance use. *Journal of abnormal child psychology*, 40(8), 1265–1276.

Jester, J.M., Wong, M.M., Cranford, J.A., Buu, A., Fiztgerald, H.E., Zucker, R.A. (2015). Alcohol expectancies in childhood: Change with the onset of drinking and ability to predict adolescent drunkenness and binge drinking. *Addiction*, 110(1), 71–79.

Jones, A.L., Perera-Diltz, D.M., Salyers, K.M., Laux, J.M., Cochrane, W.S. (2007). Testing hypothesized differences between adult children of alcoholics (ACOAs) and non-ACOAs in a college student sample. *Journal of College Counseling*, 10(1), 19–27.

Kachadourian, L.K., Homish, G.G., Quigley, B.M., Leonard, K.E. (2012). Alcohol expectancies, alcohol use, and hostility as longitudinal predictors of alcohol-related aggression. *Psychology of Addictive Behaviors*, 26(3), 414–422.

Kareken, D.A., Dzemidzic, M., Wetherill, L., Eiler, W., Oberlin, B.G., Harezlak, J., Wang, Y., O'Connor, S.J. (2013). Family history of alcoholism interacts with alcohol to affect brain regions involved in behavioral inhibition. *Psychopharmacology*, 228(2) 335–345.

Kashdan, T.B., Adams, L.M., Kleiman, E.M., Pelham, W.E., Lang, A.R. (2013). Stress-induced drinking in parents of boys with attention-deficit-hyperactivity disorder: Heterogeneous groups in an experimental study of adult-child interactions. *Journal of Abnormal Child Psychology*, 41(6) 919–927.

Keller, P.S., Cummings, E.M., Davies, P.T. (2005). The role of marital discord and parenting in relations between parental problem drinking and child adjustment. *Journal of Child Psychology and Psychiatry*, 46(9), 943–951.

Keller, P.S., Cummings, E.M., Davies, P.T., Lubke, G. (2007). Children's behavioral reactions to marital conflict as a function of parents' conflict behaviors and alcohol problems. *European Journal of Developmental Psychology*, 4(2), 157–177.

Keller, P.S., Cummings, E.M., Davies, P.T., Mitchell, P.M. (2008). Longitudinal relations between parental drinking problems, family functioning, and child adjustment. *Development and Psychopathology*, 20, 195–212.

Keller, P.S., El-Sheikh, M., Keiley, M., Liao, P.J. (2009). Longitudinal relations between marital aggression and alcohol problems. *Psychology of Addictive Behaviors*, 23(1), 2–13.

Keller, P.S., Gilbert, L.R., Koss, K.J., Cummings, E.M., Davies, P.T. (2011). Parental problem drinking, marital aggression, and child emotional security: A longitudinal investigation. *Journal of Studies on Alcohol and Drugs*, 72(5) 711–722.

Kelley, M.L., Fals-Stewart, W. (2002). Couples- versus individual-based therapy for alcohol and drug abuse: Effects on children's psychosocial functioning. *Journal of Consulting and Clinical Psychology*, 70(2), 417–427.

Kelley, M.L., French, A., Bountress, K., Keefe, H.A., Schroeder, V., Steer, K., Fals-Stewart, W., Gumienny, L. (2007). Parentification and family responsibility in the family of origin of adult children of alcoholics. *Addictive Behaviors*, 32(4), 675–685.

Kelley, M.L., Linden, A.N., Milletich, R.J., Lau-Barraco, C., Kurtz, E.D., D'Lima, G.M., Bodkins, J.A., Sheehan, B.E. (2014). Self and partner alcohol-related problems among ACOAs and non-ACOAs: Associations with depressive symptoms and motivations for alcohol use. *Addictive Behaviors*, 39(1), 211–218.

Kendler, K.S., Gardner, C.O., Edwards, A., Hickman, M., Heron, J., Macleod, J., Lewis, G., Dick, D.M. (2013). Dimensions of parental alcohol use/problems and offspring temperament, externalizing behaviors, and alcohol use/problems. *Alcoholism: Clinical and Experimental Research*, 37(12) 2118–2127.

Khafi, T.Y., Yates, T.M., Luthar, S.S. (2014). Ethnic differences in the developmental significance of parentification. *Family Process*, 53, 267–287.

Kim, S.H., Koo, M.S., Oh, D.Y., Park, I.H., Lee, K.S., Kim, J.Y., Song, J. (2011). Parental alcohol problems and children's behavior and psychosocial characteristics. *Journal of the Korean Academy of Child and Adolescent Psychiatry*, 22(3), 162–168.

Kim, H.K., Lee, M.H. (2011). Factors influencing resilience of adult children of alcoholics among college students. *Journal of Korean Academy of Nursing*, 41(5) 642–651.

Klostermann, K., Chen, R., Kelley M.L., Schroeder, V.M., Braitman, A.L., Mignone, T. (2011). Coping behavior and depressive symptoms in adult children of alcoholics. *Substance Use and Misuse*, 46, 1162–1168.

Knudsen, A.K., Ystrom, E., Skogen, J.C., Torgersen, L. (2015). Maternal heavy alcohol use and toddler behavior problems: A fixed effects regression analysis. *European Child and Adolescent Psychiatry*, 24(10), 1269–1277.

Kushner, M.G., Abrams, K., Thuras, P., Hanson, K.L., Brekke, M., Sletten, S. (2005). Follow-up study of anxiety disorder and alcohol dependence in comorbid alcoholism treatment patients. *Alcoholism: Clinical and Experimental Research*, 29(8), 1432–1443.

Lahti, J., Raikkonen, K., Ekelund, J., Peltonen, L., Raitakari, O.T., Keltikangas-Jarvinen, L. (2010). Novelty seeking: Interaction between parental alcohol use and dopamine D4 receptor gene exon III polymorphism over 17 years. *Personality and Temperament: New and Alternative Perspectives*, 8(2), 294–300.

Lam, W.K.K., Fals-Stewart, W., Kelley, M.L. (2008). Effects of parent skills training with behavioral couples therapy for alcoholism on children: A randomised clinical pilot trial. *Addictive Behavior*, 33(8), 1076–1080.

Lee, E.S., Bong, E.J. (2014). Impact of parents problematic drinking on the problematic drinking of their collegiate children: Mediating effects of alcohol outcome expectancy and depression. *Journal of the Korean Academic Society of Nursing*, 20(3) 392–401.

Lee, J., Kweon Y.R. (2014). Factors affecting social competence in school-aged children according to alcohol consumption by parents. *Journal of the Korean Academy of Nursing*, 44(5), 495–503.

Lee, H., Williams, R.A. (2013). Effects of parental alcoholism, sense of belonging, and resilience on depressive symptoms: A path model. *Substance Use and Misuse*, 48(3), 265–273.

Leonard, K.E., Eiden, R.D. (2007). Marital and family processes in the context of alcohol use and alcohol disorders. *Annual Review of Clinical Psychology*, 3, 285–310.

Lewis, C.E., Siegel, J.M., Lewis, M.A. (1984). Feeling bad: Exploring sources of distress among pre-adolescent children. *American Journal of Public Health*, 74(2), 117–122.

Lyvers, M., Onucha, R., Thorberg, F.A., Samios, C. (2012). Alexithymia in relation to parental alcoholism, everyday frontal lobe functioning and alcohol consumption in a non-clinical sample. *Addictive Behaviors*, 37(2), 205–210.

Marmorstein, N.R., Iacono, W.G., McGue, M. (2009). Alcohol and illicit drug dependence among parents: associations with offspring externalizing disorders. *Psychological medicine*, 39(1), 149–155.

Martin, J.I. (1995). Intimacy, loneliness, and openness to feelings in adult children of alcoholics. *Health & social work*, 20(1), 52–59.

McKelvey, L.M., Burrow, N.A., Mesman, G.R., Pemberton, J.L., Bradley, R.H., Fitzgerald, H.E. (2012). Supportive fathers lessen the effects of mothers' alcohol problems on children's externalizing behaviors. *Family Science*, 3(3–4), 189–200.

Morgan, P.T., Desai, R.A., Potenza, M.N. (2010). Gender-related influences of parental alcoholism on the prevalence of psychiatric illnesses: Analysis of the National Epidemiologic Survey on alcohol and related conditions. *Alcoholism: Clinical and Experimental Research*, 34(10), 1759–1767.

Morjaria-Keval, A., Orford, J. (2002). The role of religion and spirituality in recovery from drink problems: A qualitative study of alcoholics anonymous members and South Asian men. *Addiction Research and Theory*, 10(3), 225–256.

McEwen, B.S. (1998). Stress, adaptation, and disease: Allostasis and allostatic load. *Annals of the New York Academy of Sciences*, 840(1), 33–44.

Meyers, R.J., Miller W.R. (Eds) (2001). *A community reinforcement approach to addiction treatment*, International Research Monograph in the Addictions (IRMA). Cambridge: Cambridge University Press.

Meyers, R.J., Miller, W.R., Hill, D., Tonigan, J. (1999). Community reinforcement and family training (CRAFT): Engaging unmotivated drug users in treatment. *Journal of Substance Abuse*, 10, 291–308.

Moe, J., Johnson, J.L., Wade, W. (2007). Resilience in children of substance users: In their own words. *Substance Use and Misuse*, 42, 381–398.

Morgan, P.T., Desai, R.A., Potenza, M.N. (2010). Gender-Related Influences of Parental Alcoholism on the Prevalence of Psychiatric Illnesses: Analysis of the National Epidemiologic Survey on Alcohol and Related Conditions. *Alcoholism: Clinical and Experimental Research*, 34(10), 1759–1767.

Murphy, E.M., Kelley, M.L. (2015). Examining the risk for developing alcohol-related problems among adult children of alcoholics. *Drug and Alcohol Dependence*, 147, e47–e48.

National Institute on Alcohol Abuse and Alcoholism, n.d., Drinking levels defined. Available from www.niaaa.nih.gov/alcohol-health/overview-alcohol-consumption/moderate-binge-drinking (accessed 21 February 2015).

Ohannessian, C.M. (2013). Parental problem drinking and adolescent psychological problems: The moderating effect of adolescent-parent communication. *Youth and Society*, 45(1), 3–26.

Ohlmeier, M.D., Peters, K., Te Wildt, B.T., Zedler, M., Ziegenbein, M., Wiese, B., Emrich, H.M., Schneider, U. (2008). Comorbidity of alcohol and substance dependence with attention-deficit/hyperactivity disorder (ADHD). *Alcohol and Alcoholism*, 43(3), 300–304.

Pasternak, A., Schier, K. (2012). The role reversal in the families of adult children of alcoholics. *Archives of Psychiatry and Psychotherapy*, 3, 51–57.

Pearson, M.R., D'Lima, G.M., Kelley, M.L. (2012). Maternal and paternal alcohol misuse and alcohol-related outcomes among college students. *Substance Use and Misuse*, 47(6), 708–717.

Peleg-Oren, N., Hospital, M., Morris, S.L., Wagner, E.F. (2013). Mechanisms of association between paternal alcoholism and abuse of alcohol and other illicit drugs among adolescents. *Journal of Child & Adolescent Substance Abuse*, 22(2), 133–149.

Rangarajan, S. (2008). Mediators and moderators of parental alcoholism effects on offspring self-esteem. *Alcohol and alcoholism*, 43(4), 481–491.

Roberts, L., McCrady, B. (2003). *Alcohol problems in intimate relationships: Identification and intervention: A guide for marriage and family therapists*. Washington, DC: National Institute on Alcoholism and Alcohol Abuse.

Roth, J.D., Tan, E.M. (2008). Spirituality and recovery from familial aspects of alcohol and other drug problems: Analysis of an online Al-Anon meeting. *Alcoholism Treatment Quarterly*, 26(4), 399–426.

Rounsaville, D., O'Farrell, T.J., Andreas, J.B., Murphy, C.M., Murphy, M.M. (2014). Children's exposure to parental conflict after father's treatment for alcoholism. *Addictive Behaviors*, 30(7), 1168–1171.

Schuckit, M.A., Smith, T.L., Radziminski, S., Heyneman, E.K. (2000). Behavioral symptoms and psychiatric diagnoses among 162 children in nonalcoholic or alcoholic families. *The American Journal of Psychiatry*, 157(11), 1881–1883.

Serec, M., Svab, I., Kolsek, M., Svab, V., Moesgen, D., Klein, M. (2012). Health-related lifestyle, physical and mental health in children of alcoholic parents. *Drug and Alcohol Review*, 31(7), 861–870.

Shaji, T.D. (2012). Problems faced by children of alcoholics admitted in selected de-addiction centers in Mangalore. *International Journal of Nursing Education*, 4(2), 4–8.

Substance Abuse and Mental Health Services Administration 2014, The NSDUH Report. Available from http://store.samhsa.gov/shin/content//NSDUH14-0904/NSDUH14-0904.pdf (accessed 21 February 2015).

Substance Abuse and Mental Health Services Administration. (2012a). The NSDUH Report. Available from: http://store.samhsa.gov/product/Results-from-the-2012-National-Survey-on-Drug-Use-and-Health-NSDUH-/SMA13-4795 (accessed 21 February 2015).

Substance Abuse and Mental Health Services Administration. (2012b). Data spotlight: More than 7 million children live with a parent with alcohol problems. Available from: www.samhsa.gov/data/sites/default/files/Spot061ChildrenOfAlcoholics2012/Spot061ChildrenOfAlcoholics2012.pdf (accessed 21 February 2015).

Timko, C., Young L.B., Moos, R.H. (2012). Al-Anon Family Groups: Origins, conceptual basis, outcomes, and research opportunities. *Journal of Groups in Addiction and Recovery*, 7(2–4), 279–296.

Ullman, S.E., Filipas, H.H., Townsend, S.M., Starzynski, L.L. (2006). Correlates of comorbid PTSD and drinking problems among sexual assault survivor. *Addictive Behaviors*, 31(1), 128–132.

Vernig, P.M. (2011). Family roles in homes with alcohol-dependent parents: An evidence based review. *Substance Use and Misuse*, 46, 535–542.

Waldron, M., Martin, N.G., Heath, A.C. (2009) Parental alcoholism and offspring behavior problems: Findings in Australian children of twins. *Twin Research and Human Genetics*, 12(5), 433–440.

Wang, J.C., Kapoor, M., Goate, A.M. (2012). The genetics of substance dependence. *Annual Review of Genomics and Human Genetics*, 13, 241–261.

Wegscheider-Cruse, S. (1989). *Another chance: Hope and health for the alcoholic family.* Palo Alto, CA: Science and Behavior Books.

Wegscheider-Cruse, S., Cruse, J. (2012). *Understanding codependency, updated and expanded: The science behind it and how to break the cycle.* Deerfield Beach, FL: Health Communications Inc.

Windle, M., Windle, R.C. (2012). Intergenerational relations for drinking motives: Invariant for same- and opposite-sex parent-child dyads? *Journal of Studies on Alcohol and Drugs*, 73(1), 63–70.

World Health Organization. (2010). ATLAS on Substance Use (2010): Resources for prevention and treatment of substance use disorders. Available from: www.who.int/substance_abuse/publications/treatment/en/ (accessed 21 February 2015).

Yarosh, H.L., Hyatt, C.J., Meda, S.A., Jiantonio-Kelly, R., Potenza, M.N., Assaf, M., Pearlson, G.D. (2014). Relationships between reward sensitivity, risk-taking and family history of alcoholism during an interactive competitive fMRI task. *PLoS One*, 9(2), e88188.

CHAPTER 7

Parental cancer

Cynthia W. Moore and Paula K. Rauch

INTRODUCTION

Among medical conditions, cancer is the leading cause of death for adults in their prime parenting years (ages 21–55) (Centers for Disease Control and Prevention, 2013), and is one of the most variable illnesses in its many presentations, treatments and prognoses. Many children have had some personal experience of cancer in their extended family or community prior to a parent's diagnosis. Even children who have not themselves witnessed the impact of cancer may have expectations about what it means to have cancer from a multitude of other sources. For example, information about cancer regularly appears in news and entertainment media, and includes reports on medical breakthroughs, newly identified risk factors or the cancer diagnosis or death of a celebrity or public figure. School curricula in both science and literature also frequently incorporate information about cancer, and cancer is a common focus of community or school-based fundraisers in which children may participate. This is the multifaceted and challenging backdrop against which a parent with cancer must negotiate his or her own reaction to the diagnosis of cancer, and try to support the well-being of each child in the family.

LITERATURE REVIEW

Fortunately, there is a growing, albeit nascent, literature on the impact of a parent's cancer on a child's emotional health that may help guide parents and health providers in supporting children. At least 18% of US patients diagnosed with cancer in the past two years have minor children living at home (Weaver et al., 2010). Living with parental cancer is a not-uncommon experience for children; in Finland, almost 7% of a cohort of children born in 1987 had a parent with cancer (Niemela et al., 2012) and about 3% of minor children and 8% of young adults in Norway have a parent who has been diagnosed (Syse et al., 2012).

Patients who are parenting minor children experience the range of challenges common to others living with cancer, as well as some that are unique, resulting in increased strain for patients and their children (Bell and Ristovski-Slijepcevic, 2011; Bultmann et al., 2014; Nilsson et al., 2009). Compared to survivors without children, young mothers report more fear of cancer recurrence and a sense that the illness intrudes more in their lives, with mothers of adolescents reporting the most stress (Ares et al., 2014). Parents reporting high levels of distress about the impact of their illness on children also have more symptoms of depression and anxiety, worse quality of life (Muriel et al., 2012) and poorer parenting role satisfaction (Cho et al., 2015).

Concerns about dependent children are prominent, and distressing in this group. Specific concerns commonly identified include the impact of the parent's own altered physical and emotional functioning on the child's day-to-day routine and emotional well-being, as well as how to simultaneously protect children from distress and keep them informed about the illness. Even in the early stages of illness, many parents consider how children would cope in the event of their death and are aware that children worry about that possibility as well (Asbury et al., 2014; Muriel et al., 2012).

Children experience a range of concerns about the parent's cancer. Youth of all ages may miss activities they are unable to continue to engage in, as well as contact with peers, and as a result may feel angry or guilty. Latency-age children (e.g. 6–11 years old) report worries about the side effects of treatment to the parent, the parent's possible death, changes in the parent's appearance and the potential for separation from the parent. Adolescents also express concerns about making mistakes in the parent's care, the well parent's functioning, their own risk of cancer and how to accept and find meaning in the parent's illness, for example in valuing the importance of family relationships or by recognising personal growth in response to adversity (Bradbury et al., 2012; Grabiak et al., 2007; Thastum et al., 2009; Visser et al., 2004). Having a parent with breast cancer poses particular challenges for adolescent girls; they may fear developing breast cancer themselves (Visser et al., 2004), and 11- to 19-year-old girls with a first- or even second-degree relative with breast cancer perceive themselves at higher risk of cancer, and report more generalised anxiety and more tobacco use than girls at population risk of breast cancer

(Bradbury et al., 2012). This suggests that perception of cancer risk may relate both to adolescents' distress and health-related behaviour.

Children's adjustment is affected by parental cancer as well. The need for support is one indication of heightened distress; over a 21-year period, children of cancer patients in Finland used more specialised psychiatric care than peers, with the presence of psychiatric illness in either parent further increasing the child's use of these services (Niemela et al., 2012). While children with a parent with cancer seem not to be more likely to meet criteria for a clinical diagnosis of depression or an anxiety disorder than peers with parents who are cancer-free, they are at-risk for symptoms of anxiety and depression, irritability, intrusive thoughts, somatic complaints, difficulty concentrating in school and poorer school performance (Nelson and While, 2002; Rainville et al., 2012; Visser et al., 2005; Watson et al., 2006). Evidence is mixed about whether these children show more externalising behaviour, with some studies suggesting that they do (Visser et al., 2005; Watson et al., 2006) and others finding that parental illness is unrelated to externalising or problem behaviour (Hoke, 2001; Jantzer et al., 2013).

Qualities of an individual child, such as coping strategies typically employed, help predict youth adjustment to parental cancer. In a study of Hispanic adolescents with a parent with cancer, teen depression was related to denial and behavioural disengagement as coping strategies, and anxiety was associated with acceptance, substance use and behavioural disengagement (Costas-Muniz, 2012). Another cross-sectional study of adolescents in Germany found that problem-focused or approach-oriented coping strategies were generally associated with better mental health, while avoidance-oriented coping was associated with worse mental health (Krattenmacher et al., 2013).

Children's adjustment has also been studied in relation to parent functioning. While type or stage of a parent's cancer do not predict children's distress, cancer-related disability predicts worse adjustment in children (Bultmann et al., 2014; Krattenmacher et al., 2012; Osborn, 2007). Reduced health-related quality of life in the cancer-free parent was also associated with worse adjustment in children in a study that did not find this association for ill parents (Krattenmacher et al., 2014). Thus, it is important to assess functioning across all affected family members, because children are affected not only by the well-being of the parent with cancer, but also by the emotional health of the cancer-free parent.

Both cross-sectional and longitudinal research indicate that having a parent with both cancer and symptoms of depression or anxiety heightens a child's risk for adjustment problems and poorer quality of life (Bultmann et al., 2014; Gotze et al., 2014; Krattenmacher et al., 2012; Lewis and Darby,

2003). Depression in a parent with cancer was the most significant factor in predicting impaired family functioning in a sample of 381 European families (Schmitt et al., 2008), and having a depressed mother and poorly defined family roles created particular risk for internalising problems in children, particularly for girls (Watson et al., 2006).

Other family-level processes show potential to clarify which youth are most at-risk for poorer adjustment, as well as suggesting possible targets for intervention. Lower family cohesion predicted more depression, anxiety and externalising behaviour in adolescents (Lindqvist et al., 2007; Osborn, 2007; Watson et al., 2006). In addition, a family's flexibility in problem solving predicted less adolescent distress, and warm and supportive parenting was associated with fewer internalising symptoms in 8- to 16-year-old children in families dealing with parental cancer, but not in families without cancer in a parent (Lindqvist et al., 2007; Vannatta et al., 2010). While improvement in family functioning is likely to promote better youth adjustment in all families, regardless of parental health status, these findings highlight promising areas to focus on, specifically in families with a parent with cancer.

Communication and children's adjustment

Family communication style also relates to children's adjustment to parental cancer. Adolescents who feel there is open communication between family members have less anxiety and fewer externalising problems (Lindqvist et al., 2007; Watson et al., 2006). Adolescents with negative feelings about family communication, or who tend not to share feelings with parents, reported more intrusive thoughts about the parent's illness, greater efforts to avoid thinking about it and more overall distress. Further, communication was poorer when the parent had recurrent disease or was receiving more intensive treatment (Huizinga et al., 2005). In contrast, mothers' report of poorer communication, or children's report of ability to ask questions or satisfaction with information provided, were not associated with adjustment in 8- to 16-year-olds a year after completion of the mother's treatment (Nelson and While, 2002).

A study that applied cluster analysis to measures of family functioning found distinct groups based on levels of family cohesion, expressiveness and conflict resolution. Two groups were characterised by low expressiveness but differed in other ways. 'Low communicating' families, who comprised about 20% of the sample, had high cohesiveness and high ability to resolve conflict, while another 6% of families were 'hostile', with low cohesion and low conflict resolution. The contrast between these two low expressive groups suggests that only measuring communication in the absence of other factors may limit our understanding of the family process, and that lack of open communication likely feels quite different in families that are otherwise well-functioning vs much less well-functioning (Schuler et al., 2014).

Cultural differences may also be reflected in communication patterns. In a sample of Korean women with and without breast cancer, closed communication was more typical than open communication in both groups of mothers, and was higher among children of women with breast cancer than in children with healthy mothers (Cho et al., 2015).

Content of family communication about illness

Interviews with parents further clarify the communication challenges they face. Choosing whether, when and how to share news of a cancer diagnosis with children is one of parents' first, and most difficult, decisions. Studies suggest that parents base these decisions on their wish to protect children and maintain a sense of normality (Asbury et al., 2014) and that there is variability in the extent to which children are told about the illness. In a group of children whose mothers had breast cancer, 19% were unaware of the diagnosis even after the mother's surgery or radiation therapy (Barnes et al., 2002). Older children received more information sooner. Families particularly tend to avoid communication about their feelings or other emotional aspects of illness (Shands et al., 2000), focusing instead on its practical impact. Mothers who talked more openly believed the child had a right to know, wanted to keep the child's trust and hoped that talking would alleviate the child's anxiety. Those who disclosed less wanted to avoid facing difficult questions, including questions about death, wished to protect the child, to preserve special family occasions, and believed that the child would not understand the illness (Barnes et al., 2000).

While parents want very much to protect children from worrisome news, children themselves seem to want information. A qualitative study of 8–15 year olds indicated their desire for a clear understanding of their parent's illness, even though they realised such conversations could be difficult (Thastum et al., 2008). Interviews with adolescents with a mother with breast cancer indicated that they valued the opportunity to talk with parents about it, and in particular, they wanted to know whether she would survive (Kristjanson et al., 2004). Bereaved adolescents overwhelmingly believe they should have been told that a parent was going to die imminently, within hours or days. Strikingly, 43% of this group had not realised that a parent's death was imminent up to a couple of hours before the loss (Bylund-Grenklo et al., 2015). A finding that children using a web-based peer support system experienced a lack of communication in their direct environment (Giesbers et al., 2010) highlights interesting questions. Do children rely more on peers for support and information if parents are not forthcoming? If so, what does that mean for the child's understanding of the illness and ability to cope?

These studies together emphasise the value that parents and children place on open communication about illness. However, the fact that individual adolescents' need for information varied, depending on family and personal characteristics, poses a challenge in translating these results to family interventions. It may be that an individualised parent or family guidance approach may be better suited to meeting the unique needs of each child in a family, than a group 'one size fits all' model.

There also seems to be an increasingly recognised need for professional support for parents about how best to talk to children about cancer. Nurses expressed a desire for more information about the impact of parental cancer on children and how to help families communicate more openly (Turner et al., 2007), and helping children to understand the parent's somatic illness and medical treatments was a consistent priority for a number of interventions reviewed (Diareme et al., 2007). However, this need is not yet fully met; for example, healthy parents in Norway who wanted to talk with a health professional about how and when to tell children when an ill parent would die, rarely experienced the opportunity for such a conversation (Aamotsmo and Bugge, 2014).

INTERVENTIONS

A variety of interventions, both peer support and family-based, have been developed to mitigate the negative impact of parental cancer on children's functioning. Parents' aims for seeking counselling vary, but include problems with communication, experiencing a high level of conflict and a change of roles (Thastum et al., 2006). Stated goals across interventions often include increasing the child's knowledge about the parent's illness and treatment, providing a supportive environment in which feelings and concerns can be shared and normalised, and facilitating healthy coping (Diareme et al., 2007). Interventions for a subset of families in palliative care have also focused on parenting competence, anticipatory grief, active coping and communication (Kuhne et al., 2012). The impact of these interventions has often remained unevaluated, or evaluated in ways that preclude full confidence in the results. Interested readers are referred to reviews by Diareme et al. (2007), Niemela et al. (2010) and Kuhne et al. (2012) for excellent summaries of this history. Several relatively recent efforts to measure the effectiveness of very disparate interventions are described here in more detail to provide a sense of the 'state of the art'.

In the European COSIP (Children of Somatically Ill Parents) consortium, a family-based counselling programme has been developed and preliminarily tested with encouraging results. Thastum et al. (2006) report that in their group of 24 families who participated in the 3–8 session intervention, mothers and children, but not fathers, experienced a decrease in depression, and parents reported improvement in communication and effective responsiveness. Changes did not occur in children's anxiety, peer relations or self-concept over the course of the study. Parents and children described what they gained from the counselling at the end of the study; common themes from this qualitative portion of the intervention assessment included confirmation in being a 'good-enough' parent, better understanding of emotions and reactions of other family members, heightened intimacy and cohesion and normalisation of feelings.

A peer-support programme developed in the United States, Children's Lives Include Moments of Bravery (CLIMB) was implemented in a cancer charity organisation in Northern Ireland. Group meetings lasting one and a half hours per session were held over six consecutive weeks for children aged 5–12. Participating children had to be already aware of the parent's cancer diagnosis. The programme's qualitative assessment used focus groups for parents (n=6) and children (n=7), as well as interviews with the two professionals who delivered the intervention (Semple and McCaughan, 2013). Parents expressed a lack of confidence and skills in communicating about cancer, and were eager for professional input related to changes in children's behaviour. They described some gains in children's understanding of cancer, and improvements in their mood and behaviour. Children were able to describe misunderstandings about cancer that had changed as a result of the intervention, such as the illness being contagious, or somehow their fault, and also expressed a sense of relief in having correct information. In addition, children seemed to appreciate the connection to peers in similar circumstances.

Another pilot intervention study assessed the impact of a three-week inpatient programme on 116 mothers with breast cancer and their 3- to 14-year-old children, which combined rehabilitative treatment for mothers and child-centred psychosocial interventions (John et al., 2013). Pre-school and school-age children participated separately in four peer-group meetings over their stay, and mothers in two sessions focused on family communication. Mothers completed questionnaires at three time points: before a wait period prior to the intervention, at the beginning of the treatment and at the end of the programme. Changes during the intervention period were significantly greater than during the wait period on 3 out of 20 scales: mothers' emotional functioning, children's psychological health and children's emotional symptoms. However, the authors note that the study design did not permit conclusions about whether the changes were caused by the group meetings or other factors such as the reprieve from usual daily obligations while staying in the seaside rehabilitation centre.

The challenge of engaging families with different cultural backgrounds was addressed by Davey et al. (2013) in their evaluation of a family intervention for African-American parents coping with cancer and their school-age children. Twelve parent-child dyads recruited over a two-year period participated in a family intervention or a psycho-educational control group. The family intervention consisted of three child support group sessions and two multi-family group sessions, with content focused on mood monitoring, increasing pleasant activities, relaxation and communication. It was culturally adapted to fit the needs of African-American families by facilitating a sense of community among participants, being highly interactive and drawing on Afrocentric coping skills such as relying on faith, promoting kin support, highlighting positives and encouraging flexibility in family roles. The control group received the same number of sessions, covering the same psycho-educational content, but using a lecture and video format.

Results suggested that communication with school-age children was significantly better for parents who completed the culturally adapted family intervention than for the psychoeducation group, and children in this intervention were more satisfied with it. However, the communication measure used had internal consistency below the usual standard, making interpretation of this result somewhat more difficult. No changes in parent or in child depression, or in child anxiety were found following the intervention.

The most promising indication that a psychosocial intervention can have a measurable positive impact on family functioning comes from a multi-site study of 176 married mothers with breast cancer and their 8- to 12-year-old children, randomised into experimental or control groups (Lewis et al., 2015). The Enhancing Connections Program included five scripted one-hour counselling sessions for the mother, a booklet about breast cancer for mothers to read to the child, a mother's workbook and a child activity booklet focused on ways of dealing with stress. Mothers in the control group received a booklet about how they could support her child about breast cancer, and a brief phone call from a patient educator who reviewed the contents of the booklet. Outcomes based largely on standardised questionnaires with good validity and reliability were assessed at 2 and 12 months post-intervention, and included both mother and child reports.

At 2 months but not 12 months, mothers in the experimental group showed significant improvements compared to controls in depressed mood and self-report of parenting skills. Children in the experimental group had significantly lower depression at 2 and 12 months compared to controls, using both mother and child report measures. In addition, children had fewer behavioural problems compared to controls at 2 months. The intervention did not significantly affect parenting self-efficacy or maternal anxiety.

Taken together, these studies reveal both the promise and challenges of quantifying the impact of psychosocial interventions for families facing parental cancer. Two family-based interventions (Lewis et al., 2015; Thastum et al., 2006) showed promise in decreasing depression in both mothers and children, and another intervention study that did not measure depression specifically found improvements in children's emotional functioning (John et al., 2013). However, reductions in mother's or child's anxiety were not apparent (Davey et al., 2013; Lewis et al., 2015). Children's externalising behaviour was less frequently assessed, but participation in the Enhancing Connections intervention resulted in its decrease. Family interventions improved family communication (Davey et al., 2013; Semple and McCaughan, 2013; Thastum et al., 2006) and parent report of parenting skills (Lewis et al., 2015).

These successful interventions share an emphasis on improving communication and the normalisation of emotions. The variability among promising programmes suggests that a range of possibilities can be helpful to families; different interventions meet different needs, and face different implementation challenges. For example, family-focused interventions allow the treatment to be tailored to the family's unique needs, and a direct focus on communication patterns, but do not provide peer support for parents or children, and can be extremely difficult to schedule, given family members' other obligations and interests. Child focus groups offer peer support and normalise children's experiences, but have notoriously low turnout, can increase worries about potential bad outcomes a child had not yet considered, and may not readily allow parents to receive specific feedback on their child's unique challenges that they report wanting (Semple and McCaughan, 2013). Parent guidance sessions do allow this kind of individual feedback, may be more easily scheduled around other medical appointments since children are not involved, and can promote improvements in children's functioning, but relying on parents to assess and describe children's experiences may mean that important information is lost to the clinician.

One of the challenges in building upon this research is that so many disparate outcomes are arguably reasonable targets of change. Intervention studies have measured outcomes at the family, parent and individual child levels, and have focused on clinically significant symptoms like depression, and also normative adjustment, such as children feeling supported or not alone in their experiences of coping with a parent's cancer. In addition, functional improvements in one family member have been targeted both directly, as when children are included in family sessions, and indirectly, as in the Enhancing Connections intervention. Both can be effective, and indeed, some of the most robust decreases in children's depressive symptoms resulted from direct intervention with the mother and not the child (Lewis et al., 2015). The goals of intervention programmes must be explicit, so that future research can continue to clarify the goodness of fit between family functioning and intensity of distress, goals of care and the applied intervention.

Obstacles encountered in these intervention studies highlight factors that should be considered in choosing intervention strategies. Recruitment and retention posed a significant challenge across several studies. Davey et al. (2013) provided transportation, babysitting and remuneration to participants, yet still had difficulty recruiting families to participate. They concluded that while their culturally adapted intervention was highly acceptable to families, its feasibility was uncertain. Thastum et al. (2006) saw families for 3–8 sessions, suggesting that families have preferences about the intervention's dosage that may or may not match the study design. Improving the feasibility of interventions may require offering them in locations to which participants already travel, such as the clinic (or at home) and allowing choice in duration of participation.

Parents with cancer, even the same type of cancer, are a clinically heterogeneous population. They vary in post-diagnosis lifespan, in cognitive, physical and emotional symptoms, and in functional status. Children's experience of the parent's illness is correspondingly variable. This is difficult to account for in assessment of interventions that frequently create seemingly homogenous groups based on type of cancer.

IN PRACTICE

Unlike the healthcare provider's sophisticated understanding of cancer treatment and prognosis, a diagnosis of 'cancer' is frequently undifferentiated in the minds of patients and families, as if cancer were a single entity. The need for a parent and co-parent to have an accurate understanding of the primary cancer diagnosis, its staging and treatment requires significant education from the healthcare team. This individualised information permits parents to communicate with their children, correct misinformation and anticipate the demands of treatment, expected symptoms and disability that will have a direct impact on their parenting capacities.

Healthcare providers can also support parents in thinking through how to talk with children about cancer. How the child initially learns of the parent's diagnosis, whether through direct communication or overhearing adult conversations, sets the stage for future communication. Providers can encourage patients to reflect on what they would like to communicate, then to make active choices about how to do so. Parents may want help framing an acute event, such as a seizure, in a way that helps a child understand how it connects to the cancer diagnosis, and also reassures the child that there is a plan in place should more seizures occur.

Healthcare providers can also remind parents that children will be affected by both positive and negative outcomes of the cancer treatment; for example, fluctuations in parental mood, the arrival of extended family or calls from concerned friends. Both routine cancer treatment and unplanned complications often affect children through cancelled vacations, or parents missing special school or after-school events, or being too fatigued to engage in usual daily routines. Being mindful of these potential disruptions to children allows healthcare providers to describe treatment side effects in terms of impact on functionality, which is particularly useful to parents.

Cancer care and its impact will intersect with the child's stage of development, and will be understood and integrated anew as the child gets older and brings new cognitive understanding, emotional reactions and social circumstances to the meaning of the parent's disease, recurrence or death. While an in-depth description of the relationships among a child's developmental stage, likely reactions to parental illness and age-appropriate responses is beyond the scope of this chapter, Table 7.1 summarizes key points to be considered by healthcare providers. The interested reader is also referred to Moore and Rauch (2015). It is easy to understand why parents need and want sophisticated, developmentally informed input about how to support their children's coping. At times of high anxiety, it is difficult to translate generic parent guidance such as 'be honest' or 'maintain regular daily routines' into an individualised plan that is responsive to the particular children in the family and the parent's clinical course. The practice guidelines presented below are based on the authors' decade-plus experience providing parent guidance using the Parenting At a Challenging Time (PACT) model. This evidence-informed intervention is based on the literature focused on supporting child resilience. The PACT model stresses the value of stable, caring and supportive relationships between children and the important adults in their lives, parental attunement and an engaged, supportive community and school environment (National Scientific Council on the Developing Child, 2015). The programme provides a collaborative intervention between a cancer centre-based child mental health clinician and a parent to approximately 275 families per year in

TABLE 7.1 Developmental stage and typical illness-related challenges, expressions of distress, and recommended support

Typical characteristics and goals of stage	*Major parental illness-related challenges for child*	*Typical expressions of distress*	*Age-appropriate support*
Infants and toddlers (birth to 2 years)			
Developing secure attachments to caregivers, allowing the child's confident exploration of the environment and trust in being soothed when distressed	Unpredictable or long separations, changes to routines or caregivers, unfamiliar environments, intense adult distress	Fussiness, picky eating, separation distress, regression in newly learned behaviour (toileting, sleeping through night)	Limited number of caregivers who are made familiar with predictable routines, protection from intense emotions in adults
Pre-school children (3–5 years)			
Developing verbal skills, learning through play, mixing fantasy and fact about how events relate to each other ('magical thinking'); working on self-control of impulses	Long or unpredictable separations from caregivers, loss of control over routines and choices, imagined explanations for parent's illness or withdrawal may lead to a sense of personal responsibility	Irritability, questions that reflect guilty feelings, changes in imaginative play, separation distress, emotional outbursts seeming out of proportion to the current situation	Knowing name and simple explanation of illness and treatment, that nothing the child thought or did caused the illness or side effects, having choices, when possible, about changes in routines, keeping consistent routines despite protests to limit setting
Latency-age children (6–11 years)			
Mastering more complex physical skills, developing close friendships and navigating group dynamics, learning to read and reading to learn, using familiar rules to manage new situations, regulating own emotions	May experience illness as intensely unfair, concrete thinking can create misperceptions and self-blame for the illness or changes in parent, loss of activities and friendships due to scheduling challenges, fearing parent's death	Somatic complaints, trips to school nurse, changes in sleep or eating pattern, anger at unfairness of the situation, often coping by staying busy and distracted so reduced engagement signals distress	Provide concrete description of illness (e.g. non-contagious, not caused by anything the child did), distinguish between symptoms of illness and treatment side effects, maintain consistent involvement in activities and friendships, avoid euphemisms (easily misunderstood), share information with educators and request that they monitor the child's adjustment

Adolescents (12–18 years)

- Balancing individuation/independence with connectedness to family, developing intimate relationships – both romantic and platonic, using abstract thinking skills to understand the world and their place in it
- New roles and responsibilities posing emotional challenges or interfering with normative activities and relationships, witnessing parent's physical and emotional suffering, being seen as different from peers due to parent's illness or death, balancing time with friends and time at home, concern about own risk for illness
- Sadness, irritability, worry about impact of cancer on selves and family and future, avoidance of ill parent due to distress about suffering or ongoing conflictual relationship, risk-taking behaviour, withdrawal from friends, needing to be 'too good'
- Provide clear information about diagnosis and treatment, discourage independent internet research, offer choices about communication with school, consider genetic counselling for parent for factual information, reassurance and realistic screening plans, acknowledge the love that exists even in challenging relationships, challenge guilt, give choices about new responsibilities and be sure needed skills are already present

a busy cancer centre (Moore, 2014). Parents share their knowledge of a child's temperament and reactions to previous smaller challenges and transitions, while learning about how children at their child's phase of development are likely to understand cancer and be affected by the challenges of cancer care.

While resources and expertise in child development vary widely across settings, it is recommended that, at a minimum, healthcare providers be able to guide parents to written, web-based or in-person resources. Written and web-based parent resources developed by PACT programme clinicians are mentioned at the end of this chapter. Provided resources should support parents in talking to their children about cancer, prioritising the maintenance of regular schedules and routines, fostering child-focused family time, and engaging the child's school community and other community resources. Support for open communication should help parents decide on age-appropriate words to use to describe cancers and treatments to children.

Assessing concerns

As suggested by the literature, patients coping with cancer share many of the same general concerns, and parents have additional, often pressing, concerns about the impact on children. Thus routine cancer care must include asking if a patient is a parent, and what parenting concerns are present. This can be achieved as part of a general psychosocial assessment or using a screening tool. One recently developed tool is the 15-item Parenting Concerns Questionnaire (PCQ: Muriel et al., 2012), which assesses a parent's parenting concerns about the practical and emotional impact of the illness on children, and the level of support from a co-parent to the ill parent and children. Higher parenting concerns corresponded to more symptoms of depression and anxiety, more overall distress and worse quality of life in parents. The PCQ may be used in conjunction with a psychosocial interview or as a means of identifying the most distressed parents.

Both parents' mental health affects children and should be included in the clinician's overall conceptualisation of a family's strengths and challenges. Assessment of parental depression and anxiety is assumed to be part of the cancer centre's routine patient assessment, so is not elucidated here. Given the interrelationship of the psychological health of parents and children, mental health resources need to be available not only to the parent with cancer, but also to the co-parent in order to best support the well-being of the children at home. While cancer centres routinely provide mental healthcare for the designated patient, they are less likely to have clinicians available to treat a co-parent's depression or anxiety. Facilitating co-parent referral is helpful.

In a general psychosocial interview, five simple parenting questions may include: (i) Tell me about your children (ii) What have you told them about your diagnosis? (iii) What specific words have you used? (iv) Do you have specific concerns about any of your children? (v) Who might you talk with if you had parenting concerns? Next, information can be offered about available parenting resources.

Parents often welcome the opportunity to describe each child's personality or temperament along with their ages. Interest in one's children can be alliance building. Learning about a child's usual style of coping with past challenges or transitions likely informs how a child will react initially and how easy or difficult it may be for that child to adapt to the many disruptions that accompany cancer treatment. The clinician doing the psychosocial assessment may share basic child development information relevant to understanding the diagnosis and adaptation to the treatment (see Table 7.1), or may direct the parent to age-appropriate written resources with a plan to discuss further at a later appointment. Hearing what a parent has already shared with each child and what actual words, if any, have been used to describe the cancer diagnosis helps the clinician appreciate the parent's style of communication, and identify where assistance in age-appropriate explanations may be needed and what might be productive next steps to advance the parent-child conversation. This approach recognises the importance of open communication between parent and child in facilitating child coping.

Enquiring about concerns related to an individual child may elicit information about pre-existing mental health issues such as anxiety or depression, developmental challenges such as autism or learning disabilities, or relevant past experiences such as the death of a grandparent or a friend's parent to cancer. Asking a parent to whom she might turn for parenting advice or support helps the clinician learn about the ways a patient may feel well supported in their parenting with cancer, or somewhat isolated. This opens the door to talking about the resources at the hospital, clinic or in the community. It may also provide an opportunity to share a brochure or web-based resources, such as the PACT website (www.mghpact.org).

In an initial assessment, a parent's immediate questions and concerns need to be addressed, but parents should be assured that parenting issues will be an ongoing consideration throughout care. There is often so much information being shared at the time of a diagnosis, that parents may benefit from help prioritising immediate parenting concerns, such as what to say to the children that day, or what additional childcare may be needed to enable the patient and co-parent to complete medical tests and appointments. Discussion about longer-term adjustment challenges are usually better left to future interactions.

Communication basics for parents

Healthcare providers should encourage parents to identify the cancer by name, for example as breast cancer or leukaemia, and not use a euphemism such as a 'bump' or 'boo-boo' or a vague description, such as 'Daddy is sick'. For young children, hearing the name of the cancer helps the child differentiate the parent's serious illness from common words used to describe their own minor injuries or routine childhood conditions. For older children, this open communication about the diagnosis ensures that the child will hear the information from a loving parent first, rather than overhearing it or learning the diagnosis from another adult or child. Direct communication is respectful of the importance of this news to the child and allows the child to ask questions. For children of any age, identifying cancer by name invites the child into the discussions about the parent's illness. It is an 'error of kindness' to imagine that excluding a child from conversations about difficult news is protective. On the contrary, it may increase the likelihood of the child being confused, misinformed and ultimately mistrustful of the parent.

Healthcare providers can encourage parents to welcome each of their child's questions warmly and try to help the child describe more fully what may underlie a particular question. It may help to remind parents who are anxious about having correct information, that children's questions do not necessarily need to be answered immediately. Parents can take their time to understand a child's question and offer to ask others, such as the doctor, nurse, co-parent or the child's teacher or a clergy member, depending on what has been asked. When parents feel less pressured to have a good answer immediately, they are often better listeners and more relaxed. This can be felt by the child and often leads to greater comfort with asking questions and thinking aloud. Parents should be encouraged to remind their children not to worry alone, but rather to share worries with the parents and other designated adults. Older children may imagine that keeping their worries to themselves is protecting the parent or a stressed co-parent. It may be helpful for the parent to communicate that he will be worrying about the child if the child is not forthcoming, and that they can face the challenges together if the parent is not left to guess what is troubling the child.

Stability at home

During times of uncertainty, children benefit from regular routines and a predictable schedule. They will look to parents and other familiar adults for the emotional cues about how worried to be and whether the 'new normal' feels secure. Parents should try to maintain as many of the familiar routines as possible, but inevitably there will be some changes mandated by the demands of the work-up, time in hospital, treatment and limitations caused by advanced disease. Focusing on regular mealtimes and bedtimes and making sure the child knows who will be present during daily transitions (such as waking up, going to school, getting to an after-school activity or when returning home) supports stability. Ideally, a parent can prioritise some quiet time at home, when a young child can have some contact comfort and an older child can spend time talking or just being together. Setting aside some time at the weekend to review the child's past and upcoming week at school or after-school activities can help a busy parent stay more attuned to challenges unrelated to the parent's health. Turning off mobile phones at mealtimes and bedtime and limiting visitors also signal to children that they are a parent's priority.

Extended family members or friends may be called upon to help with childcare or transportation during a parent's cancer treatment. These additional adults may provide valuable assistance to the parent, but sometimes children experience these non-parental adults as unwelcome additions to the family, and want only their parents to be providing this support. Parents may be stressed by a child's irritability with these helpers, and may need guidance to appreciate the child's perspective and to set appropriate expectations about a child's behaviour.

Sometimes, parents may need to rely on a relative, often a grandparent to the children or an aunt, whose rules and routines may be at odds with the parent's preferences, but which are hard to change or complain about because this person's help is needed. Parent-child conversations about the benefits of the support, and also the challenges, can help a child feel less alone with frustrations about necessary compromises in the context of treatment. The same principles may apply to the attention of a co-parent, who a child may feel is attending to the ill parent at the expense of availability to the child. Since feeling part of a positive family unit helps children cope, it is useful to identify what can be adjusted to balance the child's experience and the parent's support needs. Problem solving together as a family is itself a positive skill to develop.

Engaging the community

Parents may be encouraged to be thoughtful about what they share about their cancer, treatment and prognosis with their community and how it is shared. This includes sharing how the parent or co-parent is feeling or things that the child may be experiencing. Many families will use web-based communities to connect with their friends and family members. Parents should assume that if information is being shared with a large number of adults, some of those adults will share what they read with their children. This information is likely to find its way back to all but the youngest children.

Parents should talk with someone from each child's school to update them about the parent's diagnosis and treatment plan. Parents do not need to disclose more than they feel comfortable sharing, but it is best for the child's teacher to know that the family is experiencing the challenges of the cancer care so that if the child needs additional support or accommodation at school this can be arranged. The parent should be direct with the school contact about what should or should not be shared with the school community.

Many children experience school as a welcome escape from the changes imposed by the parent's cancer and medical care. They may not want to talk about the parent's cancer or treatment during the school day. Ideally, each child would have a designated person at school to talk with at their own initiative if the child feels particular distress. Teachers should be asked to speak with parents if the child is struggling academically or socially or shares particular worries related to the parent's health. Parents should also request that the teachers let the parent know if there will be things in the curriculum that may be especially challenging; for example, a reading assignment with a character who is seriously ill, or a science class studying the genetics of cancer.

Neighbours, friends and other community members may want to offer assistance to the family during the parent's cancer treatment. It can be exhausting to try to manage the many individuals who want to be of assistance. Designating a close friend or family member as the first point of contact enables someone other than the parent to guide individuals who want to help in ways to be genuinely helpful. This also allows the parent to turn her attention to her children rather than answering the many questions and often burdensome reactions of well-intended community members. Children may resent having their fatigued parent engaged by many adults rather than feeling the focus of the parent's attention.

Especially for younger children, but for children of all ages, it is helpful to remind the parents of a child's friends and other adults not to talk about the parent's cancer during times such as school drop-off, or during an event where the focus should be on the child. This may particularly occur when the co-parent is with the child, and community members are eager for an update on the parent with cancer. Some parents will refer questioners to their web-based posting or to a contact who is dealing with community communication for them. Others may choose to have a standard statement such as 'we're all doing well and taking it day by day' in the hope of not being rude, but also ending an unwelcome conversation with the child present.

RECOMMENDATIONS FOR FUTURE RESEARCH

There is still much to be learned about *how* the identified risk factors for poorer adjustment in children exert their effects, and how illness-related factors (such as limited lifespan or physical function) interact with family-process variables (like communication and cohesion) and child factors (like stage of development, temperament and roles in the family). For example, a child's roles in the family and her priorities may shift as the parent's health deteriorates (Kennedy and Lloyd-Williams, 2009) so the effect of parental cancer on the child's functioning may appear different depending on whether the parent is expected to survive or is facing end-of-life challenges.

Further studies on communication about parental cancer are needed to clarify how the family's general communication style, most often measured, relates to communication about cancer in particular, and how that varies according to children's ages. In addition, both too little and too much information about cancer might negatively affect children. Practice recommendations could be informed by taking a closer look at exactly what is shared, how soon in the treatment course, and with what emotional tone, as a factor in children's adjustment.

The literature on children's coping and effective interventions would benefit from studies that include multiple assessments of constructs from multiple reporters, have controlled study designs, ideally with randomisation into treatment arms, and include longitudinal follow-up assessments. Clear thinking about the feasibility of interventions, including their potential to reach many families based on practicalities in everyday family life, will also aid the design of new interventions and the assessment of their utility. Little is known about the efficacy of online support groups and other web-based interventions for children. While use of the internet can enhance access to support, more needs to be learned about what is gained and what is lost in trading in-person group meetings for a virtual support group, for children at different developmental stages.

Finally, building on existing intervention studies, it will be helpful for future research to explore how healthcare providers with different competencies can be best trained to serve as resources to parents with cancer. For example, what kind of targeted education would allow mental health clinicians working in non-medical settings most easily to learn enough about cancer treatment so they can provide support around parenting with cancer? And what educational content, and delivery method, would most efficiently teach oncology nurses and social workers accustomed to treating adults about child development as it relates to adjusting to a parent's illness? How best to employ the ever-increasing range of media available for teaching content and skills remains an important question for researchers interested in making a positive difference in the lives of families affected by cancer.

CONCLUSION

Parenting is challenging in the best of circumstances. Parenting while managing the physical and emotional tolls on each family member imposed by a life-threatening illness, such as cancer, poses challenges that can feel overwhelming to children and adults. Parents want, and deserve, guidance around the range of concerns experienced in all stages of cancer survivorship, including how to talk about a cancer diagnosis and genetic risk with children, how to recognise and facilitate healthy coping in children, and how to support children even as a parent is nearing the end of life. Basic research has succeeded in identifying targets for interventions, such as open communication, as well as populations at particular risk, such as children whose parent suffers from depression in addition to cancer. Research on interventions, while still in its early stages, suggests that families benefit from a range of supportive programmes, and holds the promise of clarifying best practices to form the basis of future advocacy efforts.

RESOURCES FOR PATIENTS

- www.mghpact.org: This website, developed by the clinicians of the Marjorie E. Korff Parenting At a Challenging Time (PACT) Program at Massachusetts General Hospital, offers information about supporting children when a parent has cancer, including communication, signs a child needs additional support, and common concerns at different developmental stages.

- Rauch, P.K., Muriel, A.C. (2006) *Raising an emotionally healthy child when a parent is sick.* New York: McGraw-Hill: 2006.

REFERENCES

Aamotsmo, T., Bugge, K.E. (2014). Balance artistry: The healthy parent's role in the family when the other parent is in the palliative phase of cancer: Challenges and coping in parenting young children. *Palliative and Supportive Care*, 12, 317–329.

Ares, I., Lebel, S., Bielajew, C. (2014). The impact of motherhood on perceived stress, illness intrusiveness and fear of cancer recurrence in young breast cancer survivors over time. *Psychology and Health*, 29(6), 651–670.

Asbury, N., Lalayiannis, L., Walshe, A. (2014). How do I tell the children? Women's experiences of sharing information about breast cancer diagnosis and treatment. *European Journal of Oncology Nursing*, 18(6), 564–570.

Barnes, J., Kroll, L., Burke, O., Lee, J., Jones, A., Stein, A. (2000). Qualitative interview study of communication between parents and children about maternal breast cancer. *British Medical Journal*, 321(7259), 479–482.

Barnes, J., Kroll, L., Lee, J., Burke, O., Jones, A., Stein, A. (2002). Factors predicting communication about the diagnosis of maternal breast cancer to children. *Journal of Psychosomatic Research*, 52(4), 209–214.

Bell, K., Ristovski-Slijepcevic, S. (2011). Metastatic cancer and mothering: Being a mother in the face of a contracted future. *Medical Anthropology*, 30(6), 629–649.

Bradbury, A.R., Patrick-Miller, L., Egleston, B. Schwartz, L., Tuchman, L., Moore, C., Rauch, P., Sands, C., Shorter, R., Rowan, B., Malhotra, S., van Decker, S., Schmidheiser, H., Sicilia, P., Bealin, L., Daly, M. (2012). Perceptions of breast cancer risk, psychological adjustment and behaviors in adolescent girls at high-risk and population-risk for breast cancer. *Cancer Research*, 72(24a), 1931–1932.

Bultmann, J.C., Beierlein, V., Romer, G., Moller, B., Koch, U., Bergelt, C. (2014). Parental cancer: Health-related quality of life and current psychosocial support needs of cancer survivors and their children. *International Journal of Cancer*, 135(11), 2668–2677.

Bylund-Grenklo, T., Kreicbergs, U., Uggla, C., Valdimarsdóttir, U.A., Nyberg, T., Steineck, G., Fürst, C.J. (2015). Teenagers want to be told when a parent's death is near: A nationwide study of cancer-bereaved youths' opinions and experiences. *Acta Oncologica*, 54(6), 944–950.

Centers for Disease Control and Prevention. (2013). Detailed tables for the National Vital Statistics Report (NVSR) 'Deaths: Final Data for 2013.' www.cdc.gov/nchs/data_access/Vitalstatsonline.htm.

Cho, O.H., Yoo, Y.S., Hwang, K.H. (2015). Comparison of parent-child communication patterns and parental role satisfaction among mothers with and without breast cancer. *Applied Nursing Research*, 28(2), 163–168.

Costas-Muniz, R. (2012). Hispanic adolescents coping with parental cancer. *Support Care Cancer*, 20(2), 413–417.

Davey, M., Kissil, K., Lynch, L., Harmon, L., Hodgson, N. (2013). A culturally adapted family intervention for African American families coping with parental cancer: Outcomes of a pilot study. *Psycho-Oncology*, 22, 1572–1580.

Diareme, S., Tsiantis, J., Romer, G., Tsalamanios, E., Anasontzi, S., Paliokosta, E., Kolaitis, G. (2007). Mental health support for children of parents with somatic illness: A review of the theory and intervention concepts. *Families, Systems, and Health*, 25(1), 98–118.

Giesbers, J., Verdonck-de Leeuw, I.M., van Zuuren, F.J., Kleverlaan, N., van der Linden, M.H. (2010). Coping with parental cancer: Web-based peer support in children. *Psycho-Oncology*, 19(8), 887–892.

Gotze, H., Ernst, J., Brahler, E., Romer, G., von Klitzing, K. (2014). Predictors of quality of life of cancer patients, their children, and partners. *Psycho-Oncology*, 24(7),787–795.

Grabiak, B.R., Bender, C.M., Puskar, K.R. (2007). The impact of parental cancer on the adolescent: An analysis of the literature. *Psycho-Oncology*, 16(2), 127–137.

Hoke, L.A. (2001). Psychosocial adjustment in children of mothers with breast cancer. *Psycho-Oncology*, 10, 361–369.

Huizinga, G.A., Visser, A., van der Graaf, W.T., Hoekstra, H.J., Hoekstra-Weebers, J.E. (2005). The quality of communication between parents and adolescent children in the case of parental cancer. *Annals of Oncology*, 16, 1956–1961.

Jantzer, V., Gross, J., Stute, F., Parzer, P., Brunner, R., Willig, K., Schuller-Roma, B., Keller, M., Herzog, W., Romer, G., Resch, F. (2013). Risk behaviors and externalizing behaviors in adolescents dealing with parental cancer: A controlled longitudinal study. *Psycho-Oncology*, 22(11), 2611–2616.

John, K., Becker, K., Mattejat, F. (2013). Impact of family-oriented rehabilitation and prevention: An inpatient program for mothers with breast cancer and their children. *Psycho-Oncology*, 22(12), 2684–2692.

Kennedy, V., Lloyd-Williams, M. (2009). How children cope when a parent has advanced cancer. *Psycho-Oncology*, 18(8), 886–892.

Krattenmacher, T., Kühne, F., Ernst, J., Bergelt, C., Romer, G., Möller, B. (2012). Parental cancer: Factors associated with children's psychosocial adjustment: A systematic review. *Journal of Psychosomatic Research*, 72(5), 344–356.

Krattenmacher, T., Kühne, F., Führer, D., Beierlein, V., Brähler, E., Resch, F., Klitzing, Kv., Flechtner, H.H., Bergelt, C., Romer, G., Möller, B. (2013). Coping skills and mental health status in adolescents when a parent has cancer: A multicenter and multi-perspective study. *Journal of Psychosomatic Research*, 74(3), 252–259.

Krattenmacher, T., Kühne, F., Halverscheid, S., Wiegand-Grefe, S., Bergelt, S., Bergelt, C., Romer, G., Möller, B. (2014). A comparison of the emotional and behavioral problems of children of patients with cancer or a mental disorder and their association with parental quality of life. *Journal of Psychosomatic Research*, 76(3), 213–220.

Kristjanson, L.J., Chalmers, K.I., Woodgate, R. (2004). Information and support needs of adolescent children of women with breast cancer. *Oncology Nursing Forum*, 31(1), 111–119.

Kühne, F., Krattenmacher, T., Beierlein, V., Grimm, J.C., Bergelt, C., Romer, G., Möller, B. (2012). Minor children of palliative patients: A systematic review of psychosocial family interventions. *Journal of Palliative Medicine*, 15(8), 931–945.

Lewis, F.M., Brandt, P.A., Cochrane, B.B., Griffith, K.A., Grant, M., Haase, J.E., Houldin, A.D., Post-White, J., Zahlis, E.H., Shands, M.E. (2015). The Enhancing Connections Program: A six-state randomized clinical trial of a cancer parenting program. *Journal of Consulting and Clinical Psychology*, 83(1), 12–23.

Lewis, F.M., Darby, E.L. (2003). Adolescent adjustment and maternal breast cancer: A test of the 'Faucet Hypothesis'. *Journal of Psychosocial Oncology*, 21, 81–104.

Lindqvist, B., Schmitt, F., Santalahti, P., Romer, G., Piha, J. (2007). Factors associated with the mental health of adolescents when a parent has cancer. *Scandinavian Journal of Psychology*, 48, 345–351.

Moore, C.W. (2014). Supporting children when a parent has cancer: The Parenting At a Challenging Time Program. Memorial Sloan Kettering Cancer Center, Department of Psychiatry Grand Rounds. New York. 17 Oct 2014. Lecture.

Moore, C.W., Rauch, P.K. (2015). Addressing the needs of children when a parent has cancer. In J.C. Holland, W.S. Breitbart, P.B. Jacobsen, M.J. Loscalzo, R. McCorkle, P.N. Butow (Eds) *Psycho-oncology* (3rd edn) (pp. 579–584). New York. Oxford University Press.

Muriel, A.C., Moore, C.W., Baer, L., Park, E.R., Kornblith, A.B., Pirl, W., Prigerson, H., Ing, J., Rauch, P.K. (2012). Measuring psychosocial distress and parenting concerns among adults with cancer: The Parenting Concerns Questionnaire. *Cancer*, 118, 5671–5678.

National Scientific Council on the Developing Child. (2015). Supportive relationships and active skill-building strengthen the foundations of resilience: Working paper 13. www.developingchild.harvard.edu.

Nelson, E., While, D. (2002). Children's adjustment during the first year of a parent's cancer diagnosis. *Journal of Psychosocial Oncology*, 20(1), 15–36.

Niemela, M., Hakko, H., Rasanen, S. (2010). A systematic narrative review of the studies on structured child-centred interventions for families with a parent with cancer. *Psycho-Oncology*, 19(5), 451–461.

Niemela, M., Paananen, R., Hakko, H., Merikukka, M., Gissler, M., Rasanen, S. (2012). The prevalence of children affected by parental cancer and their use of specialized psychiatric services: The 1987 Finnish Birth Cohort study. *International Journal of Cancer*, 131(9), 2117–2125.

Nilsson, M.E., Maciejewski, P.K., Zhang, B., Wright, A.A., Trice, E.D., Muriel, A.C., Friedlander, R.J., Fasciano, K.M., Block, S.D., Prigerson, H.G. (2009). Mental health, treatment preferences, advance care planning, location, and quality of death in advanced cancer patients with dependent children. *Cancer*, 115(2), 399–409.

Osborn, T. (2007). The psychosocial impact of parental cancer on children and adolescents: A systematic review. *Psycho-Oncology*, 16(2), 101–126.

Rainville, F., Dumont, S., Simard, S., Savard, M.H. (2012). Psychological distress among adolescents living with a parent with advanced cancer. *Journal of Psychosocial Oncology*, 30(5), 519–534.

Schmitt, F., Piha, J., Helenius, H., Baldus, C., Kienbacher, C., Steck, B., Thastum, M., Watson, M., Romer, G. (2008). Multinational study of cancer patients and their children: Factors associated with family functioning. *Journal of Clinical Oncology*, 26(36), 5877–5883.

Schuler, T.A., Zaider, T.I., Li, Y., Hichenberg, S., Masterson, M., Kissane, D.W. (2014). Typology of perceived family functioning in an American sample of patients with advanced cancer. *Journal of Pain and Symptom Management*, 48(2), 281–288.

Semple, C.J., McCaughan, E. (2013). Family life when a parent is diagnosed with cancer: Impact of a psychosocial intervention for young children. *European Journal of Cancer Care*, 22(2), 219–231.

Shands, M.E., Lewis, F.M., Zahlis, E.H. (2000). Mother and child interactions about the mother's breast cancer: An interview study. *Oncology Nursing Forum*, 27(1), 77–85.

Syse, A., Aas, G.B., Loge, J.H. (2012). Children and young adults with parents with cancer: A population-based study. *Clinical Epidemiology*, 4, 41–52.

Thastum, M., Johansen, M.B., Gubba, L., Olesen, L.B., Romer, G. (2008). Coping, social relations, and communication: A qualitative exploratory study of children of parents with cancer. *Clinical Child Psychology and Psychiatry*, 13(1), 123–138.

Thastum, M., Watson, M., Kienbacher, C., Piha, J., Steck, B., Zachariae, R., Baldus, C., Romer, G. (2009). Prevalence and predictors of emotional and behavioural functioning of children where a parent has cancer: A multinational study. *Cancer*, 115, 4030–4039.

Thastum, M., Munch-Hansen, A., Wiell, A., Romer, G. (2006). Evaluation of a focused short-term preventive counselling project for families with a parent with cancer. *Clinical Child Psychology and Psychiatry*, 11(4), 529–542.

Turner, J., Clavarino, A., Yates, P., Hargraves, M., Connors, V., Hausmann, S. (2007). Oncology nurses' perceptions of their supportive care for parents with advanced cancer: Challenges and educational needs. *Psycho-Oncology*, 16(2), 149–157.

Vannatta, K., Ramsey, R.R., Noll, R.B., Gerhardt, C.A. (2010). Associations of child adjustment with parent and family functioning: Comparison of families of women with and without breast cancer. *Journal of Developmental and Behavioral Pediatrics*, 31(1), 9–16.

Visser, A., Huizinga, G.A., Hoekstra, H.J., Van der Graaf, W.T., Klip, E.C., Pras, E. (2005). Emotional and behavioral functioning of children of a parent diagnosed with cancer. *Psycho-Oncology*, 14, 746–758.

Visser, A., Huizinga, G.A., van der Graaf, W.T., Hoekstra, H.J., Hoekstra-Weebers, J.E. (2004). The impact of parental cancer on children and the family: A review of the literature. *Cancer Treatment Reviews*, 30, 683–694.

Watson, M., St James-Roberts, I., Ashley, S., Tilney, C., Brougham, B., Edwards, L., Baldus, C., Romer, G. (2006). Factors associated with emotional and behavioural problems among school age children of breast cancer patients. *British Journal of Cancer*, 94(1), 43–50.

Weaver, K., Rowland, J., Alfano, C., McNeel, T. (2010). Parental cancer and the family: A population-based estimate of the number of US cancer survivors residing with their minor children. *Cancer*, 116, 4395–4401.

CHAPTER 8

Parental HIV/AIDS: from psychopathology to resilience

Peilian Chi and Xiaoming Li

INTRODUCTION

As of 2013, an estimated 17.7 million children worldwide had lost one or both parents to AIDS, with the majority living in resource-poor settings (UNICEF, 2015). Furthermore, there are millions of children whose parents are living with HIV/AIDS, given that 36.9 million people were living with the condition at the end of 2014 (WHO, 2015). With the introduction of antiretroviral therapy (ART), HIV in resource-rich regions is slowly becoming a chronic disease. However, there is a considerable treatment gap in resource-limited settings, with only 58% of treatment eligible adults receiving appropriate therapy (UNAIDS, 2012). The deleterious effects of HIV/AIDS, however, are not limited to people living with the virus; they also extend to their family members, especially their children. Parental HIV/AIDS-related illness and deaths have far-reaching and lasting consequences on children's physical and psychosocial well-being. How to provide developmentally and culturally appropriate psychosocial support, alongside interventions to promote the well-being of these children, remains a significant social and global health concern.

During the early years of the global HIV epidemic, the importance of the psychosocial well-being of children affected by parental HIV/AIDS was overshadowed by medical research into treating those affected by the condition. The recognition of, and rigorous studies concerning, the psychosocial well-being of children affected by parental HIV/AIDS only began to emerge some two decades later (Wild, 2001). Early research focused mainly on parental

HIV status and children's psychosocial well-being in resource-rich settings, such as the United States. Subsequently, research extended to regions with a high incidence of HIV (e.g. Sub-Saharan countries) and some HIV-endemic centres in resource-limited countries, such as India, China and Eastern Europe.

Studies over the past two decades have consistently demonstrated that, compared to children from HIV-free families, children affected by parental HIV/AIDS are more likely to suffer internalising and externalising problems, and other negative health outcomes (Betancourt et al., 2013; Chi and Li, 2013). Parental AIDS-related deaths generate a fundamental alteration at almost every level of the socio-ecological system of children. In addition to grieving processes, children orphaned by parental AIDS may experience additional challenges such as stigmatisation, disruption in caregiving and financial hardship (Chi and Li, 2013). Children of parents living with HIV may experience anticipatory grief, uncertainty about the future and pressure to cope with family secrecy and stigma (Rotheram-Borus et al., 2004). These findings are not surprising considering the adversities that are associated with HIV-related illness and death. However, although in less volume, the existing literature also suggests that some of these children do not report elevated or persistent levels of mental health problems (Li et al., 2015), which indicates the possibility of increased resilience in response to parental HIV/AIDS (Chi et al., 2013). Over the past decade, research frameworks among children affected by parental HIV/AIDS have shifted toward a resilience paradigm, with a focus on promoting or cultivating children's resilience so that they can live more healthily and happily in the face of parental HIV/AIDS (Betancourt et al., 2013; Li et al., 2015).

This chapter expands upon the issues introduced above. It opens with a summary of the significant body of research that has focused on the broad impact of parental HIV/AIDS on children's well-being. A number of systematic reviews are available in this area (e.g. Chi and Li, 2013; Cluver and Gardner, 2007; Li et al., 2008), and readers may wish to consult these reviews for further details. Subsequently, with the marked paradigm shift over recent years, the chapter takes a resilience perspective in relation to children's response to parental HIV/AIDS. Research on the development of resilience in children and youth affected by parental HIV/AIDS is reviewed in terms of conceptual perspectives and current research findings. The chapter continues with a discussion of interventions that have been developed and implemented to promote resilience among children affected by parental HIV/AIDS, followed by recommendations for researchers and practitioners working with these children.

LIVING WITH PARENTAL HIV/AIDS: EFFECTS AND DEVELOPMENTAL TRAJECTORIES

In the broad developmental literature, it has been recognised that problems tend to escalate as the frequency and severity of adversities increase, while remarkable individual differences have been noted among individuals sharing similar levels of risk or adversity (Masten, 2006). Research evidence supports the general expectation that the greater the losses and adversities associated with parental HIV/AIDS experienced by children, the higher the impact on their cognitive, emotional, behavioural and social adjustment. In terms of social and emotional development, children affected by HIV/AIDS report higher levels of depression, traumatic stress, anxiety, loneliness and suicidal ideation, and lower levels of school interest, self-esteem, and social competence (e.g. Chi and Li, 2013; Cluver, 2011; Du et al., 2015b; Li et al., 2009; Onuoha and Munakata, 2010; Rotheram-Borus et al., 2005). Children affected by HIV/AIDS also demonstrate an increase in behavioural/externalising problems such as delinquency, conduct problems, disruptive behaviour and high-risk sexual activities (Atwine et al., 2005; Cluver et al., 2009; Nyamukapa et al., 2008). With regard to cognitive development, HIV-exposed but uninfected children have no significant global developmental delay in infancy, while subtle shortcomings in pre-schoolers have been found in resource-rich settings. However, in resource-limited settings, children exposed to HIV show greater cognitive, motor and expressive language impairment than children who have no exposure to HIV (Le Doaré et al., 2012). Studies on the cognitive development of children whose parents have been infected by the HIV virus after their births have been rare. A recent study in China reported that children affected by parental HIV had lower scores in verbal comprehension and perceptual reasoning ability (Han et al., 2014). Even though the negative effects of parental HIV/AIDS on their uninfected children have been consistently observed, there is growing interest in untangling the effects of parental HIV/AIDS to identify the underlying determinants and pathways that mediate the observed negative effects, thus providing accurate evidence for intervention programmes.

HIV-related illness and death of parents

The effect of HIV-related parental illness and death on children is a complex process. The existing literature has provided data suggesting some general patterns of such effects. First, HIV-related parental *illness* and parental *death* seem to have similar deleterious effects on children's psychosocial well-being. Although children affected by parental HIV/AIDS show poorer physical and mental health when compared to children from HIV-free families, studies reveal that children who have lost at least one parent to HIV/AIDS and children of parents living with HIV demonstrate similar levels of psychosocial adjustment in terms of loneliness, self-esteem, future expectations, hopefulness and externalising problems (e.g. Doku, 2010; Fang et al., 2009). These findings may suggest that although the actual parental death has a negative impact on a child's well-being, the anticipatory grief and the prolonged illness and multiple losses might have a similar negative impact on children (Chi and Li, 2013). Second, parental HIV/AIDS may evoke additional risks that threaten children's normal development. Parents are children's most important guardians and companions in achieving critical developmental milestones. The loss of parents threatens core attachment relationships, upon which a child develops personal and social competence. Children who have lost parents to HIV/AIDS may experience additional stress associated with the shame, secrecy, and fear of disclosure surrounding the cause of parental illness and death. Studies from different geographical regions consistently show that even where environmental risks (e.g. poverty) are similar, AIDS-orphaned children, compared to children orphaned by other causes, demonstrate higher levels of depression, anxiety, traumatic stress, anger, problematic sleeping and behavioural patterns and peer problems, and lower levels of self-esteem (Atwine et al., 2005; Bhargava, 2005; Cluver et al., 2012; Doku, 2009; Onuoha et al., 2009). Third, parental HIV/AIDS may lead to multiple losses that result in cumulative challenges to children's coping ability and development of resilience. Because sexual contact is one of the dominant modes of HIV transmission, the chance that both parents are infected is high. A child who has lost one parent to HIV has a significant possibility of losing the surviving parent (Belsey and Sherr, 2011). In addition to parental loss, many children affected by HIV experience multiple losses of other family members, including siblings, close relatives, step-parents, subsequent caregivers or significant others (Dane, 2002; Demmer and Rothschild, 2011; Zhao et al., 2009). Multiple losses increase children's susceptibility to unsolved bereavements. Multiple losses in families or extended families also limit children's opportunities to seek social support during the grieving process (Li et al., 2008).

Pathways of effects of parental HIV/AIDS

There are many possible pathways by which parental HIV/AIDS may affect children's health, including direct and indirect processes at multiple levels. The direct effects of parental HIV/AIDS include involuntary residence replacement, sibling separation, financial hardship in the household, disrupted schooling and compromised life stability. Indirect processes include the effects of HIV/AIDS on caregivers and, consequently, the quality of care, parenting capability and caregiver distress. At the societal level, stigmatisation, abuse and bullying can constitute indirect pathways. The stress response process plays a role in the threats posed by parental HIV to children. The negative impact of perceived stigma can affect children's biological stress response systems (Chi et al., 2015). In comparison to those who perceive lower levels of stigma, children affected by HIV/AIDS who perceive higher levels of stigma have demonstrated an unhealthier diurnal cortisol rhythm. Parental HIV/AIDS also has a cumulative effect in relation to existing adversities in a child's life. In some resource-poor settings, children's basic needs, such as food, clothing, shelter, medical care and educational opportunities cannot be met even in the absence of parental HIV/AIDS (Campbell et al., 2012; Delva et al., 2009; Nyamukapa et al., 2008). These socio-economic disadvantages may accelerate the negative effects of parental HIV/AIDS on children's well-being.

Developmental stage

A child's age, or developmental stage, is also a factor when considering the effects of parental HIV/AIDS. Developmental perspectives merit consideration in relation to the influences of individual changes in children's emotional understanding, cognitive ability to interpret experiences, self-regulation skills and many other aspects of function that could affect their subjective experience related to parental illness (Masten and Narayan, 2012). Young children might exhibit a greater number of problems and symptoms of distress in response to parental illness and death because they are more dependent on the parents' caregiving than older children are. However, younger children might lack the cognitive ability to fully understand these experiences and are thus exposed to less risk. Cognitive maturity is associated with a greater awareness of parental health status, changes in life conditions and other risks such as stigmatisation, but also with greater skills for problem solving and seeking help (Masten and Narayan, 2012). A number of studies, however, report that age does not influence the impact of parental HIV/AIDS on children's psychological adjustment (Brackis-Cott et al., 2007; Li et al., 2009; Nyamukapa et al., 2008). By contrast, a longitudinal study with a large sample in South Africa found an increase in distress with age among AIDS-orphaned children (Cluver et al., 2012). Conversely, a further study in Zimbabwe found older children showed less psychological distress than the younger children who had lost both parents to AIDS (Howard et al., 2006). Such inconsistent findings may reflect the complexity of age differences in regards to the effects of parental HIV/AIDS. To reveal the interaction between age and the effects of parental HIV/AIDS, it is necessary to take account of the developmental stage of children in terms of cognitive maturity, coping ability and emotional regulation skills.

FROM PSYCHOPATHOLOGY TO RESILIENCE: A PARADIGM SHIFT

In contrast to psychopathological models, one of the unique features of resilience is the focus on strengths and positive development, pointing to pathways for interventions. A resilience framework holds specific appeal for research on children facing adversities because it provides a useful roadmap on ways to mitigate risk and promote resilience among these children (Masten and Narayan, 2012); this paradigm shift results in a transformative working approach to cultivate or enhance resilience among children affected by HIV/AIDS.

Resilience is a dynamic and longitudinal process that negotiates adversities (APA, 2012; Luthar et al., 2000; Masten and Narayan, 2012). It can be defined as the capability of an individual to resist or adapt to significant challenges that threaten their stability, sustainability and development (Masten, 2011). Studies on risk and resilience in diverse populations of children exposed to a wide range of adversities, such as war, disaster, poverty, maltreatment and parental mental illness, have indicated a consistent set of factors, such as positive future orientation, problem-solving skills, trusting relationships with caregivers and an effective school and supportive community, that are associated with enhanced physical and psychosocial outcomes (Cicchetti and Toth, 2006; Masten ad Narayan, 2012; Rutter, 1985). These factors are often referred to as supportive and protective factors, which exist at multiple levels of children's socio-ecological system (e.g. intrapersonal assets, family, school and community). Resilience occurs when one or more such factors could protect children from the negative influences of adversities. These widely reported supportive and protective factors suggest that the development of resilience depends on fundamental human adaptive systems embedded in individuals, relationships, families, communities and societies. These systems might be impaired to a certain degree by the adversities, but are theorised as supportive and protective factors for children's resilience during or after traumatic experiences (Masten and Narayan, 2012).

A recently proposed resilience framework (Li et al., 2015) delineates the mechanism of resilience in children's adaptation to parental HIV/AIDS (see Figure 8.1). The framework reflects the viewpoint that children do not necessarily develop significant developmental problems as a response to parental HIV/AIDS, but rather the relative balance of risk and protective

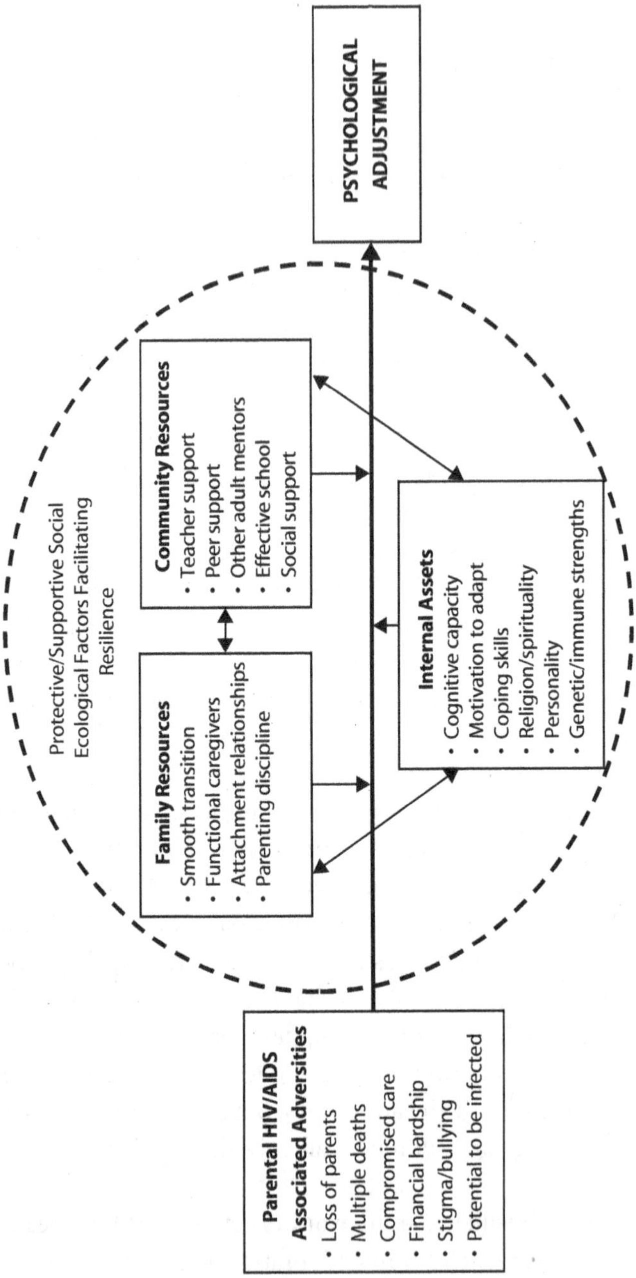

FIGURE 8.1 Conceptual Framework of Psychological Resilience among Children affected by HIV/AIDS (Adapted from Li et al., 2015)

and supportive factors in their lives predicts children's short-term and long-term physical and psychosocial functioning. The framework focuses on the propensity of the disease course to generate multiple stressful life events and dynamic processes of resilience within the context of parental HIV/AIDS; it explicitly emphasises adaptable individual and contextual factors that may alleviate the potentially deteriorating and enduring effects of parental HIV/AIDS on children. The quality of support from family and community, two critical contextual factors in positive child development in the face of parental HIV/AIDS, are expected mutually to foster the development of children's internal assets (e.g. self-esteem, self-efficacy and positive future orientation). Biological factors, such as brain function, genes and immune function, also play an important role in resilience development because some internal assets may be biological in origin.

SUPPORTIVE AND PROTECTIVE FACTORS IN RESILIENCE DEVELOPMENT

As suggested by existing theoretical perspectives (Li et al., 2015), children affected by parental HIV/AIDS might not necessarily experience prolonged psychosocial distress. With the presence of potentially supportive and protective factors, children might demonstrate substantial resilience. Potential supportive and protective factors at individual, relational and social levels identified by previous empirical studies may help children achieve a normative development and even thrive despite the presence of adversities. Although empirical research focusing on resilience factors has been limited, the recognition of resilience has been emerging in the field. This resilience perspective has been detailed in previous work (Li et al., 2015) and is briefly explained below in terms of how resilience occurs in the presence of multiple resources at various levels of children's socio-ecological systems. It should be noted that resources at multiple levels may be reciprocal and bidirectional in the process of resilience development.

Internal assets allow resilience to develop. Through the course of coping with life challenges associated with parental HIV/AIDS, children develop tenacity, hope, optimism, coping capacity and problem-solving skills based on their successful (or indeed unsuccessful) experiences. These competences continually develop during the socialisation process through the interaction of inborn traits and opportunities to learn. These adaptive competences include cognitive abilities, emotional and behavioural regulation, the motivation to adapt and specific personality traits. HIV-affected children higher in these competences may have greater internal assets to adapt flexibly, persistently and resourcefully to stressful situations while perceiving less stress and therefore enjoy better developmental outcomes (Chi et al., 2015).

Family resources facilitate resilience. Among the range of family resources, a trusting relationship with current caregivers is critical for a child's resilience development. Resilience in HIV-affected children is more likely to occur when an adult reliably satisfies the child's physical and emotional needs. For example, positive parental bonds have been shown to reduce children's emotional distress and increase future positive expectations in a US urban sample (Rotheram-Borus et al., 2006). A trusting relationship with current caregivers is the most proximal protective factor for children affected by HIV/AIDS (Wang et al., 2012). In addition, positive parenting, including positive communication, effective monitoring, mutual understanding and reliable support provide valuable resources for children to develop their self-esteem and life skills (Allen et al., 2014; Chi et al., 2015; Lachman et al., 2014; Zhao et al., 2011).

Community resources nurture children's resilience. Perceived and received social support is the prominent protective factor for the healthy development of children affected by HIV/AIDS. Individual support from peers, teachers and adult mentors can also provide supplementary resources in addition to parental support to satisfy children's needs (Du et al., 2015a; Fawzi et al., 2012; Qiao et al., 2014). Child-nurturing institutions, such as schools, can re-establish routines in a child's life and also afford opportunities for peer interaction, connections to competent adults, leadership and agency experiences. For example, when the HIV pandemic emerged, effective schools were able to promote resilience among children by establishing school-based networks that function across systems to support children and other vulnerable members of the community (Ebersöhn and Ferreira, 2011).

INTERVENTION EFFORTS TO PROMOTE RESILIENCE

The accumulating research findings on effects of supportive and protective factors have many implications for programmes devised to promote resilience and support children affected by parental HIV/AIDS. Intervention research, however, remains limited. The dearth of evidence-based interventions to mitigate the negative effects of parental HIV/AIDS has been noted by several recent reviews (Betancourt et al., 2015; Chi and Li, 2013; King et al., 2009). The scarcity of high-quality intervention programmes based on sound psychological or other theories is particularly worrying given the scope of problems and urgent need to support children affected by HIV/AIDS in various populations and across different cultural contexts. It is clear that greater effort is needed in the conceptualisation, research design, research methodology and implementation in order to build a better evidence base to help practitioners and stakeholders move forward in their efforts to assist children affected by parental HIV/AIDS. In this section, we highlight exemplary studies of interventions focusing on resilience development at different socio-ecological levels; children's individual assets, family resources or community resources.

Interventions that focus on empowering children

There are several interventions that focus on individual child agency and empowerment (Kumakech et al., 2009; Mueller et al., 2011; Ssewamala et al., 2009, 2012). Most of these interventions were designed and delivered in peer-group format, consisting of a set of developmentally appropriate activities to enhance children's resilient coping abilities and self-efficacy. Three interventions with rigorous research design and efficacy evaluation are highlighted.

In South Africa, Mueller et al. (2011) evaluated the efficacy of an art programme, *Make a Difference*. This programme aimed to increase children's self-esteem, self-efficacy and HIV insight, thereby improving their psychosocial health and resilience. The intervention was guided by social learning theory and principles of art therapy. In the quasi-experimental design, 177 out of 297 participating children, aged 8–18 years, attended more than 50 group sessions led by a team of trained and supervised 'youth ambassadors' for six months. The programme ran school-based activities with children creating 'hero' art books about their life, while HIV education sessions focused on self-advocacy and empowerment. Immediately after the intervention, children who attended the intervention displayed significantly higher levels of self-efficacy than children who did not. The benefits remained after controlling for a set of psychosocial and demographic confounders. An association between programme exposure and increased self-esteem and decreased depression or emotional and behavioural problems was not found in the study. However, the authors suggested that the increased self-efficacy and resilience might have an effect on other psychological outcomes over time.

Ssewamala et al. (2012) examined an *Economic Empowerment Intervention* to reduce the risk of poverty and depression among children who had lost at least one parent to HIV/AIDS in Uganda. The programme, named SUUBI ('hope' in the local language), incorporated a combined microfinance youth empowerment and health-promotion approach to enhance family-level economic security by using child savings accounts along with financial planning training. Using a cluster-randomised experimental design, 286 orphaned adolescents from 15 primary schools in a district in Uganda were recruited to participate in the study. Children in the intervention condition received economic empowerment consisting of three components: (i) 12 one- to two-hour school-based workshops over a period of 10 months which focused on asset building and financial planning, led by trained local university students; (ii) a monthly mentorship programme for adolescents with peer mentors on future planning; (iii) a matched child savings account, dedicated to paying for secondary schooling or a small family business. The child savings account was a matched savings account with a match rate of 2:1 as an incentive for participants to save, but with a limit on the maximum savings that could be matched (US$10 a month). If a child in the SUBBI programme saved US$10 each month for a year, the family's US$120 savings would be matched by US$240 from the programme. Children in the intervention group exhibited a significant decrease in depression and an increase in self-concept 10 and 20 months after the intervention. Although the programme demonstrated robust efficacy, funding availability is a crucial factor in sustaining such economic empowerment programmes.

In southwestern Uganda, Kumakech et al. (2009) evaluated the efficacy of an after-school *Peer-group Support Intervention* among children orphaned by AIDS. The intervention was guided by participatory psychosocial approaches, which focus on the transformation of repressive experiences into liberating ones. In this intervention approach, participants have opportunities to reflect and challenge adverse experiences as a means of developing effective coping strategies. The intervention comprised 16 psychosocial exercises, led by trained primary school teachers over a period of 10 weeks. In addition, children in the intervention were offered a monthly healthcare visit. Following a general physical examination during these visits, somatic symptoms were discussed and treated by physicians. Each exercise was approximately one hour long and took the form of a semi-structured game or play. In the first sessions, children were encouraged to introduce themselves and share emotional reactions about orphanhood. In subsequent sessions, children were involved in exercises such as trust-building within the group, problem solving and emotion regulation. The last set of group exercises was aimed at enhancing self-esteem and social support. As a cluster-randomised controlled trial, 326 children orphaned by AIDS, aged 10–15 years, were assigned to either an intervention group or a control group. In the 10-week follow-up, children in the intervention group showed significant improvement in levels of depression, anger and anxiety, but not in self-concept. One of the limitations of the study was the difficulty in differentiating the intervention effects of peer-group activities from those of monthly somatic care.

Interventions that focus on enhancing family functioning

A number of researchers agree that intervention at the family level is crucial in the context of parental HIV/AIDS. Several studies have based their interventions within family system theories and the principles of family therapy. These interventions usually contain three sets of intervention sessions: sessions for children, sessions for parents living with HIV and joint parent-child sessions. The purposes of family-based interventions are typically multifaceted; increasing a child's well-being, enhancing coping skills of people living with HIV and improving the parent-child relationship and family functioning. The fundamental rationale of family-based intervention is that adaptation and resilience occur in the entire family system. That is, if a family as an integrated adaptive system functions well, the individual members in the family system should also function well.

The earliest, and probably most comprehensive, family-based group intervention for children affected by parental HIV was developed by Rotheram-Borus et al. in the 1990s. The intervention, *Teaching Adolescents Learning Communication (TALC)*, included separate and joint meetings for HIV-affected families in small groups for both HIV-infected mothers and their children (Rotheram-Borus et al., 2001, 2003, 2004). TALC included 12 sessions for HIV-infected parents focusing on self-care and positive parenting. Another 12 sessions for children focused on stress coping. The four mother-and-child joint sessions focused on parent-child communication, conflict resolution and parental monitoring. The first efficacy trial of TALC was conducted in New York City, USA in the 1990s. Results indicated that adolescents attending the intervention were significantly less depressed and anxious, reported fewer conduct problems, delayed sexual debut, had fewer sexual partners over time, used fewer drugs and had higher levels of self-esteem. HIV-positive parents attending the intervention reported significantly lower levels of emotional distress and problem behaviour. It is noteworthy that TALC was successfully adapted and implemented in Central Haiti, a resource-limited setting (Fawzi et al., 2012). However, the recent implementation trial of TALC in Los Angeles, USA reported a null intervention effect in an 18-month follow-up (Rotheram-Borus et al., 2012). The authors suggested the contrasting findings in their two studies in the US might be due to sampling bias and the changing dynamics of how HIV affects families in the country, concluding that family-based HIV interventions should be targeted at people living with HIV who are experiencing substantial problems.

A recent *Parent-Child Group Intervention* was developed by Eloff et al. (2014) to promote resilience in young children, aged 6–10 years, living with their HIV-infected mothers in South Africa. The intervention design was guided by resilience theory and family relationship theories. The intervention consisted of 24 weekly group sessions led by two trained community care workers. Mothers and children were in separate groups for 14 sessions, followed by 10 interactive joint sessions, each lasting 75 minutes. The first seven mother-only sessions focused on the mother's issues relating to living with HIV, which were followed by sessions addressing parenting. The children's sessions focused on building self-esteem and enhancing both interpersonal and life skills. The mother-child joint sessions were designed to promote healthy parent-child interaction and the modelling of positive parenting behaviour and included activities such as compiling a family legacy box. Because children in the intervention group were young, the HIV disclosure rate in the study was very low. The focus of the intervention was on overarching skills rather than HIV-specific themes. There were 390 mother-child dyads that participated in the efficacy trial. Mothers attending the intervention reported significant improvements in children's externalising behaviour, communication and daily living skills, but did not report significant improvement in internalising behaviour and socialisation at least 12 months later.

Betancourt et al. (2014) developed the *Family-Strengthening Intervention (FSI)*, which focused on reducing mental health problems and promoting resilience among HIV-affected children in Rwanda. The FSI is a structured intervention with four core components: building parenting skills and improving family communication; developing a family narrative to increase family connectedness and hope; providing psycho-education on HIV transmission, prevention and normative responses to HIV diagnosis; and strengthening problem-solving skills and social support. Trained, local bachelor-level psychologists led the therapy sessions under the close supervision of the programme developers and experienced clinical psychologists in local universities. In their feasibility trial, 39 pairs of HIV-infected caregivers and children aged 7–17 years participated in the FSI. Caregiver-reported improvements in family connectedness, good parenting, social support and children's prosocial behaviour were sustained and strengthened from post-intervention to a six-month follow-up. There were also improvements in caregiver-reported child self-esteem, depression, anxiety and irritability at the follow-up. Decreases in child-reported harsh punishment were also observed at post-intervention and the follow-up.

Interventions that target resources at multiple levels

Interventions that target multiple levels of children's socio-ecological systems have also been developed. These programmes have been guided by the integration of different theoretical perspectives, including social ecological models, attachment theories, family functioning theories and community coalition perspectives. The focus of such programmes is to take advantage of all available intrapersonal and interpersonal resources to promote resilience of children in the context of parental HIV/AIDS.

Together for Empowerment Activities (TEA) is a multi-level intervention that focuses on the capacity of the family and community to overcome the impact of living with HIV (Li et al., 2014). The programme was designed to promote positive mental health in people living with HIV, to improve parent-child communication and interactions, and promote community resilience. The TEA intervention constitutes three levels of intervention activities: (i) TEA Gathering consists of six small group sessions for people living with HIV and their family members; (ii) TEA Time includes six home-based family activities with all family members, including children after each TEA Gathering session; and (iii) TEA Garden has three community events that aim to build community integration. In an efficacy trial for the intervention, 79 families were recruited to participate in the study and followed up at three and six months. Positive results relating to children's psychosocial well-being (i.e. self-esteem, perceived parental care, externalising problems), accompanied by an improvement in mental health indicators of people living with HIV and their family members (i.e. depression, family functioning) were observed following the intervention. The study highlights the importance of empowering the family and community as integrated systems to confront HIV-related challenges.

The *Child-Caregiver-Advocacy Resilience (ChildCARe)* intervention was developed to promote child, family, and community resilience in a rural HIV epicentre in China (Li et al., 2015). The intervention focuses on three distinct levels: child, caregiver and community. The child intervention includes 10 sessions of peer-group activities that aim to promote individual resilience in six components: positive thinking, emotional regulation, positive coping skills, problem solving, support seeking, future orientation and self-esteem. Caregivers receive four sessions of positive parenting training. At the community level, trained community ambassadors (i.e. teachers, village nurses) conduct monthly home visits and organise a set of community activities to promote the cohesion and strengths of the local village community. Seven hundred and ninety children aged from 6 to 17 were recruited to participate in the study. Participants were randomly assigned to one of three intervention conditions (i.e. child intervention, child + caregiver intervention, child + caregiver intervention + community advocacy) or a control group. Preliminary short-term efficacy of the ChildCARe intervention in a 6-month and 12-month follow-up was demonstrated through an improvement in resilience-related competences and enhanced psychosocial well-being of those children in the intervention groups.

RECOMMENDATIONS FOR PRACTITIONERS AND RESEARCHERS

Based on the existing literature the authors emphasise four pertinent areas for researchers and practitioners who work with, or are in a position to help, children affected by parental HIV/AIDS.

HIV as a family issue

Many scholars advocate family-based interventions in order to enhance the resilience of both HIV-infected parents and their children (Pequegnat and Szapocznik, 2000). A functional family system can be protective for children in light of the adversities associated with parental HIV/AIDS. A dysfunctional family system can accelerate the negative effects of accumulated life stress associated with parental HIV. The HIV-infected parents face a double challenge of illness management and parenting. HIV may compromise family functioning and parenting practices, but decades of family studies also reveal that outside stressors (e.g. chronic illness, natural disasters) can enhance family resources and improve family cohesion (Patterson, 2002). Thus, in addition to offering professional help (e.g. medical care) for parents living with HIV, practitioners also need to provide support for parenting and family functioning and make such support available both to parents and their children. These services have the capacity to build a secure and supportive parent-child relationship, which is the most immediate and robust protective system for children and their HIV-infected parents.

Multi-level resources

Future intervention or support programmes need to incorporate resources at multiple levels of the children's social-ecological system. Structural factors, such as financial support, reduction in community-based stigma and policy advocacy, are crucial to meet the basic needs of children affected by HIV. Among the multiple levels of support, effects at macro level might exert effects through changes in individual and family adaptive systems. For example, financial subsidies at a national level for HIV-affected families might improve their quality of life and standard of living, thus providing a better and more stable family environment for children (Hong et al., 2015). Interventions targeted at reducing stigma at the community level might lessen family strain associated with external stressful events (Chi et al., 2014). Practitioners who work with children affected by HIV should work in conjunction with other relevant organisations and agencies to refer families to receive necessary support from the broader community (Hong et al., 2015).

Assessment of physiological pathways

To the best of our knowledge, the majority of studies on children affected by parental HIV/AIDS have relied on behavioural or other psychosocial outcomes. The combination of behavioural data and biomedical data ('biomarkers') will provide an opportunity to examine physiological pathways of effects of early childhood adversities on health. Psychological stress is known to undermine physical health when it results in chronic dysregulation of the biological stress response system. One such biomarker is cortisol. Cortisol is a hormone sensitive to psychological stress, released by the hypothalamic pituitary adrenocortical (HPA) axis. Constant or recurrent exposure to stressful circumstances during childhood appears to alter the HPA axis function in particular (Miller et al., 2007). Measurement of cortisol in saliva has proven to be convenient and non-invasive such that it can be gathered in large community-based samples (Adam and Kumari, 2009; Hellhammer et al., 2009). For more than two decades, salivary cortisol has been used as a biological indicator of neurobiological stress among children. Although HPA-axis responses allow the body to effectively respond to the short-term stress demands, chronic HPA activation is associated with immune suppression, inhibited growth, cognitive deficits and psychological maladjustment (Sapolsky et al., 2000; Saxbe, 2008). Future research might consider using such biomarkers to evaluate the intervention effects on children's physiological processes associated with health and resilience development.

Evidence-based programmes across cultural settings

As presented in the previous sections, efforts are increasing worldwide to develop and evaluate effective programmes to promote resilience among children affected by parental HIV/AIDS. Many of these programmes have been demonstrated to be efficacious (or to have the potential to be efficacious) in achieving their goals. Given the resources and time required to develop and evaluate effective intervention programmes, it would be expedient to adapt existing programmes that have shown evidence of efficacy or effectiveness (i.e. evidence-based programmes) through rigorous evaluation in other cultural settings, especially those which are resource-limited. In the cultural adaptation of an evidence-based intervention, developmental and cultural appropriateness should be always taken into consideration. Culture is not only related to geographical areas but also to social, economic, and cultural features. The focus of an intervention adaptation process should be: (i) the responsiveness of the intervention approach to the local culture of children and their caregivers affected by HIV; and (ii) the cultural and age appropriateness of the various intervention activities. In resource-poor settings, the lack of financial and human resources may threaten the integrity and fidelity of evidence-based programmes in new cultural settings. A number of issues should, therefore, be carefully considered in any cross-cultural adaptation of evidence-based programmes in facilitating or promoting resilience among children affected by parental HIV/AIDS. These issues include how best to equip local personnel and empower healthcare providers, how to translate research findings into the real world and provide sustained support for children and families in need, and how to effectively train paraprofessionals (e.g. teachers, community healthcare workers) in resource-poor settings.

CONCLUSION

In conclusion, this chapter has discussed the challenges of living with parental HIV/AIDS and the effects of parental HIV/AIDS on children's well-being alongside the development of resilience. Research over the past two decades has been consistent regarding the negative impact of parental HIV/AIDS on children's well-being. However, limited longitudinal studies suggest the potential for resilience among such children in the face of multiple adversities, which mirrors risk and resilience perspectives in the broad developmental literature. It may be possible to encourage and develop resilience among children in the face of adversities when internal assets and supportive resources in the family, school and community are present. Based on the review of the relevant interventions that promote resilience among children affected by parental HIV/AIDS, it is suggested that family-based interventions may have great promise in promoting resilience in HIV-affected families, thereby empowering children. Multi-level interventions should be considered where resources are available. Cross-cultural adaptation of existing evidence-based programmes and the inclusion of physiological outcomes in evaluations are to be encouraged in future research and practice. In resource-poor settings, it may also be necessary to empower the local community and train paraprofessionals to sustain efforts to support children affected by HIV/AIDS with many aspects of their lives, including a resilient response to parental illness.

ACKNOWLEDGEMENT

Preparation of this chapter was supported by National Institute of Nursing Research Grant (R01-NR13466) and a research grant from the Research Development and Administration Office of the University of Macau (SRG2014-00022-FSS).

REFERENCES

Adam, E.K., Kumari, M. (2009). Assessing salivary cortisol in large-scale, epidemiological research. *Psychoneuroendocrinology*, 34(10), 1423–1436.

Allen, A.B., Finestone, M., Eloff, I., Sipsma, H., Makin, J., Triplett, K., Ebersöhn, L., Sikkema, K., Briggs-Gowan, M., Visser, M., Ferreira, R., Forsyth, B.W. (2014). The role of parenting in affecting the behavior and adaptive functioning of young children of HIV-infected mothers in South Africa. *AIDS and Behavior*, 18(3), 605–616.

APA. (2012). What is resilience? www.apa.org/helpcenter/road-resilience.aspx (accessed 27 June 2012).

Atwine, B., Cantor-Graae, E., Bajunirwe, F. (2005). Psychological distress among AIDS orphans in rural Uganda. *Social Science and Medicine*, 61(3), 555–564.

Belsey, M.A., Sherr, L. (2011). The definition of true orphan prevalence: Trends, contexts and implications for policies and programmes. *Vulnerable Children and Youth Studies*, 6(3), 185–200.

Betancourt, T.S., Grelotti, D.J., Hansen, N.B. (2015). Mental health and resilience in children and adolescents affected by HIV/AIDS. In A. Thapar, D.S. Pine, J.F. Leckman, S. Scott, M.J. Snowling, E. Taylor (Eds) *Rutter's child and adolescent psychiatry* (pp. 599–611). Chichester, UK: John Wiley and Sons.

Betancourt, T.S., Meyers-Ohki, S.E., Charrow, A., Hansen, N. (2013). Annual Research Review: Mental health and resilience in HIV/AIDS-affected children: A review of the literature and recommendations for future research. *Journal of Child Psychology and Psychiatry*, 54(4), 423–444.

Betancourt, T.S., Ng, L.C., Kirk, C.M., Munyanah, M., Mushashi, C., Ingabire, C., Teta, S., Beardslee, W.R., Brennan, R.T., Zahn, I., Stulac, S., Cyamatare, F.R., Sezibera, V. (2014). Family-based prevention of mental health problems in children affected by HIV and AIDS: An open trial. *AIDS*, 28, S359-S368.

Bhargava, A. (2005). AIDS epidemic and the psychological well-being and school participation of Ethiopian orphans. *Psychology, Health and Medicine*, 10(3), 263–275.

Brackis-Cott, E., Mellins, C.A., Dolezal, C., Spiegel, D. (2007). The mental health risk of mothers and children: The role of maternal HIV infection. *The Journal of Early Adolescence*, 27(1), 67–89.

Campbell, C., Skovdal, M., Mupambireyi, Z., Madanhire, C., Robertson, L., Nyamukapa, C.A., Gregson, S. (2012). Can AIDS stigma be reduced to poverty stigma? Exploring Zimbabwean children's representations of poverty and AIDS. *Child: Care, Health and Development*, 38(5), 732–742.

Chi, P., Li, X. (2013). Impact of parental HIV/AIDS on children's psychological well-being: A systematic review of global literature. *AIDS and Behavior*, 17(7), 2554–2574.

Chi, P., Li, X., Barnett, D., Zhao, J., Zhao, G. (2013). Do children orphaned by AIDS experience distress over time? A latent growth curve analysis of depressive symptoms. *Psychology, Health and Medicine*, 19(4), 420–432.

Chi, P., Li, X., Tam, C.C., Du, H., Zhao, G., Zhao, J. (2015). Parenting Mediates the Impact of Caregivers' Distress on Children's Well-Being in Families Affected by HIV/AIDS. *AIDS and Behavior*, 19(11), 2130–2139.

Chi, P., Li, X., Zhao, J., Zhao, G. (2014). Vicious circle of perceived stigma, enacted stigma and depressive symptoms among children affected by HIV/AIDS in China. *AIDS and Behavior*, 18(6), 1054–1062.

Chi, P., Slatcher, R.B., Li, X., Zhao, J., Zhao, G., Ren, X., Zhu, J., Stanton, B. (2015). Perceived stigmatization, resilience, and diurnal cortisol rhythm among children of parents living with HIV. *Psychological Science*, 26(6), 843–852.

Cicchetti, D., Toth, S.L. (2006). Developmental psychopathology and preventive intervention. In W. Damon, R.M. Lerner, K.A. Renninger, I.E. Sigel (Eds) *Handbook of child psychology. Vol. 4* (6th edn) (pp. 497–547). Hoboken, NJ, US: John Wiley and Sons.

Cluver, L.D. (2011). Children of the AIDS pandemic. *Nature*, 474(7349), 27–29.

Cluver, L.D., Gardner, F. (2007). The mental health of children orphaned by AIDS: A review of international and southern African research. *Journal of Child and Adolescent Mental Health*, 19(1), 1–17.

Cluver, L.D., Operario, D., Gardner, F. (2009). Parental illness, caregiving factors and psychological distress among children orphaned by acquired immune deficiency syndrome (AIDS) in South Africa. *Vulnerable Children and Youth Studies*, 4(3), 185–198.

Cluver, L.D., Orkin, M., Gardner, F., Boyes, M.E. (2012). Persisting mental health problems among AIDS-orphaned children in South Africa. *Journal of Child Psychology and Psychiatry*, 53(4), 363–370.

Dane, B.O. (2002). Bereavement groups for children: Families with HIV/AIDS. In N.B. Webb (Ed.), *Helping bereaved children: A handbook for practitioners* (pp. 265–296). New York; London: The Guilford Press.

Delva, W., Vercoutere, A., Loua, C., Lamah, J., Vansteelandt, S., De Koker, P., Claeys, P., Temmerman, M., Annemans, L. (2009). Psychological well-being and socio-economic hardship among AIDS orphans and other vulnerable children in Guinea. *AIDS Care*, 21(12), 1490–1498.

Demmer, C., Rothschild, N. (2011). Bereavement among South African adolescents following a sibling's death from AIDS. *African Journal of Aids Research*, 10(1), 15–24.

Doku, P.N. (2009). Parental HIV/AIDS status and death, and children's psychological wellbeing. *International Journal of Mental Health Systems*, 3(1), 26.

Doku, P.N. (2010). Psychosocial adjustment of children affected by HIV/AIDS in Ghana. *Journal of Child and Adolescent Mental Health*, 22(1), 25–34.

Du, H., Li, X., Weinstein, T.L., Chi, P., Zhao, J., Zhao, G. (2015a). Links between teacher assessment and child self-assessment of mental health and behavior among children affected by HIV/AIDS. *AIDS Care*, 27(7), 876–884.

Du, H., Li, X., Chi, P., Zhao, J., Zhao, G. (2015b). Relational self-esteem, psychological well-being, and social support in children affected by HIV. *Journal of Health Psychology*, 20(12), 1568–1578.

Ebersöhn, L., Ferreira, R. (2011). Coping in an HIV/AIDS-dominated context: Teachers promoting resilience in schools. *Health Education Research*, 26(4), 596–613.

Eloff, I., Finestone, M., Makin, J.D., Boeving-Allen, A., Visser, M., Ebersöhn, L., Ferreira R, Sikkema, K.J., Briggs-Gowan, M.J., Forsyth, B.W. (2014). A randomized clinical trial of an intervention to promote resilience in young children of HIV-positive mothers in South Africa. *AIDS*, 28, S347–S357.

Fang, X., Li, X., Stanton, B., Hong, Y., Zhang, L., Zhao, G., Zhao, J., Lin, X., Lin, D. (2009). Parental HIV/AIDS and psychosocial adjustment among rural Chinese children. *Journal of Pediatric Psychology*, 34 (10), 1053–1062.

Fawzi, M.C.S., Eustache, E., Oswald, C., Louis, E., Surkane, P.J., Scanlan, F., Hook, S., Mancuso, A., Mukherjee, J.S. (2012). Psychosocial support intervention for HIV-affected families in Haiti: Implications for programs and policies for orphans and vulnerable children. *Social Science and Medicine*, 74(10), 1494–1503.

Han, T., Li, X., Chi, P., Zhao, J., Zhao, G. (2014). The impact of parental HIV/AIDS on children's cognitive ability in rural China. *AIDS Care*, 26(6), 723–730.

Hellhammer, D.H., Wüst, S., Kudielka, B.M. (2009). Salivary cortisol as a biomarker in stress research. *Psychoneuroendocrinology*, 34(2), 163–171.

Hong, Y., Chi, P., Li, X., Zhao, G., Zhao, J., Stanton, B., Li, L. (2015). Community-based family-style group homes for children orphaned by AIDS in rural China: An ethnographic investigation. *Health Policy and Planning*, 30(7), 928–937.

Howard, B., Matinhure, N., McCurdy, S.A., Johnson, G.A. (2006). Psychosocial disadvantage: Preparation, grieving, remembrance and recovery for orphans in eastern Zimbabwe. *African Journal of AIDS Research*, 5(1), 71–83.

King, E., De Silva, M., Stein, A., Patel, V. (2009). Interventions for improving the psychosocial well-being of children affected by HIV and AIDS. *Cochrane Database of Systematic Reviews*, 2, CD006733.

Kumakech, E., Cantor-Graae, E., Maling, S., Bajunirwe, F. (2009). Peer-group support intervention improves the psychosocial well-being of AIDS orphans: Cluster randomized trial. *Social Science and Medicine*, 68(6), 1038–1043.

Lachman, J.M., Cluver, L.D., Boyes, M.E., Kuo, C., Casale, M. (2014). Positive parenting for positive parents: HIV/AIDS, poverty, caregiver depression, child behavior, and parenting in South Africa. *AIDS Care*, 26(3), 304–313.

Le Doaré, K., Bland, R., Newell, M.L. (2012). Neurodevelopment in children born to HIV-infected mothers by infection and treatment status. *Pediatrics*, 130(5), e1326–1344.

Li, L., Liang, L.-J., Ji, G., Wu, J., Xiao, Y. (2014). Effect of a family intervention on psychological outcomes of children affected by parental HIV. *AIDS and Behavior*, 18(11), 2051–2058.

Li, X., Barnett, D., Fang, X., Lin, X., Zhao, G., Zhao, J., Hong, Y., Zhang, L., Naar-King, S., Stanton, B. (2009). Lifetime incidence of traumatic events and mental health among children affected by HIV/AIDS in rural China. *Journal of Clinical Child and Adolescent Psychology*, 38(5), 731–744.

Li, X., Chi, P., Sherr, L., Cluver, L.D., Stanton, B. (2015). Psychological resilience among children affected by parental HIV/AIDS: A conceptual framework. *Health Psychology and Behavioral Medicine*, 3(1), 217–235.

Li, X., Naar-King, S., Barnett, D., Stanton, B., Fang, X., Thurston, C. (2008). A developmental psychopathology framework of the psychosocial needs of children orphaned by HIV. *Journal of the Association of Nurses in AIDS Care*, 19(2), 147–157.

Luthar, S.S., Cicchetti, D., Becker, B. (2000). The construct of resilience: A critical evaluation and guidelines for future work. *Child Development*, 71(3), 543–562.

Masten, A.S. (2006). Competence and resilience in development. *Annals of the New York Academy of Sciences*, 1094(1), 13–27.

Masten, A.S. (2011). Resilience in children threatened by extreme adversity: Frameworks for research, practice, and translational synergy. *Development and Psychopathology*, 23(2), 493–506.

Masten, A.S., Narayan, A.J. (2012). Child development in the context of disaster, war, and terrorism: Pathways of risk and resilience. *Annual Review of Psychology*, 63, 227–257.

Miller, G.E., Chen, E., Zhou, E.S. (2007). If it goes up, must it come down? Chronic stress and the hypothalamic-pituitary-adrenocortical axis in humans. *Psychological Bulletin*, 133(1), 25–45.

Mueller, J., Alie, C., Jonas, B., Brown, E., Sherr, L. (2011). A quasi-experimental evaluation of a community-based art therapy intervention exploring the psychosocial health of children affected by HIV in South Africa. *Tropical Medicine and International Health*, 16(1), 57–66.

Nyamukapa, C.A., Gregson, S., Lopman, B., Saito, S., Watts, H.J., Monasch, R., Jukes, M.C.H. (2008). HIV-Associated orphanhood and children's psychosocial distress: Theoretical framework tested with data from Zimbabwe. *American Journal of Public Health*, 98(1), 133–141.

Onuoha, F.N., Munakata, T. (2010). Inverse association of natural mentoring relationship with distress mental health in children orphaned by AIDS. *BMC Psychiatry*, 10, 6.

Onuoha, F.N., Munakata, T., Serumaga-Zake, P.A.E., Nyonyintono, R.M., Bogere, S.M. (2009). Negative mental health factors in children orphaned by AIDS: Natural mentoring as a palliative care. *AIDS and Behavior*, 13(5), 980–988.

Patterson, J.M. (2002). Integrating family resilience and family stress theory. *Journal of Marriage and Family*, 64(2), 349–360.

Pequegnat, W., Szapocznik, J. (2000). *Working with families in the era of HIV/AIDS*. Thousand Oaks, CA: Sage Publications.

Qiao, S., Li, X., Zhao, G., Zhao, J., Stanton, B. (2014). The role of perceived social support in loneliness and self-esteem among children affected by HIV/AIDS: A longitudinal multilevel analysis in rural China. *AIDS*, 28, S369–S377.

Rotheram-Borus, M.J., Lee, M., Leonard, N., Lin, Y.Y., Franzke, L., Turner, E., Lightfoot, M., Gwadz, M. (2003). Four-year behavioral outcomes of an intervention for parents living with HIV and their adolescent children. *AIDS*, 17(8), 1217–1225.

Rotheram-Borus, M.J., Lee, M., Lin, Y.Y., Lester, P. (2004). Six-year intervention outcomes for adolescent children of parents with the human immunodeficiency virus. *Archives of Pediatrics and Adolescent Medicine*, 158(8), 742–748.

Rotheram-Borus, M.J., Lee, M.B., Gwadz, M., Draimin, B. (2001). An intervention for parents with AIDS and their adolescent children. *American Journal of Public Health*, 91(8), 1294–1302.

Rotheram-Borus, M.J., Rice, E., Comulada, W.S., Best, K., Elia, C., Peters, K., Li, L., Green, S., Valladares, E. (2012). Intervention outcomes among HIV-affected families over 18 months. *AIDS and Behavior*, 16(5), 1265–1275.

Rotheram-Borus, M.J., Stein, J.A., Lester, P. (2006). Adolescent adjustment over six years in HIV-affected families. *Journal of Adolescent Health*, 39(2), 174–182.

Rotheram-Borus, M.J., Weiss, R., Alber, S., Lester, P. (2005). Adolescent adjustment before and after HIV-related parental death. *Journal of Consulting and Clinical Psychology*, 73(2), 221–228.

Rutter, M. (1985). Resilience in the face of adversity. Protective factors and resistance to psychiatric disorder. *British Journal of Psychiatry*, 147(6), 598–611.

Sapolsky, R.M., Romero, L.M., Munck, A.U. (2000). How do glucocorticoids influence stress responses? Integrating permissive, suppressive, stimulatory, and preparative actions. *Endocrine Reviews*, 21(1), 55–89.

Saxbe, D.E. (2008). A field (researcher's) guide to cortisol: Tracking HPA axis functioning in everyday life. *Health Psychology Review*, 2(2), 163–190.

Ssewamala, F.M., Han, C.K., Neilands, T.B. (2009). Asset ownership and health and mental health functioning among AIDS-orphaned adolescents: Findings from a randomized clinical trial in rural Uganda. *Social Science and Medicine*, 69(2), 191–198.

Ssewamala, F.M., Neilands, T.B., Waldfogel, J., Ismayilova, L. (2012). The impact of a comprehensive microfinance intervention on depression levels of AIDS-orphaned children in Uganda. *Journal of Adolescent Health*, 50(4), 346–352.

UNAIDS. (2012). *Report on the Global AIDS Epidemic*. Geneva, Switzerland: UNAIDS.

UNICEF. (2015). Statistics by Area/HIV/AIDS. http://data.unicef.org/hiv-aids/care-support#sthash.El8i5Wnx.dpuf (accessed 15 January 2013).

Wang, B., Li, X., Barnett, D., Zhao, G., Zhao, J., Stanton, B. (2012). Risk and protective factors for depression symptoms among children affected by HIV/AIDS in rural China: A structural equation modeling analysis. *Social Science and Medicine*, 74(9), 1435–1443.

WHO. (2015). HIV/AIDS Fact Sheets. www.who.int/mediacentre/factsheets/fs360/en/ (accessed 23 July 2015).

Wild, L. (2001). The psychosocial adjustment of children orphaned by AIDS. *Southern African Journal of Child and Adolescent Mental Health*, 13(1), 3–22.

Zhao, J., Li, X., Barnett, D., Lin, X., Fang, X., Zhao, G., Naar-King, S., Stanton, B. (2011). Parental loss, trusting relationship with current caregivers, and psychosocial adjustment among children affected by AIDS in China. *Psychology, Health and Medicine*, 16(4), 437–449.

Zhao, Q., Li, X., Lin, X., Fang, X., Zhao, G., Zhao, J. (2009). Knowing kids dying of HIV: A traumatic event for AIDS orphans. *Journal of the Association of Nurses in AIDS Care*, 20(4), 275–282.

CHAPTER 9

Underinvestigated parental conditions: an overview

Laura Kelly and David Morley

INTRODUCTION

Previous chapters have detailed parental conditions where significant research has been conducted. If a parental condition has a relatively high profile and supporting evidence, this means that children and young people's needs are more likely to be recognised in clinical guidelines as seen with, for example, multiple sclerosis (National Institute for Health and Care Excellence, 2014). This chapter gives an overview of parental conditions where there is little available evidence to support inclusion in such guidelines, although initial attempts have been made to quantify their effects on children and young people. These conditions include, but are not restricted to, amyotrophic lateral sclerosis/motor neurone disease (ALS/MND), arthritis, chronic back pain, chronic pain, epilepsy, inflammatory bowel disease (IBD), leprosy, obsessive-compulsive disorder (OCD), schizophrenia and spinal cord injury (SCI). The limited degree of research into these conditions means that specific recommendations or practical guidance in their management would be unwise. The chapter will, however, give the reader an insight into some of the potential challenges faced by children and young people with a parent experiencing these less well investigated conditions.

AMYOTROPHIC LATERAL SCLEROSIS

ALS is the most common form of motor neurone disease, and is a chronic degenerative neurological condition characterised by progressive degeneration of upper and lower motor neurons in the brain and spinal cord. The majority of people with ALS die of respiratory muscle weakness less than three years from the onset of symptoms (Gordon, 2013). Calvo et al. (2015) have recently provided the first assessment of the impact of parental ALS through a comparison of children and young people with a parent with ALS and an aged-matched control group of children with healthy parents. Both groups contained 23 children aged 5–17 who were administered the Youth Self-Report Questionnaire (YSR; Achenbach and Rescorla, 2001) and the Rorschach Comprehensive System (Exner and Erdberg, 2005). Additionally, healthy parents completed the Child Behaviour Checklist (Achenbach, 1991). Results indicated that children of parents with ALS are at significantly higher risk of emotional and behavioural disturbances than children of healthy parents, with approximately 40% in the clinical range for depression. Whilst the sample size for this study limits what can reasonably be concluded, the authors suggest that families may require support to deal with a condition such as ALS.

ARTHRITIS

Arthritis is a common condition characterised by pain and inflammation in the joints. The two most common forms of the condition are rheumatoid arthritis and osteoarthritis, although a range of other types and related conditions exist. The worldwide prevalence of arthritis is significant (Sokka et al., 2010). For example, in the United Kingdom 33% of people aged 45 years and over have sought treatment for osteoarthritis, rising to 49% of women and 42% of men aged 75 years and over (Arthritis Research UK, 2013).

The condition can lead to a number of deleterious consequences. From the affected individual's perspective these can include persistent pain, fatigue, functional disability and mental health problems (Pollard et al., 2005). Whilst the impact of arthritis on carers has been well demonstrated (Brouwer et al., 2004; das Chagas Medeiros et al., 2000; Jacobi et al., 2003; Riemsma et al., 1999), the effect on children is largely limited to studies focusing on parental reports of how their condition affects their ability to fulfil a parenting role (e.g. Barlow et al., 1999; Katz et al., 2003; Ostenson and Rugelsjoen, 1992; Reisine et al., 1987). For example, in the study of Barlow et al. (1999) parents reported feelings of guilt, anger and frustration at their perceived inability to fulfil their parental role. More positively, they emphasised the advantage of being able to spend a greater amount of time with their children as a result of their condition. Mothers also reported that their children showed a greater awareness of the effects of the disability, and demonstrated greater independence and were more caring and sensitive than other children.

A more recent study by Zelkowitz et al. (2013) aimed to assess perceived parenting disability and stress, alongside children's behaviour (as measured by the CBCL) in early inflammatory arthritis, i.e. in parents diagnosed within 6 weeks to 18 months. The authors identified a number of associations between the variables assessed and suggest a reciprocal relationship between symptoms of arthritis, parental disability and parent and child distress. As the authors recognise, the study is extremely limited due to a sample size of just 29 affected parents. In addition, as with previous research focusing on parental arthritis, the study is limited to parental reports of their child's behaviour. There is a clear need to include data from children themselves in future work in this area.

CHRONIC BACK PAIN

Chronic back pain is a common condition, with the costs of its treatment estimated to be as much as $100 billion in the United States alone (Dreisinger, 2014). People with chronic back pain can experience both physical and psychological distress and disability. Although no research has directly involved children of parents with chronic back pain, Strunin and Boden (2004) provide some evidence of its impact through qualitative analyses of telephone interviews with 414 affected parents. In their study of males and females absent from work for one month or longer, parents discussed the effects of their condition on both their physical and emotional relationships with their children. Themes included increased responsibility for children, changes in parental behaviour such as increased irritability, and the inability to be involved in activities with children. These are perceived as a loss on the part of both mothers and fathers. Although the children were not directly involved in the study, the authors speculate that the children would also experience this loss. Whilst the study makes a valuable initial contribution to understanding the impact of parental chronic back pain on children, further research is required to assess directly the views of children themselves.

CHRONIC PAIN

Chronic pain is commonly defined as any pain lasting more than 12 weeks. Chronic pain may be the result of trauma from an injury or be the result of an ongoing illness. The impact on the individual may be a multitude of health problems such as fatigue, disturbed sleep, mood changes and loss of appetite. A person suffering with chronic pain may also have reduced mobility and stamina (NIH, 2011). Limited research has been undertaken to explore specifically the impact of parental chronic pain on children. However, some qualitative work has recently been carried out with the aim of developing theory around how children understand and experience parental chronic pain.

Umberger et al. (2013, 2014, 2015) have published a number of articles using primary and secondary qualitative analysis of interview data collected among a sample of 30 adolescents, aged 18–21. The analyses have a common underlying theme of aiming to better understand how adolescents manage living with parental chronic pain. In their primary analysis (Umberger et al., 2013), findings indicated that the manner in which parents experience chronic pain, and the extent to which they are open about how their pain affects them, can directly influence how offspring manage their own feelings and day-to-day activities. This study highlighted the importance of both the parent's and child's ability to communicate their thoughts, feelings and needs in relation to living with parental chronic non-cancer pain (CNCP).

The second analysis of Umberger et al. (2014) aimed to understand how adolescents manage the experience of living with a parent suffering with CNCP and investigate the environmental factors that help or hinder the management process. Findings indicated that adolescents can struggle to understand and make sense of their parents' experiences and the consequences of chronic pain. Six themes relating to adolescent understanding of parental pain were identified: (i) noticing something is different and changes in their parent's behaviour, functioning and mood; (ii) struggling with understanding and knowing what is happening; (iii) not receiving clear information about the parent's condition; (iv) questioning the validity of pain; (v) developing insight into the complexity of pain; and (vi) being 'better off' for learning important life lessons.

In subsequent work, Umberger et al. (2015) aimed to understand the challenges and needs of children living with parental CNCP. The adolescent dataset described above was used in this analysis in addition to four focus groups with parents or partners. The authors identified key challenges which both the children and parents face when affected by parental CNCP. These challenges include: (i) understanding the parent's pain and related disability; (ii) enduring hardships, such as taking on parental responsibilities and coping with changes in parental moods; (iii) grieving losses in relation to parental absences from significant childhood events and loss of 'childhood'; (iv) communicating effectively with the parent; and (v) feelings of isolation from the child's peer group. The authors particularly highlight how these children are faced with adult responsibilities at a younger age when compared to their peers, a process referred to as 'parentification', as first described by Jurkovic (1997). Potential positive and negative outcomes of the parentification process are discussed, such as the benefits of building independence and the possible adverse effects of parent/child role reversal. The authors conclude that three areas in relation to the child's needs should be addressed in cases of parental CNCP: knowledge, skills and supervised interaction.

A number of analyses (Hoftun et al., 2013; Kaasbøll et al., 2012, 2014) have been carried out using data from a large population based project, the Nord-Trøndelag Health Study (HUNT 3), conducted in central Norway. Data collection for HUNT 3 was collected using a cross-sectional survey during 2006–2008. In addition to parents completing a self-administered health and lifestyle questionnaire, adolescents aged 13–18 took part in the Young-HUNT 3, enabling data to be matched.

Kaasbøll et al. (2012, 2014) identified matching cases where both parents took part in the study (n=3227). Children who had one or both parents reporting chronic pain were identified (n=1333) from the matched sample while the remainder were treated as a general population reference group (n=1740) or missing (n=154). The authors investigated the association of parental chronic pain and psychological symptoms in adolescent offspring. Adolescents who had two parents with chronic pain were found to be at more than twice the risk of having symptoms of anxiety and depression when compared with the reference group. Girls also had an increased risk of conduct problems in school if their mother experienced chronic pain.

In their later analysis, Kaasbøll et al. (2014) investigated links between parental chronic pain and substance use in adolescents. Outcome variables included smoking, alcohol intoxication and drug use. Symptoms of anxiety and depression among adolescents were assessed using a short version of the Hopkins Symptom Checklist SCL-25, the symptom checklist-5 (SCL-5; Tambs and Moum, 1993). After adjusting for confounding factors, boys whose parents both experienced chronic pain were more likely to engage in smoking and alcohol intoxication than those who had parents who did not experience chronic pain. Although symptoms of anxiety and depression, as measured by the SCL-5, among this group of boys were significantly associated with smoking and alcohol intoxication, adjusting for anxiety and depression only minimally influenced the association between parental chronic pain and substance abuse. No association between substance abuse and parental chronic pain was identified.

Hoftun et al. (2013) performed an analysis on 5370 adolescents for whom one or both parents participated in the HUNT 3 adult survey. The authors examined the association of parental chronic pain with chronic pain in their adolescent offspring. Results indicated that parental chronic pain was associated with non-specific chronic pain in adolescents and was particularly strong among cases where both parents experience chronic pain. Family structures were also shown to influence the relationship as chronic pain was associated with the parent with whom they primarily lived.

Limitations of the results using the HUNT 3 data include the need to match parental and respective adolescent data for inclusion in analyses, as this may compromise the internal and external validity of the sample (Kaasbøll et al., 2012, 2014). In addition, underrepresentation of those in poorer health is a potential limitation of this dataset (Hoftun et al., 2013; Kaasbøll et al., 2012, 2014).

EPILEPSY

Epilepsy is an overarching term for a number of disorders that result in recurrent seizures of varying types. Causes of the condition can include genetic predisposition, brain injury, structural brain anomalies and specific epilepsy syndromes. Regardless of aetiology, the risk for recurrent seizures is common to all patients diagnosed with epilepsy (Bates, 2015). Concerns regarding the impact of epilepsy on the children of affected individuals first became evident in the mid-1980s (Lechtenberg, 1984; Lechtenberg and Akner, 1984) and were further reiterated by Lannon (1992), who concluded that the needs of children with parents with epilepsy required far greater attention. A review conducted by Ellis et al. (2000) highlighted how little research had been undertaken specifically on the needs of these children, although a body of literature had emerged that addressed the impact on the family unit as a result of childhood epilepsy (e.g. Camfield et al., 2001; Ryan et al., 2003; Shore et al., 2002) and epilepsy in adulthood (e.g. Anderson and Barton, 1990; Thompson and Upton, 1992).

Particular themes emerge from the publications of Lannon (1992) and Lechtenberg and Akner (1984). The latter places particular emphasis on issues surrounding parental disclosure of their condition to offspring, an issue discussed in more depth in Chapter 10 of this book. Although limited by sample size (12 families were studied), the authors conclude that 'the least disruptive to children at any age is a frank discussion of what the neurologic problem is and what is being done to control it. Efforts to conceal the problem breed distrust.'

Lannon (1992) reported on one of the first family interventions of its type, developed at the Oregon Comprehensive Epilepsy Program. The basis for this programme was centred around the main issues raised by Lechtenberg and Akner (1984), i.e. learning about epilepsy, fear of abandonment, transfer of dependence and fear of developing epilepsy. The programme developed by Lannon and her colleagues attempts to address each of these four areas. First, an individual assessment of each family's needs is made, with the family offered a range of services from education and counselling, through to medication reviews. There is an emphasis on the need to develop a close relationship with the family, and to discuss children's reactions to their parent's epilepsy, even if they are not present. Following an initial meeting the family is invited to prioritise their needs for themselves. As Lannon states, 'this empowers them, making them participants in care rather than recipients, and shows respect for their concerns and opinions.' Based on this, families are provided with education, guidance and support to help them adjust and deal with the many issues that a diagnosis of epilepsy can bring. As with a number of interventions developed for children previously discussed in this book, there appears to be no data regarding the long-term effectiveness of the programme outlined by Lannon.

More recently, Gauffin and Landbolm (2014) focused on three case studies investigating physical trauma in children of a parent with epilepsy. They demonstrate that parental epilepsy can result in offspring being vulnerable to violence, particularly when the parent is in difficult psychosocial circumstances. The authors highlight the importance of targeting support to parents in challenging circumstances.

INFLAMMATORY BOWEL DISEASE

IBD is a chronic illness of unknown aetiology, although there is increasing evidence of a genetic component (Karantanos and Gazouli, 2011). The condition is characterised by recurrent abdominal pain, diarrhoea, constipation, fatigue and weight-loss, frequently linked with stress or anxiety. Investigation into the impact of parental IBD is sparse with just two reported studies, both by Mukherjee et al. (2002a; 2002b). In the first of their publications (2002a) they report on a relatively small exploratory qualitative study in which they assess the experiences, both positive and negative, of 24 parents with IBD. On a positive note, parents reported the development of closer relationships with their children, and a heightened sense of compassion and understanding towards those who are unwell. Amongst the more negative findings, parents experienced feelings of worry and guilt, and, in a small number of cases, bouts of depression as a result of the constraints placed upon them by their symptoms. Parents reported their children as reacting with frustration and anger to constraints such as restrictions in social activities, and anxiety when the parent was experiencing IBD symptoms or in hospital. The authors concluded by highlighting the importance of health professionals providing support for patients and their families.

The second study by Mukherjee et al. (2002b) again took a qualitative approach and explored directly how children themselves viewed their parent's IBD, its impact on their daily life, coping strategies employed and what support their family required. Twenty-three children, aged 6–20 years, took part. Whilst some children appeared relatively unaffected by their parent's illness, others reported feelings of sadness, worry, anger and guilt. The negative impact on daily life included restricted social activities, having to maintain good behaviour and withdrawal and irritability on the part of the affected parent. Positive effects included heightened independence, family closeness and spending time with the parent when the parent was unwell. Whilst most did not feel additional support was necessary, some expressed a desire for more information and the opportunity to meet others in a similar situation. It must be stressed that these conclusions are based on a relatively small qualitative study, and consequently it would be unwise to generalise about the authors' findings.

LEPROSY

A condition most commonly associated with areas in tropical Africa and Asia, leprosy is a contagious disease affecting the skin, mucous membranes and nerves. The condition causes discolouring and ulcers on the skin and, in severe cases, disfigurement and deformities (Britton and Lockwood, 2004). Research involving young people and leprosy has primarily focused on the impact of leprosy on affected children in endemic areas (Madarasingha and Senaviratne, 2011; Sachdeva et al., 2011). The impact of parental leprosy on offspring has received little attention. Few studies have been conducted which aim to assess directly the well-being of the children of affected parents.

A scholarship programme reported by Saylan et al. (2000) was implemented in Turkey at the end of the 1990's to encourage parents with leprosy (n=223) to have no further children and to keep sending their existing children (n=445) to school. Parents were provided with an income if enrolled in this project, which had a strong element of family planning. The programme did succeed in increasing affected parents' motivation for practising methods of family planning and ensuring their children's school attendance. While these programme evaluation results were promising, the study provided little or no evidence on the underlying impact of parental leprosy.

A more recent study (Yamaguchi, 2013) has investigated the impact of parental leprosy on adolescents in Nepal. Health-related quality of life (HRQOL), depression and self-esteem were assessed in adolescents (n=102) with leprosy-affected parents and compared with those of adolescent offspring (n=115) of non-affected parents. Measures used included the KINDL (Ravens-Sieberer and Bullinger, 1998) to assess HRQOL, the Center for Epidemiological Studies-Depression Scale (CES-D; Radloff, 1977) to investigate depression and the Rosenberg Self-Esteem Scale (RSES; Rosenberg, 1989) to assess self-esteem. Results indicated that adolescents with parents affected by leprosy had higher levels of symptoms associated with depression compared to those with non-affected parents. Lower levels of self-esteem and HRQOL were also reported among the affected cohort. Poor scores were particularly evident in cases where both parents had leprosy. The authors cite several contextual factors in Nepal which may contribute to poor scores among adolescents, including stigma, poverty, education and parents' economic situation. As with a number of studies discussed in this chapter, the authors acknowledge the relatively small sample size.

OBSESSIVE-COMPULSIVE DISORDER

OCD is a common anxiety disorder, characterised by intrusive, repetitive thoughts or images (obsessions) and repetitive behaviours or mental acts (compulsions; Seibell and Hollander, 2014). Black et al. (2003) report on the only study to date to assess specifically the impact of parental OCD on children's behavioural and emotional competence. Previous work by this group had highlighted the significant impact of OCD on both family and marital life (Black et al., 1998) and particular problems of communication within families.

In their second study Black et al. (2003) included a group of 21 parents with OCD and 43 of their children. A group of 22 healthy parents and 35 of their children acted as a control group. Through the use of a range of clinical diagnostic tools and validated measures the authors report some potentially important findings. First, they highlight the possibility of genetic transmission in relation to the early development of anxiety and mood disorder observed in their sample of children, which may or may not develop into OCD. Second, and potentially of more interest to service providers, they highlight the possible influence that living with an OCD parent might have on a child's emotional well-being, in terms of the parent providing a model of dysfunctional behaviour. The authors reported higher scores on the Child Behaviour Checklist (Achenbach, 1991) as predictive of the child developing

OCD. Other predictors included inappropriate affective responsiveness and poor behavioural control on the part of the OCD parent. Black et al. reported female gender as a further predictive factor, although they were unable to offer any explanation for this finding. The robustness of results from this study is limited by the small sample size and potential sample bias.

SCHIZOPHRENIA

Schizophrenia is a long-term mental health condition which has a variety of symptoms such as lack of insight, hallucination, delusions, thought disorder, social withdrawal and self-neglect. These experiences can be distressing not only to the affected individual but also to their relatives (Picchioni and Murray, 2007). Early research reported that birth rates were markedly lower in people with schizophrenia, but an increase in rates was observed as a result of the wide-scale process of deinstitutionalisation that took place throughout the latter half of the twentieth century (Erlenmeyer-Kimling et al., 1969). Research has now emerged that demonstrates not only the increased risk of psychopathology in children of parents with schizophrenia (Ross and Compagnon, 2001), but also the social, emotional and developmental consequences of having a schizophrenic parent.

Although limited by sample size (39 participants), the retrospective study of Caton et al. (1998) provides valuable insight into the potential effects of growing up with a schizophrenic parent, the majority in this particular sample being a schizophrenic mother. Children reported experiences of being frightened, embarrassed and in many cases, the subject of excessive physical punishment as a manifestation of their parent's schizophrenia. In addition, a number of children reported having to care for their schizophrenic parent, helping with daily household activities, and giving up work or school activities.

Caton and her colleagues make some key recommendations based on their findings. First, although virtually all the children in the study were brought up by their schizophrenic parent at some stage during their childhood, on average they were raised in three different settings, grandparents and aunts being the most common providers of alternative care. The authors therefore recommend involvement of the extended family in any rehabilitation programme. Second, the authors emphasise that whilst the children in their study were aware of their parent's illness, their degree of understanding and contact and access to health professionals differed greatly, a finding common to other parental conditions (e.g. Schrag et al., 2004). The authors suggest education regarding psychiatric illness should be made available to children of affected parents as and when they express an interest.

Many of Canon's findings have been supported through subsequent research. For example, Somers (2007) investigated the impact on parental schizophrenia on children's daily lives and experiences. Offspring (n=37) were matched with a control group and, while findings largely supported low disruption to family life among children of parents with schizophrenia compared to those of healthy parents, children were more emotionally distressed, upset and sad that their parents were unwell. Children had less contact with extended family, more problems at school and had poor experiences of health services. Findings supported the importance of the role of the well parent in relation to providing support, advice, help and discipline. Although only a small number in the study sample were living with a single parent, their particular vulnerability was emphasised.

Herbert et al. (2013) examined resilience in children (n=45) of parents with a diagnosis of schizophrenia. The authors devised a semi-structured interview schedule to collect socio-demographic data on parents and their offspring, family details and experiences of living with the parent with schizophrenia. Resilience was assessed using the Connor–Davidson Resilience Scale (CD-RISC; Connor and Davidson 2003). Offspring reported negative experiences in social and emotional aspects of life and took on more financial and emotional responsibilities. Results indicated however that despite negative experiences, children of parents with schizophrenia demonstrated resilience and were satisfied with parenting due to the support and care they received from other sources (for example, other family members, friends and relatives). The authors conclude that the negative impact of parental illness may be moderated through protective factors such as good relationships with other family members and other environmental factors such as positive distractions, reappraisal and religious practices, enabling them to cope and increase resilience.

A larger-scale study has been carried out in Brazil to assess the impact of parental schizophrenia on the social adjustment of adult offspring compared to those in the general population (Terzian et al., 2007). Data reported by parents with schizophrenia (or other family members) were collected for offspring (n=431) in relation to their education, employment and marital status. Data was collected using a structured questionnaire developed by the authors. Results indicated lower employment among offspring of patients with schizophrenia when compared to the general population and lower marital rates in adult males compared to adult males in the general population. The authors found no significant difference between education among the study sample when compared to the general population; however, they do acknowledge other studies which report more school adjustment problems among parental schizophrenia offspring (Ayalon and Merom 1985; Janes et al., 1983).

SPINAL CORD INJURY

SCI can result in a range of short- and long-term health implications (e.g. pressure injuries, disorders of muscle tone, bowel and bladder problems) that may have long-lasting effects on independence and psychological well-being (Bragge et al., 2015). While a number of studies report the impact of SCI on children as patients and their long-term outcomes (e.g. Anderson and Vogel, 2002; Lee et al., 2009; Russell et al., 2015; Spoltore et al., 2000), the impact of parental spinal cord injury on children is less well investigated. Buck and Hohmann (1981) were the first to investigate parental SCI through a retrospective study of 45 adult children of fathers with SCI. Children were aged 18–30 at the time of the study and had been raised by their father from age 2 or younger. They were compared to a matched control group of 36 children of able-bodied fathers. All participants completed a battery of self-report questionnaires assessing factors such as parent-child relationship, personality and gender role type. Results indicated that children with spinally injured fathers were well-adjusted and emotionally stable and that family relationships were not negatively affected by the disability status of the father. The authors recognised a number of limitations in their study, including its retrospective nature and potentially biased sample. The relatively small sample size is a further potential limitation.

A further study by Alexander et al. (2002) investigated the impact of maternal spinal cord injury on marital, family and child adjustment. A comparison of two groups was made; an experimental group with 88 spinally injured mothers, 46 partners and 31 children and a matched control group of 84 able-bodied mothers, 33 partners and 28 children. Participants completed a range of self-report instruments assessing child adjustment, self-esteem, gender role identity, family adjustment and parental stress and satisfaction. From their results the authors drew similar conclusions to those of Buck and Hohmann: maternal SCI 'does not appear to affect children adversely in terms of individual adjustment, attitudes towards their parents, self-esteem, gender roles, and family functioning'. The authors acknowledged, however, that mothers in their study came from higher than average socio-economic, educational and employment backgrounds, and therefore may have had access to more resources to help cope with the demands of parenting.

Two further studies have focused specifically on the challenges of parenting with SCI. Westgren and Levi (1994) assessed the effects of SCI on a mother's ability to provide adequate care for her children. Twenty-six spinally injured mothers participated in a standardised interview that spanned a range of topics including their own level of independence, the daily care of their children and the schooling of their children. The authors concluded that there are no grounds to question the ability of mothers with SCI to fulfil their parenting role. As noted by Westgren and Levi, the study was limited by its small sample size and by its descriptive nature. A more recent study by Duvdevany et al. (2008) focuses on the parenting experience of fathers with SCI. A small, and therefore limited, sample of 12 fathers participated in in-depth semi-structured interviews. Results from these interviews indicate that fathers with SCI take an active role in influencing their children's attitude towards disability. SCI does not appear to undermine the bond between father and child or the child's perception of the father's role as a parent.

CONCLUSION

This chapter has presented a range of parental conditions where less is known about their impact on children than those conditions with dedicated chapters in this book. What is striking about the conditions discussed is that many of them are relatively common. Also of particular note is the apparent similarity between the impact of these parental conditions on children and the impact of those more substantially investigated. Issues surrounding mental health, behavioural difficulties, experiences of grief and sadness, communication problems and isolation from peers are evident from the reported studies. Positive implications are also apparent; some children demonstrate greater independence, empathy and resilience as a consequence of the parent's illness.

The consequences for parenting are similarly diverse. Some conditions, for example SCI, appear to have little impact on the parenting, although this appears somewhat counterintuitive. The conditions discussed also highlight potentially negative implications for the parenting role (e.g. feelings of guilt, anger and frustration) alongside those that are significantly more positive, such as parents being able to spend more time with their children and developing closer relationships with them.

There remains a heavy note of caution with the majority of these less well investigated parental conditions. A number are limited by small sample sizes, some alarmingly so, and many are qualitative in nature. Generalising their results would, therefore, be unwise. In addition, none have been the subject of longitudinal investigation that would facilitate an understanding of how children adjust to their parent's condition over time, rather than the snapshot provided by the cross-sectional studies discussed. One can only conclude that significantly more research is required into these parental conditions.

REFERENCES

Achenbach, T.M. (1991). *Achenbach behavior checklist.* Burlington, VT: University of Vermont.

Achenbach, T., Rescorla, L. (2001). *The Manual for the ASEBA School-Age Forms and Profiles.* Burlington, VT: University of Vermont, Research Center for Children, Youth, and Families.

Alexander, C.J., Hwang, K., Sipski, M.L. (2002). Mothers with spinal cord injury: Impact on marital, family, and children's adjustment. *Archives of Physical Medicine and Rehabilitation*, 83, 24–30.

Anderson, C.J., Vogel, L.C. (2002) Employment outcomes of adults who sustained spinal cord injuries as children or adolescents. *Archives of Physical Medicine and Rehabilitation*, 83, 791–801.

Anderson, E., Barton, R. (1990). Epilepsy: A family burden? *Clinical Psychology Forum*, 25, 3–5.

Arthritis Research UK. (2013). Osteoarthritis in general practice.

Ayalon, M., Merom, H. (1985). The teacher interview. *Schizophrenia Bulletin*, 11(1), 117–120.

Barlow, J., Cullen, L., Foster, N., Harrison, M., Wade, M. (1999). Does arthritis influence perceived ability to fulfil a parenting role? Perceptions of mothers, fathers and grandparents. *Patient Education and Counselling*, 37, 141–151.

Bates, K. (2015). Epilepsy: Current evidence-based paradigms for diagnosis and treatment. *Primary Care*, 42(2), 217–232.

Black, D.W., Gaffney, G.R., Schlosser, S., Steven, M.A.T., Gabel, J. (1998). The impact of obsessive compulsive disorder on the family: Preliminary findings. *Journal of Nervous and Mental Diseases*, 186, 440–442.

Black, D.W., Gaffney, G.R., Schlosser, S., Gabel, J. (2003). Children of parents with obsessive compulsive disorder: A 2-year follow up study. *Acta Psychiatrica Scandinavica*, 107, 305–313.

Bragge, P., Piccenna, L., Middleton, J.W., Williams, S., Creasey, G., Dunlop, S., Brown, D., Gruen, R.L. (2015). Developing a spinal cord injury research strategy using a structured process of evidence review and stakeholder dialogue. Part I: Rapid review of SCI prioritisation literature. *Spinal Cord*, [Epub ahead of print].

Britton, W.J., Lockwood, D.N.J. (2004). Leprosy. *The Lancet*, 363(9416), 1209–1219.

Brouwer, W.B., van Exel, N.J., van de Berg, B., Dinant, H.J., Koopmanschap, M.A., van den Bos, G.A. (2004). Burden of caregiving: Evidence of objective burden, subjective burden, and quality of life impacts on informal caregivers of patients with rheumatoid arthritis. *Arthritis and Rheumatism*, 51, 570–577.

Buck, F.M., Hohmann, G.W. (1981). Personality, behavior, values, and family relations of children of fathers with spinal cord injury. *Archives of Physical Medicine and Rehabilitation*, 62, 432–438.

Calvo, V., Bianco, F., Benelli, E., Sambin, M., Monsurrò, M.R., Femiano, C., Querin, G., Soraru, G., Palmieri, A. (2015). Impact on children of a parent with ALS: A case-control study. *Frontiers in Psychology*, 6, 288.

Camfield, C., Breau, L., Camfield, P. (2001). Impact of pediatric epilepsy on the family: A new scale for clinical and research use. *Epilepsia*, 42, 104–112.

Caton, C.L.M., Cournos, F., Felix, A., Wyatt, R.J. (1998). Childhood experiences and current adjustment of offspring of indigent patients with Schizophrenia. *Psychiatric Services*, 49, 86–90.

Connor, K.M., Davidson, J.R. (2003). Development of a new resilience scale: The Connor-Davidson Resilience Scale (CD-RISC). *Depression and Anxiety*, 18(2), 76–82.

das Chagas Medeiros, M., Ferraz, M., Quaresma, M. (2000). The effect of rheumatoid arthritis on the quality of life of primary caregivers. *Journal of Rheumatology*, 27, 76–83.

Dreisinger, T,E. (2014). Exercise in the management of chronic back pain. *The Ochsner Journal*, 14(1), 101–107.

Duvdevany, I., Buchbinder, E., Yaacov, I. (2008). Accepting disability: The parenting experience of fathers with spinal cord injury (SCI). *Qualitative Health Research*, 18(8), 1021–1033.

Ellis, N., Upton, D., Thompson, P. (2000). Epilepsy and the family: A review of current literature. *Seizure*, 9, 22–30.

Erlenmeyer-Kimling, L., Nichol, S., Rainer, J.D., Edwards-Deming, W. (1969). Changes in fertility rates in schizophrenic patients in New-York State. *American Journal of Psychiatry*, 125, 916–927.

Exner, J., Erdberg, P. (2005). *The Rorschach: A comprehensive system. Vol. II* (3rd edn). Hoboken, NJ: Wiley and Sons.

Gauffin, H., Landtblom, A.M. (2014). Epilepsy and violence: Case series concerning physical trauma in children of persons with epilepsy. *Neuropsychiatric Disease and Treatment*, 10, 2183–2189.

Gordon, P.H. (2013). Amyotrophic Lateral Sclerosis: An update for 2013 Clinical Features, Pathophysiology, Management and Therapeutic Trials. *Aging and Disease*, 4(5), 295–310.

Herbert, H.S., Manjula, M., Philip, M. (2013). Growing up with a parent having schizophrenia: Experiences and resilience in the offsprings. *Indian Journal of Psychological Medicine*, 35, 148–153.

Hoftun, G.B., Romundstad, P.R., Rygg, M. (2013). Association of parental chronic pain with chronic pain in the adolescent and young adult: Family linkage data from the HUNT Study. *JAMA Pediatrics*, 167(1) 61–69.

Jacobi, C.E., van den Berg, B., Boshuizen, H., Rupp, I., Dinant, H.J., van den Bos G. (2003). Dimension-specific burden of caregiving among partners of rheumatoid arthritis patients. *Rheumatology*, 42, 1226–1233.

Janes, C.L., Weeks, D.G., Worland, J. (1983). School behavior in adolescent children of parents with mental disorder. *The Journal of Nervous and Mental Disease*, 171(4), 234–240.

Jurkovic, G.J. (1997). *Lost childhoods: The plight of the parentified child*. New York: Brunner Routledge.

Kaasbøll, J, Lydersen, S., Indredavik, M.S. (2012) Psychological symptoms in children of parents with chronic pain: The HUNT study. *Pain*, 153(5), 1054–1062.

Kaasbøll, J., Lydersen, S., Indredavik, M.S. (2014). Substance use in children of parents with chronic pain: The HUNT study. *Journal of Pain Research*, 21(7), 483–494.

Karantanos, T., Gazouli, M. (2011). Inflammatory bowel disease: Recent advances on genetics and innate immunity. *Annals of Gastroenterology*, 24, 164–172.

Katz, P., Pasch, L., Wong, B. (2003). Development of an instrument to measure disability in parenting activity among women with rheumatoid arthritis. *Arthritis and Rheumatism*, 48, 935–943.

Lannon, S.L. (1992). Meeting the needs of children whose parents have epilepsy. *Journal of Neuroscience Nursing*, 24, 14–18.

Lechtenberg, R. (1984). *Epilepsy and the family*. Harvard University Press.

Lechtenberg, R., Akner, L. (1984). Psychological adaptation of children to epilepsy in a parent. *Epilepsia*, 25, 40–45.

Lee, J.H., Sung, I.Y., Kang, J.Y., Park, S.R. (2009). Characteristics of pediatric-onset spinal cord injury. *Pediatrics International*, 51(2), 254–257.

Madarasingha, N.P., Senaviratne, J.K. (2011). A study of household contacts of children with leprosy. *The Ceylon Medical Journal*, 56(3), 112–114.

Mukherjee, S., Sloper, P., Turnbull, A. (2002a). An insight into the experiences of parents with inflammatory bowel disease. *Journal of Advanced Nursing*, 37(4), 355–363.

Mukherjee, S., Sloper, P., Lewin, R. (2002b). The meaning of parental illness to children: The case of inflammatory bowel disease. *Child: Care, Health and Development*, 28(6), 479–485.

National Institute for Health and Care Excellence. (2014). *Management of multiple sclerosis in primary and secondary care*. London: National Clinical Guideline Centre.

NIH. (2011). Chronic Pain: Symptoms, Diagnosis, and Treatment. *NIH Medline plus* 6(1), 5–6.

Ostensen, M., Rugelsjoen, A. (1992). Problem areas of the rheumatic mother. *American Journal of Reproductive Immunology*, 28(3–4), 254–255.

Picchioni, M.M., Murray, R.M. (2007). Schizophrenia. *British Medical Journal*, 335(7610), 91–95.

Pollard, L., Choy, E.H., Scott, D.L. (2005). The consequences of rheumatoid arthritis: Quality of life measures in the individual patient. *Clinical and Experimental Rheumatology*, 23(5 Suppl 39), S43–S52.

Radloff, L.S. (1977). The CES-D scale: A self-report depression scale for research in the general population. *Applied Psychological Measurement*, 1(3), 385–401.

Ravens-Sieberer, U., Bullinger M. (1998). Assessing health-related quality of life in chronically ill children with the German KINDL: First psychometric and content analytical results. *Quality of Life Research*, 7(5), 399–407.

Reisine, S.T., Goodenow, C., Grady, K.E. (1987). The impact of rheumatoid arthritis on the homemaker. *Social Science and Medicine*, 25, 89–95.

Riemsma, R., Taal, E., Rasker, J., Klein, G., Bruyn, G., Wouters, J., Wiegman, O. (1999).

The burden of care for informal caregivers of patients with rheumatoid arthritis. *Psychology and Health*, 14, 773–794.

Rosenberg, M. (1989). *Society and the adolescent self-image*. Middletown, CT: Wesleyan University Press.

Ross, R., Compagnon, N. (2001). Diagnosis and treatment of psychiatric disorders in children with a schizophrenic parent. *Schizophrenia Research*, 50(1–2), 121–129.

Russell, H.F., January, A.M., Kelly, E.H., Mulcahey, M.J., Betz, R.R., Vogel, L.C. (2015). Patterns of coping strategy use and relationships with psychosocial health in adolescents with spinal cord injury. *Journal of Pediatric Psychology*, 40(5), 535–543.

Ryan, B.L., Speechley, K.N., Levin, S.D., Stewart, M. (2003). Parents' and physicians' perceptions of childhood epilepsy. *Seizure*, 12, 359–368.

Sachdeva, S., Amin, S.S., Khan, Z., Sharma, P.K., Bansal, S. (2011). Childhood leprosy: Lest we forget. *Tropical Doctor*, 41(3),163–165.

Saylan, T., Karadeniz, A., Iyier, N., Soydan, M., Pamuk, D. (2000). A scholarship project for the children of leprosy patients in Turkey. *Leprosy Review*, 71(2), 212–216.

Schrag, A., Morley, D., Quinn, N., Jahanshahi, M. (2004). Impact of Parkinson's disease on patients' adolescent and adult children. *Parkinsonism and Related Disorders*, 10, 391–397.

Somers, V. (2007). Schizophrenia: The impact of parental illness on children. *British Journal of Social Work*, 37, 1319–1334.

Seibell, P.J., Hollander, E. (2014). Management of obsessive-compulsive disorder. *F1000Prime Reports*, 6, 68.

Shore, C.P., Austin, J.K., Huster, G.A., Dunn, D.W. (2002). Identifying risk factors for maternal depression in families of adolescents with epilepsy. *Journal for Specialists in Pediatric Nursing*, 7, 71–80.

Sokka, T., Kautiainen, H., Pincus, T., et al. (2010). Work disability remains a major problem in rheumatoid arthritis in the 2000s: Data from 32 countries in the QUEST-RA study. *Arthritis Research and Therapy*, 12, R42.

Spolotore, T., Mulcahey, M.J., Johnston, T., Kelly, K., Morales, V., Rebuck, C. (2000). Innovative programs for children and adolescents with spinal cord injury. *Orthopaedic Nursing*, 19, 55–62.

Strunin, L., Boden, L.I. (2004) Family consequences of chronic back pain. *Social Science and Medicine*, 58, 1385–1393.

Tambs, K., Moum, T. (1993). How well can a few questionnaire items indicate anxiety and depression? *Acta Psychiatrica Scandinavica*, 87(5), 364–367.

Terzian, A.C., Andreoli, S.B., de Oliveira, L.M., de Jesus Mari, J., McGrath, J. (2007). A cross-sectional study to investigate current social adjustment of offspring of patients with schizophrenia. *European Archives of Psychiatry and Clinical Neuroscience*, 257(4), 230–236.

Thompson, P.J., Upton, D. (1992). The impact of chronic epilepsy on the family. *Seizure*, 1, 43–48.

Umberger, W., Martsolf, D., Jacobson, A., Risko, J., Patterson, M., Calabro, M. (2013).

The shroud: Ways adolescents manage living with parental chronic pain. *Journal of Nursing Scholarship*, 45(4), 344–354.

Umberger, W., Martsolf, D., Jacobson, A., Risko, J., Calabro, M., Patterson, M. (2014). Ways of understanding parental chronic pain: A typology. *Pain Management Nursing*, 15(4), 854–863.

Umberger, W.A., Risko, J., Covington, E. (2015). The forgotten ones: Challenges and needs of children living with disabling parental chronic pain. *Journal of Pediatric Nursing*, 30(3), 498–507.

Westgren, N., Levi, R. (1994). Motherhood after traumatic spinal cord injury. *Paraplegia*, 32, 517–523.

Yamaguchi, N., Poudel, K.C., Jimba, M. (2013). Health-related quality of life, depression, and self-esteem in adolescents with leprosy-affected parents: Results of a cross-sectional study in Nepal. *BMC Public Health*, 13, 22.

Zelkowitz, P., Looper, K.J., Mustafa, S.S., Purden, M., Baron, M; McGill Early Arthritis Research Group. (2013). Parenting disability, parenting stress and child behaviour in early inflammatory arthritis. *Chronic Diseases and Injuries in Canada*, 33(2), 81–87.

CHAPTER 10

Disclosure of parental illness to children: examples from HIV/AIDS

Shan Qiao and Xiaoming Li

INTRODUCTION

HIV (human immunodeficiency virus), the virus that causes AIDS (acquired immunodeficiency syndrome), has presented one of the most serious health and developmental challenges for society since it was first reported in 1981 (Fauci and Whitescarver, 2011). With the global commitment to combating the HIV epidemic and scientific advances in both medical treatment and behavioural prevention intervention, new HIV infections have decreased by 38% globally since 2001 (UNAIDS, 2014). Still, HIV is a leading cause of death worldwide and the number-one cause of death in Africa (UNAIDS, 2014). In 2013, there were approximately 2.1 million new infections worldwide, 35 million people were living with HIV and 1.5 million people died of AIDS around the world (UNAIDS, 2014).

HIV/AIDS not only affects the physical and psychological well-being of those who are infected, but also impacts their community and family, including children. Worldwide, over 18 million children under the age of 18 have lost one or both parents to HIV/AIDS and millions more are living with HIV-infected parents (UNAIDS, 2013). Compared to children living with parents with other diseases, children of HIV-infected parents may have to face additional psychosocial challenges including stigma, discrimination and social isolation (Li et al., 2008).

The manner in which parents disclose their HIV status to their children (parental HIV disclosure) has a tremendous impact on children's response to their parents' illness, psychological adjustment to parental HIV infection and self-protection from HIV infection (Qiao et al., 2013a). Disclosure, or self-disclosure, is a process in which personal information is verbally communicated to another person (Chelune, 1979). Disclosure is not a single event but a process of gradual and selective delivery of information, embedded in the context of a relationship (Lesch et al., 2007; Wiener et al., 2007; Moses and Tomlinson, 2013). A discloser needs to make decisions about when, what, where, to whom, how much to disclose and how to disclose (Cozby, 1973).

A recent concept analysis revealed that HIV disclosure is a complex process involving the following: experiencing an event, communicating, timing, contextual environment, protecting someone, relationship status and improving health or undergoing treatment (Eustace and Ilagan, 2010). Disclosure is the result of an individual experiencing a certain life event; in this instance HIV infection. In HIV disclosure, the HIV-infected people are faced with a HIV-positive diagnosis, which is seen as shameful and life-threatening. The process of communication in HIV disclosure includes the act of telling others about HIV infection. Making the decision to communicate is a difficult and personal process. Timing of HIV disclosure refers to when and why people decide to disclose their HIV infection to others. The contextual environment is the setting within which disclosure occurs, and is made up of individuals, families and communities, as well as socio-cultural and political norms. HIV-infected people choose to disclose/not disclose their serostatus (i.e. the state of either having or not having detectable antibodies against a specific antigen, as measured by a blood test) because they have a sense of responsibility to protect others (e.g. partners, family, and social networks), and in some sense to protect themselves. Disclosure practice is characterised by the social relationship between the discloser and the potential targets of the disclosure. For example, a discloser may not tell his/her HIV serostatus to everyone he/she has known, but to several persons selected depending on his/her personal relationship with them (selective disclosure). The therapeutic effect of disclosure has been commonly reported as a reason or impact of HIV disclosure. For example, disclosure to significant others is associated with gaining social support, initiating HIV treatment and adhering to HIV medications (Eustace and Ilagan, 2010).

THEORETICAL PERSPECTIVES ON PARENTAL HIV DISCLOSURE

Although there is increasing interest in HIV disclosure, empirically tested and validated theories specific to parental HIV disclosure are limited (Qiao et al., 2013a). Some theoretical models of HIV disclosure have been developed, which can be used to enhance our understanding of parental HIV disclosure (see Table 10.1). In general, the theoretical resources in relation to parental HIV disclosure can be categorised into four types: (i) theories focusing on the decision making of disclosure – these theories aim to explain and predict why, how and when HIV-infected individuals will decide to disclose their status (Qiao et al., 2013b); (ii) theories focusing on the disclosure process – these theories intend to identify and interpret different stages during the process of disclosure; (iii) theories focusing on the role of healthcare workers during the disclosure process; and (iv) theories focusing on children's development stages in understanding illness.

Disease progression theory posits that HIV-infected individuals will disclose their HIV diagnosis when HIV progresses to AIDS and it becomes difficult for them to hide the symptoms (Kalichman & Hunter, 1992). Consequence theory asserts that the decision to disclose is a result of analysis and calculation of anticipated outcomes of disclosure (Derlega et al., 2004). People will choose to reveal HIV-positive status when the perceived benefits of doing so (e.g. obtaining social support) outweigh the risks or costs (e.g. being stigmatised by others). Communication privacy management theory (originally known as communication boundary management theory), is a theory about how people make decisions about revealing and concealing private information. It proposes that people maintain and coordinate privacy boundaries with others, and control the flow of private information to decide whether to reveal or conceal information (Petronio, 2000).

A common feature of these theoretical perspectives is their focus on factors at the individual level, especially an individual's expectations and cognitive appraisal of potential consequences (both benefits and risks of disclosure), assuming the individual will make decisions of disclosure based on rational analysis. This view is consistent with behavioural theories highlighting reasoned action, i.e. the theory of planned behaviour (Lo et al., 2009). Social influence theory, applying a social ecological perspective, argues that HIV disclosure decision making is nested within multiple interrelated levels of influences, including individual, interpersonal (e.g. relationship quality) and socio-cultural factors (e.g. social norms, stigma, cultural attitudes) (Zea et al., 2007).

Some theoretical models extend beyond the realm of disclosure decision-making by exploring HIV disclosure as a process. One example is the

TABLE 10.1 Selected theoretical perspectives of HIV disclosure

Theoretical perspectives	Reference	Key points
Disease progression theory	(Kalichman, 1995 ; Babcock, 1998)	HIV-infected individuals will disclose their HIV diagnosis when HIV progresses to AIDS and it becomes difficult for them to hide the symptoms.
Consequence theory	(Derlega et al., 2004)	The decision making of HIV disclosure is a result of the analysis and the calculation of anticipated outcomes of disclosure.
Communication privacy management theory	(Petronio, 2007)	Individuals control the flow of private information and use privacy rules and strategies to decide whether to reveal or conceal information.
Social influence theory	(Zea et al., 2007)	Decision making regarding HIV disclosure is nested within multiple interrelated levels of influences, including individual, interpersonal relationships (e.g. relationship quality) and socio-cultural factors (e.g. social norms, stigma, cultural attitudes).
Disclosure Process Model	(Chaudoir et al., 2011)	The decision-making process affects the disclosure event in relation to disclosure and reaction of the targets. The disclosure event influences disclosure outcomes (individual, dyadic and social outcomes) through specific mediations. The 'feedback loop', that is, the reactions to disclosure or disclosure outcomes, may have an impact on future disclosure.
Five-Stage Process Model	(Gerson et al., 2001)	Disclosure is a continuing dialogue between children, parents and healthcare workers. The five stages of this process include 'information gathering and trust building', 'education', 'determining when the time is right for disclosure', 'the actual disclosure event' and 'monitoring post-disclosure coping and managing disclosure-related bumps in the road'.
Children's developmental stages	(Piaget and Inhelder, 1969; Werner, 1948; Bibace and Walsh, 1978; Koopman et al., 2004)	Children's thoughts about illness follow a sequence corresponding to the cognitive and social development stages, including 'sensorimotor' stage (0–2 years), 'pre-operational' stage (2–7 years), 'concrete operational' stage (7–11 years) and 'formal operational' stage (11 years).

Disclosure Process Model (Chaudoir et al., 2011) which aims to predict the HIV disclosure process (decision making, the disclosure event and feedback loop toward disclosure). The decision making affects the disclosure event by determining the content of disclosure and, in turn, the reaction of the disclosure targets. The disclosure event influences disclosure outcomes (individual, dyadic relationship and public outcomes). The 'feedback loop' includes reactions to disclosure or disclosure outcomes that may impact future disclosure. The Disclosure Process Model could be useful in predicting parental HIV disclosure. However, more empirical evidence is needed to support some of the mechanisms linking the disclosure event and disclosure outcomes as depicted in the model.

Some theories also identify stages of the disclosure process with a goal of guiding healthcare workers during the process. For instance, Gerson et al. (2001) describe a stage-wise process for informing HIV-infected children about their HIV infection (i.e. paediatric disclosure), emphasising ongoing dialogue between children, their family and healthcare providers about HIV infection and its effects during the disclosure process. According to the Gerson et al. model, the five stages of disclosure include 'information gathering and trust building', 'education', 'determining when the time is right for disclosure', 'the actual disclosure event' and 'monitoring post-disclosure coping and managing disclosure-related bumps in the road' (Gerson et al., 2001). Although the psychosocial challenges associated with paediatric disclosure might be different from parental disclosure, this model may be able to inform appropriate parental HIV disclosure practice by offering insightful guidelines on the disclosure process for healthcare providers.

Because the targets of parental HIV disclosure are children whose ages and cognitive abilities will affect their parents' decisions and the consequences of disclosure, theories regarding child developmental stages in understanding illness could also be used to guide the parental HIV disclosure research and practice. Existing studies have suggested that children's understanding of the disease process, causes and prevention proceeds through a discrete series of stages characterised by different cognitive abilities (Qiao et al., 2013a; Simoni and Pantalone, 2004). Along with their physical development, children experience different cognitive development stages including 'sensorimotor' stage (0–2 years), 'pre-operational' stage (2–7 years), 'concrete operational' stage (7–11 years) and 'formal operational' stage (11 years) (Koopman et al., 2004). Their comprehension of illness follows a sequence corresponding to the cognitive stages (Simoni and Pantalone, 2004). To assist children in understanding parental HIV infection it is therefore necessary to present the HIV-related information in a developmentally appropriate manner. Parents and healthcare providers need to consider children's age and developmental stage in making a disclosure plan.

CURRENT PRACTICE AND CHALLENGES OF PARENTAL HIV DISCLOSURE

Disclosure to children is challenging for the majority of HIV-infected parents (Simoni et al., 2000). HIV/AIDS is not just a biomedical disease but a socially constructed phenomenon. Some transmission routes of HIV may represent 'deviance' from socially accepted standards of behaviour (e.g. drug use, commercial sex), therefore acquisition of HIV infection may be viewed as socially or morally wrong (Simoni et al., 2000; Zhou, 2007). HIV-infected parents have to face stigma and discrimination from the outside world and also may suffer internal negative emotions such as shame, guilt and fear (Marks et al., 1995). They may be struggling with whether, when and how to talk about the HIV infection with their children. Many parents choose not to tell their children about their HIV. According to recent empirical studies, disclosure was low worldwide, especially in low- and middle-income countries (ranging from 21% to 67% in the US, and ranging from 11% to 50% in other countries) (Qiao et al., 2013a).

In previous studies, some HIV-infected parents reported concealing their HIV infection from their children because they thought they were too young to understand HIV, they worried that disclosure might harm their children psychologically or socially, they feared the stigma and discrimination that could result if children were to disclose their HIV infection to others (secondary disclosure) or they did not know how to tell their children or how to respond to children's reactions (Clifford et al., 2013). Parents who disclosed their HIV infection to their children did so because it was hard to hide the illness due to their worsening health and psychological stress, or because they needed emotional or material support from their children (including adult children) (Qiao et al., 2013a). Some parents told their children about their illness because they believed the children had the right to know, or they hoped to educate their children about HIV in order to protect them from future infection (Qiao et al., 2013a).

The age at which parents tell their children about parental HIV infection varies widely. In recent studies, the earliest ages for disclosure ranged from 6–10 years in the US and from 5–16 years in European countries (Qiao et al., 2013a). In low- and middle-income countries, many parents waited until children reached early adolescence (12–14 years) or even adulthood (older than 18 years) before disclosing their HIV status (Qiao et al., 2013a). The scope of disclosure (i.e. how much information parents disclosed to children) can be described as a continuum from non-disclosure to partial disclosure to full disclosure. Partial disclosure occurs when children are partly told about illness without learning the nature of the illness or the name of the illness (HIV infection or AIDS) (Funck-Brentano, 1995). When children receive full disclosure, they are informed of the name and nature of the illness, and the anticipated clinical outcome (Qiao et al., 2013a).

Disclosure to children about parental HIV infection can come from a variety of sources. Children may be informed by their parents (direct disclosure), by other family members or by non-family members from the social network (indirect disclosure). The disclosure could be planned (intentional disclosure), forced or could occur accidentally (unintentional disclosure). Most parents prefer to disclose HIV infection to children by themselves (Qiao et al., 2013a). However, in collectivist cultures where family support is valued, family members may play an important role in the process of disclosure (Foster, 2000; Palin et al., 2009). The family members might conduct disclosure to children or help parents to initiate conversations about parental health or HIV (De Baets et al., 2008). In low- and middle-income countries, many parents ask for professional help with disclosure from healthcare providers or social workers (Nostlinger et al., 2004). Some parents ask their healthcare providers to conduct disclosure on their behalf so that their children can be educated about HIV and adjust to the disclosure more effectively (Lo et al., 2009).

Unintentional disclosures are common in parental HIV disclosure practice. Some disclosures occur accidentally during arguments between family members (Dematteo et al., 2002a; Vallerand et al., 2005). Some occur when children confront their parents about HIV because they already know about a parent's medication or suspect their parent's health condition (Kennedy et al., 2010; Wiener et al., 1998). Sometimes children learn about parental HIV infection by overhearing conversations between adults; sometimes they are accidently informed by other family members or community members (Dematteo et al., 2002a). In situations of unintentional disclosure, children might learn numerous relevant 'family secrets', for instance, that more than one family member is infected, or other information related to a parent's HIV infection such as the parent's drug use, sexual orientation (homosexuality), or sexual history (Woodring et al., 2005). In previous studies, unintentional disclosure was often a regrettable experience for parents and was followed by negative reactions from children (Tenzek et al., 2013).

Parents who reported disclosing HIV status to their children have made recommendations for the disclosure process. They advise HIV-infected parents to develop a plan for disclosing HIV to children, and to inform children step by step from partial disclosure to full disclosure (Kennedy et al., 2010; Murphy et al., 2003). They suggest parents read written materials (e.g. brochures, pamphlets) about HIV/AIDS and talk with professionals to obtain accurate HIV knowledge (Dematteo et al., 2002a; Murphy et al., 2003). They also suggest disclosing to children at a time when the parents and children are in a good mood and are not concerned by other stressors or with important events such as an upcoming school examination (Gachanja et al., 2014; Murphy et al., 2003). When reflecting on their HIV disclosure experiences, most parents and the children who are informed of a parent's HIV status highlight the importance of the disclosure plan and strategies surrounding a parental HIV disclosure. Parents are aware that the manner in which they disclose information can have an impact not only on themselves, but also on the wider family unit (Dematteo et al., 2002a, Qiao et al., 2014, Vallerand et al., 2005, Woodring et al., 2005).

IMPACT OF PARENTAL HIV DISCLOSURE

Three recent literature reviews have synthesised the effects of parental HIV disclosure (Krauss et al., 2013; Qiao et al., 2013a; Tenzek et al., 2013). Tenzek et al. (2013) conducted a meta-analysis on the effect of maternal HIV disclosure (i.e. a mother discloses her HIV-positive status to her children). Krauss et al. (2013) examined the impact of parental disclosure on children 12 years and under. Finally, Qiao et al. (2013a) conducted a systematic review examining the consequences of parental (either father or mother) HIV disclosure on children, parents, and family functioning. Although the findings of empirical studies are mixed, parental HIV disclosure tends to be beneficial for the well-being of children, parents and their families overall.

Impact of parental HIV disclosure on children

Most children show strong emotional reactions to parents' HIV-positive status, although a proportion of children (usually at younger ages) demonstrate no immediate reaction to parental disclosure because of a limited knowledge of HIV and its consequences (Qiao et al., 2013a). Negative reactions can include being shocked, being upset, being anxious, crying, and rejecting the news (Qiao et al., 2013a). Children fear the uncertainty of their future and worry about losing their parents (Armistead et al., 2001; Palin et al., 2009) and fear developing HIV themselves (Corona et al., 2006). Parental HIV disclosure, especially when involuntary and unplanned, seems to have negative effects on children's psychosocial well-being in the short term (Krauss et al., 2013). For example, some cross-sectional studies have found positive associations between disclosure and lower emotional and social functioning, higher depressive symptoms, and more externalising symptoms among children (Qiao et al., 2013a). The pressure to maintain the secrecy of parental HIV infection may contribute to psychological problems for children (Qiao et al., 2012). Children who are told to keep their parent's HIV status a secret tend to have more negative externalising behaviour and lower social competence scores (Kirshenbaum and Nevid, 2002; Tompkins, 2007). A recent meta-analysis has reported significant associations between disclosure and internalising and externalising behaviour (Tenzek et al., 2013).

Although there are some negative effects of disclosure in the short term for most children, the long-term benefits of disclosure outweigh the temporary negative consequences. Disclosure may create an opportunity for communication and discussion about parental health problems and/or negative moods caused by their HIV infection and so the children can understand that they are not responsible for parental illness. This may relieve some of the tension and help them to adjust to parental illness (Tenzek et al., 2013). Omission or failure to tell children about parental HIV infection may aggravate the uncertainty and concerns of children about their parents' health condition (Forsyth et al., 1996). The majority of children who are told about a parent's HIV infection express satisfaction with being told the truth, so they can prepare better for their future, make decisions affecting themselves and be less anxious (Murphy et al., 2006; Tompkins, 2007). Longitudinal studies show that most children, particularly younger children, adjust to parental HIV disclosure over time, with observed emotional reactions lasting for a limited period of time (for most children, the reactions last less than one year) (Qiao et al., 2013a). According to previous studies, problem behaviour decreases over time in the children who are disclosed to, but increases in the children who are not (Lee and Rotheram-Borus, 2002). In addition, children who are informed of parental HIV infection report a higher self-concept level over time compared to those who are not informed (Murphy et al., 2009).

It is notable that adolescents tend to show poorer psychosocial adjustment to parental HIV disclosure than younger children (Hawk, 2007). Parents' illness may result in a shift of responsibilities from parents to adolescent children and accelerate their childhood (Kennedy et al., 2010; Vallerand et al., 2005). This so called 'parentification' as detailed by Jurkovic (1997) has been associated with higher levels of depression and emotional distress as well as poorer school performance and high-risk behaviour (e.g. unprotected sex, alcohol or drug use) among adolescents (Stein et al., 1999).

Impact of parental HIV disclosure on parents and family functioning

Parental HIV disclosure has positive effects on parents' well-being and family functioning in general (Qiao et al., 2013a; Tenzek et al., 2013). By disclosing their HIV infection to their children, HIV-infected parents have the chance to openly discuss their illness and future custody plan with their children, protect children from being accidently and adversely exposed to this news, educate their children about the disease and build up mutual trust with children (Tenzek et al., 2013).

Existing studies report that most HIV-infected parents do not express regret disclosing their HIV infection to their children because disclosure alleviates the stress they experienced as a result of hiding their medical condition (Delaney et al., 2008; Murphy et al., 2003; Tompkins, 2007). Some studies indicate that disclosure to children is associated with better attendance at clinical appointments, lower anxiety and depression and higher levels of social support among HIV-infected parents (Qiao et al., 2013a). However, a cross-sectional study conducted in Guangxi, China found that parents who carried out disclosure to children reported worsened mental health and poorer medication adherence (Qiao et al., 2015). Parents may be overwhelmed and nervous after their disclosure, especially in cases of unplanned disclosure or when they do not know how to respond to negative reactions from children.

Parents who have disclosed their HIV infection to children generally report a closer and stronger relationship with the children (Schrimshaw and Siegel, 2002) and higher family cohesion compared to non-disclosers (Wiener et al., 1998). Parents also describe gaining support from children following disclosure (Murphy et al., 2001; Qiao et al., 2014). Qualitative studies among children also suggest that children who are informed of their parent's HIV infection become closer to their parents, and talk openly with them (Tenzek et al., 2013). However, caution is needed in interpreting changes in family functioning following parental HIV disclosure (Hawk, 2007). Higher family cohesion may not always positively influence children's psychosocial well-being (Hawk, 2007). Spending more time with parents and taking on more household responsibilities may be indicative of anxiety, hypervigilance and overprotectiveness (Ingram and Hutchinson, 2000; Schrimshaw and Siegel, 2002; Tompkins et al., 1999).

FACTORS INFLUENCING PARENTAL HIV DISCLOSURE

Children's characteristics

A child's age is one of the key factors affecting a parent's decision about whether or not to disclose their HIV infection. Existing studies suggest that children's age may also influence what to tell (content of disclosure) and how much to tell (scope of disclosure) during the parental HIV disclosure (Qiao et al., 2013a). Parents tend to disclose fully to older children while just using partial disclosure with their younger children (Rotheram-Borus et al., 1997; Simoni et al., 2000; Woodring et al., 2005). Children's health status and mood, as well as their emotional maturity and level of understanding about disease also seem to influence parents' disclosure practice (Gachanja et al., 2014).

Parents' characteristics

Parents' health conditions and the social support that they can access or expect to receive may affect the decision to disclose and the scope of disclosure. In general, HIV-infected parents with worse health situations tend to disclose their HIV infection to children because they find it difficult to hide their disease symptoms or progression or they want to prepare their children for an upcoming parental loss and change in custody (Qiao et al., 2013a). One study in the US showed that HIV-infected mothers with a history of drug use tended to reveal more detailed information about their HIV infection (Kirshenbaum and Nevid, 2002). Older mothers were more likely to mention their potential death from AIDS (Kirshenbaum and Nevid, 2002).

Social support may influence disclosure practice in a complex way. Empirical studies suggest that HIV-infected parents with limited social support intend to disclose their disease to their children because they need practical or emotional support from their children (Zhou et al., 2013) or need to ensure that their children are mature enough to take care of themselves (Qiao et al., 2014). A recent study among HIV-infected parents in Burkina Faso indicated that being female and being divorced or widowed was positively associated with disclosing HIV infection to children (Tiendrebeogo et al., 2013). One study among HIV-infected African immigrant parents in Sweden indicated that parents who were single and had no relatives in Sweden were more likely to disclose their HIV serostatus to children (Asander et al., 2009). A qualitative study by Qiao, Li, and Stanton (2014) indicated that single HIV-infected parents who were divorced or had lost their partners to AIDS tended to tell their children that they might die from AIDS because they hoped that this might enhance their child's development and foster a greater sense of independence. A recent study in rural South Africa found having a current partner to whom the HIV-infected mother had disclosed her

HIV infection significantly increased the odds of full disclosure to children (Rochat et al., 2014). One possible interpretation is that partner disclosure may be a proxy for increased social support to cope with potential negative reactions from children, which may facilitate a disclosure to children (Rochat et al., 2014).

Socio-cultural contexts

According to the socio-ecological perspective, the disclosure process and practices are embedded within the family, community and other larger socio-cultural contexts (Hardon et al., 2013a). For example, HIV-related stigma and discrimination is still a primary barrier to HIV disclosure. In Asia and Africa, where HIV-related stigma still persists, most HIV-infected parents do not disclose their HIV infection to children because they fear severe consequences of secondary disclosure (i.e. their children tell others of parental HIV infection). If children inadvertently disclose it to the community, the children may suffer stigma and discrimination and even be deprived of property rights (Thomas et al., 2009). In Uganda, some HIV-infected parents disclose to children to ensure every family member knows the real cause of death rather than suspecting malicious witchcraft (Rwemisisi et al., 2008). One qualitative study suggested that parents who emphasise protecting children's innocence tend to shield children from parental HIV status, while parents who value children's individuality and autonomy are willing to disclose to children (Dematteo et al., 2002a).

Parents with a different cultural background express different opinions about the appropriate age at which to disclose their HIV status to their children. A study among HIV-infected mothers in the US reports that they prefer their child to be at least 6–10 years of age before they disclose their HIV status (Murphy et al., 2003). In Thailand, HIV-infected mothers state that they prefer to tell children about parental HIV infection when they are at least 10 years (Dane, 2002). In a qualitative study from multiple sites in Canada, HIV-affected families believe parental HIV disclosure should occur when children are over 11 years old and are able to understand HIV (Dematteo et al., 2002a). Parents from some Asian countries believe that their children may understand and accept parental HIV infection at older ages. For instance, in India, 15 years is believed to be an appropriate age for parental HIV disclosure (Thomas et al., 2009). In China, some parents prefer to wait until their children reached adulthood, which occurs when they become financially independent or when they get married (Qiao et al., 2014). Further studies are needed to explore the social and cultural reasons behind these variations.

Cultural values and social norms may influence the manner and the content of disclosure. For instance, in some collectivist communities in South Africa where family is valued and older women are vital for sustaining the family network, grandmothers may play an important role in HIV disclosure to children (Madiba, 2012). A study in Zimbabwe shows that 56% of parents prefer to include a healthcare worker in their disclosure process (De Baets et al., 2008). However, a study in Canada indicates that most HIV-infected parents do not want to directly involve professionals in disclosure to children, although nearly half discuss disclosure with professionals (Dematteo et al., 2002a). In Botswana, HIV-infected parents do not discuss sexual topics related to HIV transmission and prevention when they disclose their HIV infection to children because it is thought inappropriate to talk about sexual matters with children (Nam et al., 2009).

Communication strategies

In addition to socio-cultural factors, communication strategies among HIV-infected parents may contribute to the large variation in the process and consequences of parental HIV disclosure. Effective and appropriate strategies are necessary for an appropriate parental HIV disclosure (Eustace and Ilagan, 2010). Parents need to convey correct information about HIV transmission and prevention at the same time as minimising children's anxiety. They need to be open and honest during disclosure without damaging their parental identity or losing the respect of children, and protect children from potential psychological harm while ensuring they are prepared for the parent's worsening health (Edwards et al., 2014). In general, a positive and open communication style between parents and children (especially adolescents) could facilitate an appropriate disclosure (Tenzek et al., 2013). Effective strategies described by HIV-infected parents also include addressing HIV as a chronic and manageable disease, keeping conversations educational and integrating HIV-related topics within more general conversations (Edwards et al., 2014). Some HIV-infected parents also recommend interactive conversations between parents and adolescent children in which adolescents could have a 'voice' (talk about their concerns) and a 'choice' (choose their own effective HIV prevention strategy) during HIV disclosure (Edwards and Reis, 2014).

Not all HIV-infected parents are able to use effective and appropriate communication strategies, especially in cultural contexts (e.g. China) where parents may not openly communicate with children about important issues in the family and about a parent's feelings (Xia et al., 2008). Empirical studies suggest that most HIV-infected parents require professional support in developing strategies for HIV-related conversations with their children (Nam et al., 2009; Nostlinger et al., 2004; Qiao et al., 2014; Tiendrebeogo et al., 2013).

However, qualitative interviews among healthcare workers or key informants in relevant health organisations show that the suggestions and advice from health professionals or counsellors are inconsistent due to lack of policy and training guidelines on parental HIV disclosure (Moyer et al., 2013, Rwemisisi et al., 2008). Intervention and training related to HIV disclosure are urgently needed for HIV-infected parents, healthcare workers and counsellors working closely with HIV patients (Hardon et al., 2013b).

PARENTAL HIV DISCLOSURE INTERVENTIONS

In a systematic literature review, Kennedy et al. (2015) indicated that there are very few intervention studies in low- and middle-income countries that aim to help HIV-infected parents disclose their HIV infection to their children (i.e. one of the 13 published HIV disclosure intervention studies they reviewed focused on parental disclosure). Globally, the number of these interventions is increasing but it remains relatively small, given the numerous demands in practice (WHO, 2011). This section briefly introduces four parental HIV disclosure interventions, focusing on the theories or conceptual frameworks in which they are grounded, the curriculum or intervention activities that they deliver, and their effects on parental HIV disclosure practices. See Table 10.2 for information about these interventions.

Teens and Adults Learning to Communicate (TALC) intervention

An early intervention related to parental HIV disclosure is a two-year randomised controlled trial of 307 parents living with AIDS and 412 adolescent children (11–18 years of age at baseline) in New York (Rotheram-Borus et al., 2001). The TALC intervention was initiated in 1993, targeting both parents and their adolescent children who were already aware of their parent's HIV infection. The parent-focused intervention was designed to help parents improve their coping skills, reduce risk behaviour and create positive family routines. The adolescent-focused intervention aimed to help adolescents adjust to parental illness, improve family relationships and reduce youth risk-taking behaviour. The intervention design was guided by Social Learning Theory, which provides a conceptual framework for how individuals change their behaviour and identify factors that must be changed (e.g. skills, ability, expectations of competence and efficacy, etc.) (Kelly, 1995).

The structured intervention was delivered in small groups over 12 weeks by social workers and graduate students in clinical psychology, who received five days of intensive training for each of two modules. Module 1 included eight sessions for parents alone and Module 2 included 16 sessions for both

TABLE 10.2 Summary of parental HIV disclosure interventions

Intervention, Study design, reference	Year of study	Site	Theoretical framework	Study population	Intervention approach	Intervention content	Outcomes
TALC intervention, 24-month RCT (Rotheram-Borus et al., 2001)	1993–1994	New York, USA	Social Learning theory (Kelly, 1995)	307 parents living with AIDS; 412 adolescent children (11–18 years of age at baseline)	Structured 24-session intervention organised into two modules (eight for parents alone; 16 for parents and adolescents group). Delivered by social workers and trained graduate students over 12 weeks (two sessions per week).	Parents: Coping skills with illness and disclosure, emotional management, custody plan and parenting skills. Adolescents: Adjustment to parental illness, family relationship and risky acts reduction.	Reduced emotional distress and multiple problem behaviour among both parents and adolescents, and improved adolescents' self-esteem. No difference was found between the intervention and control groups in terms of parent's coping style or scope of disclosure.
TRACK intervention, 9-month RCT (Murphy et al., 2011)	n/a	Los Angeles, USA	Disclosure Decision-Making Model (Derlega et al., 2004)	80 HIV-positive mothers and their children (6–12 years of age at baseline)	Structured three-session intervention including home visits, telephone support and educational materials. Sessions were spaced one week apart.	Parents: Children's typical development, disclosure readiness and decision making, mother-child communication, behavioural practice for disclosure (role-play exercise).	Increased disclosure rate, disclosure self-efficacy, promoted mother-child communication, and improved maternal emotional functioning. The intervention also showed initial efficacy in reducing depression and anxiety and increasing happiness feelings among children.

(*continued*)

Intervention, Study design, reference	Year of study	Site	Theoretical framework	Study population	Intervention approach	Intervention content	Outcomes
Amagugu intervention, Pre-/post-test study (Rochat et al., 2014)	2010–2012	South Africa KwaZulu-Natal province	Disclosure Decision-Making Model (Derlega et al., 2004)	281 HIV-positive mothers and their HIV-uninfected children (6–10 years of age at baseline)	Home-based structured training and counselling with six sessions, including printed materials, narrative therapeutic tools and child-friendly activities and games. Delivered in participant's house by local lay counsellors and community healthcare workers over a six- to eight-week period.	Parents: Pros and cons of disclosure, family relationship, life stories of living with HIV, planning and preparing the disclosure event, taking children to clinic visits and custody planning.	High rates of full HIV disclosure to children (60%) among the HIV-positive mothers participating in the intervention, and improved mental health conditions among the majority of the children following the intervention. For children at risk of withdrawn-depressed syndromes at baseline, disclosure, particularly the partial disclosure, was significantly beneficial for their psychological well-being.
ICOPE intervention, 36-month RCT On-going project (Li et al.)	2013–2017	China Guangxi Province	Disclosure Process Chaudoir Model (Chaudoir et al., 2011) and the Five-Stage Disclosure Process Model (Gerson et al., 2001) children's developmental stages (Piaget, 1972)	791 HIV-positive parents with children aged 6–15 years at baseline; 313 healthcare workers in HIV clinics.	Structured five-session group intervention among parents. Two-session intervention among healthcare workers. The intervention for parents was delivered by trained healthcare workers, and the intervention for healthcare workers was delivered by research staff in Guangxi CDC.	Parents: Positive coping with HIV and self-care (coping with stigma, emotional control), decision making of disclosure, developing developmentally appropriate disclosure plan and strategies, and access to social support and post-disclosure counselling. Healthcare workers: similar components in the parent curriculum and a clinical guideline for parental HIV disclosure.	The process evaluation suggested that the intervention was feasible and acceptable to HIV-positive parents and local healthcare workers.

parents and adolescents. In Module 2, each intervention activity involved some time with parents and children meeting in separate groups and some time when parents and children were together. A typical intervention activity was held at a community centre each Saturday with one two-hour session in the morning and another two-hour session in the afternoon. Transportation, breakfast, lunch and child care were provided. Each session included reviewing behavioural successes over the past week, introducing new materials and skills and setting new goals. Tools for learning emotional self-control ('feeling thermometer') and problem solving ('charting problems') were routinely used in sessions. The intervention significantly reduced emotional distress, multiple problem behaviour among both parents and adolescents and improved adolescents' self-esteem. However, no difference was found between the intervention and control groups in terms of a parent's coping style (Rotheram-Borus et al., 2001).

Teaching, Raising, and Communicating with Kids (TRACK) intervention

Murphy et al. designed and implemented a nine-month randomised controlled trial among 80 HIV-infected mothers and their children (6–12 years of age at baseline) in Los Angeles (Murphy et al., 2011). The TRACK intervention aimed to enhance family communication and parenting skills, assist mothers in preparing for disclosure, increase disclosure, improve mental health among both mothers and their children and improve the parent-child relationship and family functioning. The intervention design was grounded in the Disclosure Decision-Making Model (DDMM), which posits that individual, temporal and relational contexts and the social environment affect the decision making of disclosure (Derlega et al., 2004). The intervention design also focused on family context and family relationship (e.g. intrafamilial communication and parenting skills).

The TRACK was delivered in three sessions, which included home visits, telephone support and educational materials. The intervention sessions were spaced approximately one week apart. Session 1 addressed children's typical development. Session 2 focused on improving mother-child communication. Session 3 included behavioural practice for disclosure (i.e. role-play exercises) and a final discussion on disclosure readiness and positive reinforcement from the facilitator. This intervention successfully increased the disclosure rate and disclosure self-efficacy, promoted mother-child communication and improved maternal emotional functioning. The intervention was also effective at reducing depression and anxiety and at increasing happiness among children (Derlega et al., 2004).

The Amagugu intervention

One maternal HIV disclosure intervention conducted in rural South Africa during 2010 to 2012 enrolled 281 HIV-infected women and their uninfected children aged 6–10 years (Rochat et al., 2014). The Amagugu (a Zulu term meaning 'Treasures') intervention focused on increasing maternal HIV disclosure in order to benefit family relationships, increase children's knowledge about HIV and health, and improve the quality of custody planning for the children (Rochat et al., 2013). As with the TRACK, the Amagugu intervention was grounded in the Disclosure Decision-Making Model (Derlega et al., 2004), in addition to being informed by recent literature reviews on parental HIV disclosure (Murphy, 2008; Qiao et al., 2013a). During the implementation process, this intervention also highlighted the family-centred approach. The intervention activities were mainly conducted in participants' homes. Family members were encouraged to discuss not only HIV disclosure issues but also parenting skills, custody and care plans and challenges for family regular clinic visits.

The six session intervention package included printed materials, narrative therapeutic tools (i.e. therapeutic tools to transform personal experiences into personal stories that are given meaning and help shape a person's identity; the therapist utilises the power of people's personal stories to discover the life purpose of the narrator) and child-friendly activities and games. The intervention sessions were delivered in participants' homes by local lay counsellors and community healthcare workers over a six- to eight-week period. HIV-infected mothers and their children were supposed to receive the intervention but fathers and other family members were encouraged to join in. The sessions covered issues related to disclosure, family relationships, life stories of living with HIV, planning and preparing the disclosure event, taking children to clinic visits and custody planning. The uncontrolled pre- and post-intervention evaluation study indicated high rates of full HIV disclosure to children (60%) among the HIV-infected mothers participating in the intervention, with improved mental health among the majority of the children in the intervention. For children at risk of withdrawn-depressed symptoms at baseline, disclosure, particularly partial disclosure, was significantly beneficial for their psychological well-being (Rochat et al., 2014).

Interactive Communication with Openness, Passion and Empowerment (ICOPE) intervention

Another parental HIV disclosure intervention in low- and middle-income countries is the ICOPE intervention, developed and evaluated with an ongoing longitudinal randomised controlled trial among 791 HIV-infected parents with children aged 6–15 years and 313 healthcare workers in HIV clinics in Guangxi, China. This multi-level intervention aimed to (i) provide healthcare workers with training and guidelines so they could obtain sufficient knowledge, skills and confidence to assist HIV-infected parents with the process of disclosing their HIV infection to their children; and (ii) deliver structured intervention activities among HIV-infected parents to enhance their ability to plan and carry out parental HIV disclosure, increase the knowledge of HIV and improve communication skills needed for HIV disclosure, encourage the development of an appropriate plan for HIV disclosure and for conducting the disclosure, and improve medical adherence and clinical outcomes of parents as well as the psychological well-being of both parents and children. The ICOPE intervention design was guided by the Disclosure Process Model (Chaudoir et al., 2011) and the Five-Stage Disclosure Process Model (Gerson et al., 2001) and was also consistent with the Piaget's theory of children's development (Piaget, 1951).

Based on qualitative data collected from parents, children, local healthcare workers and community members and informed by both TALC and TRACK interventions, The ICOPE intervention package consists of five two-hour sessions for parents, focusing on positive coping (e.g. coping with stigma, emotional control), disclosure decision making, developing a developmentally appropriate disclosure plan and accessing social support and post-disclosure counselling. The intervention for healthcare workers is made up of two 45-minute sessions organised around two primary themes: knowledge of child cognitive development and effective parent-child communication skills in the context of parental disclosure (e.g. how to help children understand HIV). The intervention for parents was delivered to groups in local HIV clinics by healthcare workers who were selected as facilitators and received a three-day intensive training workshop. The intervention for healthcare workers was delivered by research staff in provisional Centres for Disease Control. A process evaluation suggested that the intervention was feasible and acceptable both to HIV-infected parents and local healthcare workers.

The design and implementation of the four sample interventions discussed here suggest a set of common components in parental HIV disclosure intervention and core principles in guiding the development and adaptation of the intervention within different cultural settings. On the one hand, informed by existing theoretical and empirical studies, these interventions specify common individual, interpersonal and socio-cultural factors influencing parental HIV disclosure. They aim to increase developmentally and culturally appropriate disclosure and to improve the well-being of parents and children. The key factors to be considered include parents' knowledge of the child's developmental stage, their communication and coping skills, the parent-child relationship and family functioning, in addition to stigma and social support. On the other hand, the different features of the interventions in terms of target populations and goals, the theoretical framework, intervention content and approach, reflect the growth of understanding of parental HIV disclosure and are consistent with the trends of HIV prevention and treatment. For instance, the TALC intervention targeted parents in New York in 1994 diagnosed with AIDS who typically only lived about 14 months on average (Rotheram-Borus et al., 2001). For their children, a sudden and unexpected parental loss resulted in more negative outcomes than one that had been prepared for. Therefore, post-disclosure coping and making custody plans were prioritised in the intervention goals.

Disclosure interventions have moved beyond a focus on one aspect of parental HIV disclosure (e.g. post-disclosure coping, decision making about disclosure), with recent interventions focusing on a series of steps covering the entire disclosure process. All the interventions discussed here employed multiple sessions and a structured intervention curriculum, but the specific content and delivery varied with different socio-cultural settings. In resource-limited settings, the disclosure interventions were mainly delivered through trained local healthcare workers/lay counsellors rather than professionals (e.g. social workers, psychiatrists, counsellors). This strategy echoes the recent recommendation by WHO about de-centralising HIV prevention and care in low- and middle-income countries by delegating the tasks of HIV prevention and care to healthcare workers with shorter training and lower skill requirement (Callaghan et al., 2010; Selke et al., 2010). Although the efficacy of parental HIV disclosure intervention needs to be proven through further evaluation studies with rigorous study designs, the existing findings suggest that it is feasible to implement interventions among HIV-infected parents to help them to conduct appropriate disclosure, and that the interventions can be effective at improving the well-being of both parents and children. Lessons from existing interventions may provide valuable implications for both research and practice in the area of parental HIV disclosure.

IMPLICATIONS

Guidelines for healthcare providers and professionals

Following a review of existing research on parental HIV disclosure, we propose a guideline for healthcare providers and professionals working closely with HIV-infected parents by positing five general considerations and specifying the content of disclosure and communication strategies for children at different cognitive developmental stages.

Consideration 1

Parental HIV disclosure is not an event but a complex and gradual process. A typical voluntary and planned parental HIV disclosure may include a series of steps: making a decision, developing a disclosure plan/strategy, conducting the disclosure and coping with the child's reactions. In addition, the scope and content of disclosure may change along with children's growth and thus disclosure may not be completed within one conversation. This nature of parental HIV disclosure requires healthcare providers and related professionals to be prepared to offer assistance, advice and counselling at each step because the details at each step may influence the consequences of disclosure and have further impact on the outcomes among parents, children and their families. Counting the number of disclosure events does not make much sense given the large variance between an involuntary and unplanned disclosure and a well-planned and developmentally appropriate one in terms of consequences and impact on children. Interventions need to target improving the quality of parental HIV disclosure, with a focus on each step of the disclosure process.

Consideration 2

Parental HIV disclosure is not isolated, but embedded in a particular social context. The meanings and behaviour related to disclosure are constructed within a person's internal, interpersonal and social context and may be changeable and reversible over time (Moses and Tomlinson, 2013). Health professionals need to help HIV-infected parents to develop a disclosure plan that fits the particular parent-child relationship, family context and social norms in local communities. The decision to disclose and strategies related to disclosure should be planned and well informed. For example, healthcare workers should not place undue pressure on the parents to disclose HIV infection to children without addressing the issues of stigma and discrimination, the stress for parents and the possible negative consequences from HIV disclosure.

Consideration 3

Parental HIV disclosure should be developmentally and culturally appropriate and meet the diverse needs of HIV-infected parents and their children. There is no 'one size fits all' intervention approach. Guidelines on disclosure to children issued by WHO and many national organisations recommend developmentally appropriate disclosure to children. This requires that disclosers fully consider and assess children's cognitive development stage, emotional maturity and their ability to understand HIV (WHO, 2011). Empirical studies have suggested that by 10–13 years it is appropriate for HIV-infected children to be informed of their parent's illness (Sahay, 2013) because by that age children are able to understand the finality of death, can define illness as a set of symptoms by age 9 and can understand multiple causes of illness and various body responses to illness by age 12 (Perrin and Gerrity, 1981). Recent interventions have focused on disclosing parental HIV infection to primary school-age children (6–12 years of age) because they have been identified as a group with particular developmental needs around understanding and coping with parental life-threatening diseases (Christ and Christ, 2006; King et al., 2009). However, healthcare workers need to respect local social norms and adapt the intervention design and approach to the local cultural context. Among HIV disclosure interventions, broad intervention approaches included cognitive behavioural support groups, home-based visits and peer/community healthcare workers (Kennedy et al., 2015). One approach rooted in one setting may not be suitable for another setting. In areas where people living with HIV still suffer severe stigma and discrimination from their neighbourhood, home visiting may not be acceptable to participants and/or their families. Resource-intense approaches in urban areas may not be feasible in resource-limited settings.

Consideration 4

Parental HIV disclosure should be an empowering process for HIV-infected parents and their families. HIV-infected parents in different settings may have different expectations of healthcare workers and professionals. In some sociocultural contexts, healthcare workers have authority due to their knowledge and expertise and make decisions related to HIV disclosure for patients (Li et al., 2007). However, a successful disclosure requires that parents do not feel coerced into disclosing to children before they are adequately prepared to do so (Dematteo et al., 2002b). Mutual respect and trust between parents and healthcare workers is the cornerstone of effective counselling and support. Healthcare workers need to recognise that it is parents who make the final decision to disclose their HIV infection to children. Collaborating with HIV-infected parents requires healthcare workers to respect and meet the parents' need for confidentiality, create a trusting and safe environment for parents in which to discuss their disclosure plan and honestly express their opinions to provide different perspectives (Gerson et al., 2001; Tasker, 1992). The role of healthcare workers is not to push HIV-infected parents to conduct a reckless disclosure, but to empower them by enhancing family communication, improving family relationships and increasing the parent's effectiveness so that they feel ready and confident for disclosure and may benefit from the disclosure in the long-term.

Consideration 5

Parental HIV disclosure interventions should be guided by ethical principles. Patients' autonomy, privacy and other rights are valued in today's legislation and social policies related to healthcare, including HIV disclosure practice (Nie, 2011). The policies and clinical guidelines need to underline the privacy and confidentiality of HIV-positive parents as a basic component of patients' rights. To safeguard the rights and well-being of HIV patients, healthcare workers need to receive training in ethics so they can develop the sensitivity to a range of ethically relevant considerations in practice; they should not initiate a parental HIV disclosure without consent from the HIV-infected parents; and they should ensure post-counselling or psychosocial support is in place to address potential adverse consequences of the disclosure.

Finally, see Table 10.3 for a clinical guide for parental HIV disclosure. This has been adapted from *Step by Step Guide for Conversation with Children (Toward Disclosure)* (Naidoo et al., 2010), developed by an interdisciplinary team of clinicians and researchers in South Africa. The South Africa Guide was originally designed for healthcare professionals and counsellors working with HIV-infected children and their caregivers. The recommended content of disclosure and communication strategies has been modified, based on preliminary qualitative studies for the ICOPE project (Qiao et al., 2014; Zhou et al., 2013).

RECOMMENDATIONS FOR FUTURE RESEARCH

Parental HIV disclosure has been emphasised as an important response to parental HIV and is a key component in efforts to prevent HIV transmission from children, promote custody planning and improve the well-being of HIV-infected parents and their children. After reviewing the rapidly increasing research and intervention work in this area, we make the following suggestions for future studies and interventions.

First, theoretical and empirical studies should be integrated and should build on each other. Although there is a growing interest in parental HIV disclosure among researchers and healthcare providers, the theoretical frameworks concerning parental HIV disclosure are limited, and the majority of existing empirical studies have not been conducted within a theoretical

TABLE 10.3 Clinical guideline for healthcare workers and counselors on parental HIV disclosure

Parental HIV disclosure readiness	• Informing parents of the benefits and risks for parental HIV disclosure • Assessing parental health condition and psychosocial well-being • Assessing child's developmental stage and emotional maturity • Assessing family context and family relationship • Providing social support and other potential resources		
Child developmental stages	**6-10 years** • Child provides illness explanations based on sequence • Child begins to understand that disease can be passed on through swallowing or inhaling	**11-12 years** • Abstract thinking and reasoning develops • Child begins to view body as a system and provides illness explanations based on interaction of a number of factors • Child can explain the cause of illness as a complex interaction between host and agent	**13-18 years** • More abstract thinking (understands future consequences of actions) • Increasingly making decisions on their own regarding identity, independence, school, career • Puberty/sexual development • Dependence on caregivers decreases • Importance of relationships with peers increases
Disclosure content	• Introduce ideas of health and illness • Briefly describe symptoms of HIV infection • Explain medicines help to keep a body healthy and strong • Introduce infections as 'germs' that can hurt or damage the body/make you sick or hurt	• Explain that the germ concerned is a virus • Naming of virus as HIV may occur but not essential • Introduce the HIV transmission routes and how children can protect themselves • May explain how parents have developed HIV infection	• Check understanding of health, medicines, sexual development and HIV infection • Explain HIV and AIDS in detail • Talk about parental HIV infection for educational purposes • Need to understand safer sex, family planning, confidentiality

(*continued*)

Disclosure content (*cont.*)	• Briefly introduce how to protect their health at home (avoid transmission through blood) • Highlight parents' ability to take care of themselves and children • Explain the information is private	• Need to explain that information is private and should only be shared with those agreed with the parents/caregiver(s) • Help the child identify who they can talk with about parental illness	• Preparation for future, encourage direct involvement in discussions and decisions • Provide potential resources for counseling or any peer support group
Disclosure scope	Partial disclosure	Partial disclosure	Full disclosure
Disclosure strategy	• Use visual aids such as drawings or media to demonstrate concepts • Use of play and more language-based communication can be more effective with age • Emphasize the concepts of health, wellness, and body • Discuss issues related to privacy, stigma, and confidentiality in an age-appropriate manner	• Use visual aids such as books or websites to demonstrate the key concepts in HIV, the immune system, and illness • Use slightly more complex language to convey the interactions between health, illness, and treatment • Discuss and explore issues regarding HIV transmission using examples of age-appropriate behaviors • Discuss issues related to privacy, stigma, and confidentiality • Explore normal sexual development and education	• Interactive conversation • Recognize and respect child's independence • Correct misconceptions of HIV and HIV prevention • Protect children from risk-taking behaviours • Integrate with reproductive health education • Engage children in discussion of any future custody plan within the family

Notes: adapted from 'Step by Step Guide for Conversation with Children (Toward Disclosure)' (Naidoo, Melvin, & Houghton, 2010) and 'Disclosure of HIV to perinatally infected children and adolescents' New York State Department of Health AIDS Institute. 2009.

framework (Qiao et al., 2013a). As a result, we do not have sufficient empirical evidence to support or question the existing theoretical models, and we also lack common conceptual systems to compare findings from diverse settings.

Second, future studies need to employ rigorous research methodology. For instance, future quantitative studies should utilise a longitudinal study design whenever possible to establish a meaningful causal relationship in the consequences of disclosure and recruit a large enough sample size of respondents to ensure statistical power to detect effects. In addition, measurement of disclosure practice in some studies was limited and did not assess the scope or approach of disclosure, such as partial disclosure/full disclosure or forced disclosure/planned disclosure. Without data on these different features of disclosure, it is difficult to determine the effects of various types of disclosure. The lack of standard measurement also makes it difficult to compare results across studies.

Third, future research and intervention concerning parental HIV disclosure needs multidisciplinary insight and collaboration. There are five important aspects to the complex process of parental HIV disclosure: international norms, national legislation and public health recommendations; household and family settings; couples' relationships; parental relationships; and relationships between health workers and HIV-infected parents (Hardon et al., 2013a). A complete understanding of how people pursue disclosure strategies in one or more of these social spaces requires various theoretical perspectives. For example, researchers from public health and health psychology may view disclosure as a health-related behaviour (Rotheram-Borus et al., 2001). Communication experts may examine disclosure through theories of information management and uncertainty (Afifi and Afili, 2009). Anthropologists may be interested in various meanings of disclosure in diverse cultural contexts (Obermeyer et al., 2011), while ethicists will discuss the dilemma between respecting a HIV-infected person's privacy and protecting people around patients (Seidel, 1996). Multidisciplinary collaboration has been rising and contributing to developing more comprehensive and culturally acceptable interventions.

Fourth, future interventions should apply a multi-level approach. Since parental HIV disclosure is embedded in social relationships and social contexts, we recommend social ecological models as the basis for intervention design. Social ecological models recognise that individuals are embedded in larger social systems and highlight interactions between individuals and their environment that underlie behaviour and health outcomes (Golden and Earp, 2012). The social-ecological approach for health promotion identifies factors to be targeted at various key levels by interventions: intrapersonal, interpersonal, organisational, community and public policy (McLeroy et al., 1988). This approach also highlights that factors at multiple levels are interactive and reinforcing (Stokols, 1996). Existing HIV disclosure interventions have focused on parents, children and families, but future interventions may extend to community and policy levels.

Fifth, future interventions should include multiple components related to HIV prevention and care. Parental HIV disclosure is closely associated with other issues in HIV prevention and treatment as well as the psychological adjustment of children affected by HIV/AIDS. Parental HIV disclosure interventions could be integrated with efforts to reduce HIV-related stigma, improve adherence to treatment and promote the resilience of children. For example, a disclosure intervention could be linked with an intervention to reduce stigma and discrimination in order to have maximum effectiveness at improving the physical and psychosocial well-being of both parents and children. A supportive environment for HIV-infected parents could facilitate their full benefit from disclosure. Disclosure to family and community could contribute to creating a trusting environment to minimise or mitigate the negative effect of HIV-related stigma (Mill, 2003).

CONCLUSION

Disclosure of parental HIV infection to children can benefit both parents and children in the long term, although it is a significant challenge for HIV-infected parents due to HIV-related stigma and other intrapersonal, interpersonal and environmental barriers. The high proportion of involuntary, unplanned disclosures highlights the importance of providing parents with appropriate disclosure-related training and counselling services. Parental HIV disclosure is a continuing conversation process between parents, children and healthcare workers, embedded in a particular family relationship and socio-cultural contexts. A successful disclosure should be developmentally, culturally and ethically appropriate, and planned, acted on and managed by empowered HIV-infected parents (which may include their adolescent children) and followed by sufficient post-disclosure counselling and social support.

Future studies need to be guided by solid theoretical frameworks, with appropriate study design and standardised measurement, and with multidisciplinary perspectives. There is no 'one size fits all' intervention approach, but we recommend a multi-level intervention integrated with other components in HIV prevention and treatment. Preliminary evaluation studies for existing intervention projects have proved it is feasible to assist HIV-infected parents in disclosing their illness to children (Qiao et al., 2013a; Rochat et al., 2014). Further efforts from multiple stakeholders are needed so that the parents, children and families can have their own 'voice' and make their informed 'choice' in disclosure practice to maximise the psychosocial and medical benefits in the long term.

REFERENCES

Afifi, T.D., Afili, W.A. (2009). *Uncertainty, information management, and disclosure decisions: Theories and applications*. New York: Routledge.

Armistead, L., Tannenbaum, L., Forehand, R., Morse, E. and Morse, P. (2001). Disclosing HIV status: Are mothers telling their children? *Journal of Pediatric Psychology*, 26, 11–20.

Asander, A.S., Bjorkman, A., Belfrace, E., Faxelid, E. (2009). HIV-infected African parents living in Stockholm, Sweden: Disclosure and planning for their children's future. *Health and Social Work*, 34, 107–115.

Babcock, J.H. (1998). Involving family and significant others in acute care. In: Aronstein, D.M., Thompson, B.J., [eds], *HIV and social work*. Harrington; Binghamton, NY, pp. 101–108.

Bibace, R., Walsh, M.E. (1978). Developmental stages in children's conceptions of illness. In: Stone, G., Cohen, F., Alder, N. [eds], *Health psychology: a handbook*. Jossey-Bass: San Francisco, pp. 285–301.

Callaghan, M., Ford, N., Schneider, H. (2010). A systematic review of task-shifting for HIV treatment and care in Africa. *Human Resources for Health*, 8, 8.

Chaudoir, S.R., Fisher, J.D., Simoni, J.M. (2011). Understanding HIV disclosure: A review and application of the Disclosure Processes Model. *Social Science and Medicine*, 72, 1618–1629.

Chelune, G.J. (1979). Measuring openness in interpersonal communication. In G.J. Chelune (Ed.) *Origins, patterns and implications of openness in interpersonal relationships*. San Francisco, CA: Jossey-Bass.

Christ, G.H., Christ, A.E. (2006). Current approaches to helping children cope with a parent's terminal illness. *CA: A Cancer Journal for Clinicians*, 56, 197–212.

Clifford, G., Craig, G.M., McCourt, C., Barrow, G. (2013). What are the benefits and barriers of communicating parental HIV status to seronegative children and the implications for Jamaica? A narrative review of the literature in low/middle income countries. *The West Indian Medical Journal*, 62, 357–363.

Corona, R., Beckett, M.K., Cowgill, B.O., Elliott, M.N., Murphy, D.A., Zhou, A.J., Schuster, M.A. (2006). Do children know their parent's HIV status? Parental reports of child awareness in a nationally representative sample. *Ambulatory Pediatrics*, 6, 138–144.

Cozby, P.C. (1973). Self-disclosure: A literature review. *Psychological Bulletin*, 79, 73–91.

Dane, B. (2002). Disclosure: The voices of Thai women living with HIV/AIDS. *International Social Work*, 45, 185–204.

De Baets, A.J., Sifovo, S., Parsons, R., Pazvakavambwa, I.E. (2008). HIV disclosure and discussions about grief with Shona children: A comparison between health care workers and community members in Eastern Zimbabwe. *Social Science and Medicine*, 66, 479–491.

Delaney, R.O., Serovich, J.M., Lim, J.Y. (2008). Reasons for and against maternal HIV disclosure to children and perceived child reaction. *AIDS Care*, 20, 876–880.

Dematteo, D., Harrison, C., Arneson, C., Goldie, R.S., Lefebvre, A., Read, S.E., King, S.M. (2002a). Disclosing HIV/AIDS to children: The paths families take to truthtelling. *Psychology, Health and Medicine*, 7, 339–356.

Dematteo, D., Wells, L.M., Salter Goldie, R., King, S.M. (2002b). The 'family' context of HIV: A need for comprehensive health and social policies. *AIDS Care*, 14, 261–278.

Derlega, V.J., Winstead, B.A., Greene, K., Serovich, J.M., Elwood, W.N. (2004). Reasons for HIV disclosure/nondisclosure in close relationships: Testing a model of HIV-disclosure decision making. *Journal of Social and Clinical Psychology*, 23, 747–767.

Edwards, L.L., Donovan-Kicken, E., Reis, J.S. (2014). Communicating in complex situations: A normative approach to HIV-related talk among parents who are HIV+. *Health Communication*, 29, 364–374.

Edwards, L.L., Reis, J.S. (2014). A five step process for interactive parent-adolescent communication about HIV prevention: Advice from parents living with HIV/AIDS. *Journal of HIV/AIDS and Social Services*, 13, 59–78.

Eustace, R.W., Ilagan, P.R. (2010). HIV disclosure among HIV positive individuals: A concept analysis. *Journal of Advanced Nursing*, 66, 2094–2103.

Fauci, A., Whitescarver, J. (2011). The 30th anniversary of the first reported cases of AIDS. *MedlinePlus* [online], 6. Available: www.nlm.nih.gov/medlineplus/magazine/issues/summer11/articles/summer11pg10-12.html (accessed 24 January 2015).

Forsyth, B.W., Damour, L., Nagler, S., Adnopoz, J. (1996). The psychological effects of parental human immunodeficiency virus infection on uninfected children. *Archives of Pediatric and Adolescent Medicine*, 150, 1015–1020.

Foster, G. (2000). The capacity of t he external family safety net for orphans in Africa. *Psychology Health and Medicine* 5, 55–59.

Funck-Brentano, I. (1995). [Informing a child about his illness in HIV infection: Words and meaning]. *La Psychiatrie de l'Enfant*, 38, 109–139.

Gachanja, G., Burkholder, G.J., Ferraro, A. (2014). HIV-positive parents, HIV-positive children, and HIV-negative children's perspectives on disclosure of a parent's and child's illness in Kenya. *PeerJ*, 2, e486.

Gerson, A.C., Joyner, M., Fosarelli, P., Butz, A., Wissow, L., Lee, S., Marks, P., Hutton, N. (2001). Disclosure of HIV diagnosis to children: When, where, why, and how. *Journal of Pediatric Health Care*, 15, 161–167.

Golden, S.D., Earp, J.A. (2012). Social ecological approaches to individuals and their contexts: Twenty years of health education and behavior health promotion interventions. *Health Education and Behavior*, 39, 364–372.

Hardon, A., Desclaux, A., Lugalla, J. (2013a). Disclosure in times of ART: A relational analysis of social practices. *SAHARA J*, 10(S1), S1–4.

Hardon, A., Gomez, G.B., Vernooij, E., Desclaux, A., Wanyenze, R.K., Ky-Zerbo, O., Kageha, E., Namakhoma, I., Kinsman, J., Spronk, C., Meij, E., Neuman, M., Obermeyer, C.M. (2013b). Do support groups members disclose less to their partners? The dynamics of HIV disclosure in four African countries. *BMC Public Health*, 13, 589.

Hawk, S.T. (2007). Disclosures of maternal HIV infection to seronegative children: A literature review. *Journal of Social and Personal Relationships*, 24, 657–673.

Ingram, D., Hutchinson, S.A. (2000). Double binds and the reproductive and mothering experiences of HIV-positive women. *Qualitative Health Research*, 10, 117–132.

Jurkovic, G.J. (1997). *Lost childhoods: The plight of the parentified child.* New York: Brunner Routledge.

Kalichman, S.C. (1995). *Understanding AIDS: A guide for mental health professionals.* American Psychological Association: Washington, DC.

Kalichman, S.C., Hunter, T.L. (1992). The disclosure of celebrity HIV infection: Its effects on public attitudes. *American Journal of Public Health*, 82, 1374–1376.

Kelly, J.A. (1995). *Changing HIV risk behavior: Practical strategies.* New York: Guilford Press.

Kennedy, D.P., Cowgill, B.O., Bogart, L.M., Corona, R., Ryan, G.W., Murphy, D.A., Nguyen, T., Schuster, M.A. (2010). Parents' disclosure of their HIV infection to their children in the context of the family. *AIDS and Behavior*, 14, 1095–1105.

Kennedy, C.E., Fonner, V.A., Armstrong, K.A., O'Reilly, K.R., Sweat, M.D. (2015). Increasing HIV serostatus disclosure in low- and middle-income countries: A systematic review of intervention evaluations. *AIDS*, 29 (S1) S7-S23.

King, E., De Silva, M., Stein, A., Patel, V. (2009). Interventions for improving the psychosocial well-being of children affected by HIV and AIDS. *Cochrane Database Systematic Reviews*, CD006733.

Kirshenbaum, S.B., Nevid, J.S. (2002). The specificity of maternal disclosure of HIV/AIDS in relation to children's adjustment. *AIDS Education and Prevention*, 14, 1–16.

Koopman, H.M., Baars, R.M., Chaplin, J., Zwinderman, K.H. (2004). Illness through the eyes of the child: The development of children's understanding of the causes of illness. *Patient Education and Counseling*, 55, 363–370.

Krauss, B.J., Letteney, S., De Baets, A.J., Baggaley, R., Okero, F.A. (2013). Caregiver's HIV disclosure to children 12 years and under: A review and analysis of the evidence. *AIDS Care*, 25, 415–429.

Lee, M.B., Rotheram-Borus, M.J. (2002). Parents' disclosure of HIV to their children. *AIDS*, 16, 2201–2207.

Lesch, A., Swartz, L., Kagee, A., Moodley, K., Kafaar, Z., Myer, L., Cotton, M. (2007). Paediatric HIV/AIDS disclosure: Towards a developmental and process-oriented approach. *AIDS Care*, 19, 811–816.

Li, L., Sun, S., Wu Z., Wu, S., Lin, C., Yan, Z. (2007). Disclosure of HIV status is a family matter: Field notes from China. *Journal of Family Psychology*, 21, 307–314.

Li, X., Naar-King, S., Barnett, D., Stanton, B., Fang, X, Thurston, C. (2008). A developmental psychopathology framework of the psychosocial needs of children orphaned by HIV. *Journal of the Association of Nurses in Aids Care*, 19, 147–157.

Lo, S.C., Zea, M.C., Poppen, P.J. (2009). Information, uncertainty, and sexual disclosures in the era of HIV/AIDS. In T.D. Afifi, W.A. Afifi (Eds) *Uncertainty, information management, and disclosure decisions: Theories and applications*. New York and London: Taylor and Francis Group.

Madiba, S. (2012). Patterns of HIV diagnosis disclosure to infected children and family members: Data from a paediatric antiretroviral program in South Africa. *World Journal of AIDS*, 2, 212–221.

Marks, G., Mason, H.R., Simoni, J.M. (1995). The prevalence of patient disclosure of HIV infection to doctors. *American Journal of Public Health*, 85, 1018–1019.

McLeroy, K.R., Bibeau, D., Steckler, A., Glanz, K. (1988). An ecological perspective on health promotion programs. *Health Education Quarterly*, 15, 351–377.

Mill, J.E. (2003). Shrouded in secrecy: Breaking the news of HIV infection to Ghanaian women. *Journal of Transcultural Nursing*, 14, 6–16.

Moses, S., Tomlinson, M. (2013). The fluidity of disclosure: A longitudinal exploration of women's experience and understanding of HIV disclosure in the context of pregnancy and early motherhood. *AIDS Care*, 25, 667–675.

Moyer, E., Igonya, E.K., Both, R., Cherutich, P., Hardon, A. (2013). The duty to disclose in Kenyan health facilities: A qualitative investigation of HIV disclosure in everyday practice. *SAHARA J*, 10 Suppl 1, S60–72.

Murphy, D.A. (2008). HIV-positive mothers' disclosure of their serostatus to their young children: A review. *Clinical Child Psychology and Psychiatry*, 13, 105–122.

Murphy, D.A., Austin, E.L., Greenwell, L. (2006). Correlates of HIV-related stigma among HIV-positive mothers and their uninfected adolescent children. *Women and Health*, 44, 19–42.

Murphy, D.A., Steers, W.N., Dello Stritto, M.E. (2001). Maternal disclosure of mothers' HIV serostatus to their young children. *Journal of Family Psychology*, 15, 441–450.

Murphy, D.A., Roberts, K.J., Hoffman, D. (2003). Regrets and advice from mothers who have disclosed their HIV + serostatus to their young children. *Journal of Child and Family Studies*, 12, 307–318.

Murphy, D.A., Marelich, W.D., Amaro, H. (2009). Maternal HIV/AIDS and adolescent depression: A covariance structure analysis of the 'Parents and Adolescents Coping Together' (PACT) model. *Vulnerable Children and Youth Studies*, 4, 67–82.

Murphy, D.A., Armistead, L., Marelich, W.D., Payne, D.L., Herbeck, D.M. (2011). Pilot trial of a disclosure intervention for HIV+ mothers: The TRACK program. *Journal of Consulting and Clinical Psychology*, 79, 203–214.

Naidoo, K., Melvin, D., Houghton, J. (2010). *Step by step guide for conversation with children (toward disclosure)*. University of KwaZulu Natal. Available at www.kznhealth.gov.za/arv/Disclosure_Poster.pdf.

Nam, S.L., Fielding, K., Avalos, A., Gaolathe, T., Dickinson, D., Geissler, P.W. (2009). Discussing matters of sexual health with children: What issues relating to disclosure of parental HIV status reveal. *AIDS Care*, 21, 389–395.

New York State Department of Health AIDS Institute. (2009). Disclosure of HIV to perinatally infected children and adolescents. Retrieved on 27 May 2015.

Nie, J.B. (2011). The 'cultural differences' argument and its misconceptions: The return of medical truth-telling in China. In A. Rudnick (Ed.) *Bioethics in the 21st century*. Rijeka, Croatia InTech.

Nostlinger, C., Jonckheer, T., De Belder, E., Van Wijngaerden, E., Wylock, C., Pelgrom, J., Colebunders, R. (2004). Families affected by HIV: Parents' and children's characteristics and disclosure to the children. *AIDS Care*, 16, 641–648.

Obermeyer, C.M., Baijal, P., Pegurri, E. (2011). Facilitating HIV disclosure across diverse settings: A review. *American Journal of Public Health*, 101, 1011–1023.

Palin, F.L., Armistead, L., Clayton, A., Ketchen, B., Lindner, G., Kokot-Louw, P., Pauw, A. (2009). Disclosure of maternal HIV-infection in South Africa: Description and relationship to child functioning. *AIDS Behavior*, 13, 1241–1252.

Perrin, E.C., Gerrity, P.S. (1981). There's a demon in your belly: Children's understanding of illness. *Pediatrics*, 67, 841–849.

Petronio, S. (Ed.) (2000). *Balancing the secrets of private disclosures*. Mahwah, NJ: Lawrence Erlbaum Associates.

Petronio, S. (2007). Translational research endeavors and the practices of communication privacy management. *Journal of Applied Communication Research*, 35(3), 218–222.

Piaget, J. (1951). *The child's conception of physical causality* London Routledge and Kegan Paul.

Piaget, J. (1972). Intellectual evolution from adolescence to adulthood. *Human Development*, 15(1), 1–12.

Piaget, J., Inhelder, B. (1969). *The psychology of the child*. New York: Basic Books.

Qiao, S., Li, X., Zhao, G., Zhao, J., Stanton, B. (2012). Secondary disclosure of parental HIV status among children affected by AIDS in Henan, China. *AIDS Patient Care and STDS*, 26, 546–556.

Qiao, S., Li, X., Stanton, B. (2013a). Disclosure of parental HIV infection to children: A systematic review of global literature. *AIDS Behavior*, 17, 369–389.

Qiao, S., Li, X., Stanton, B. (2013b). Theoretical models of parental HIV disclosure: A critical review. *AIDS Care*, 25, 326–336.

Qiao, S., Li, X., Stanton, B. (2014). Practice and perception of parental HIV disclosure to children in Beijing, China. *Qualitative Health Research*, 24, 1276–1286.

Qiao, S., Li, X., Zhou, Y.J., Shen, Z.Y., Tang, Z.Z., Stanton, B. (2015). Consequences of parental HIV disclosure and enacted stigma among HIV-positive parents in China. *AIDS Care*, (in press).

Rochat, T.J., Mkwanazi, N., Bland, R. (2013). Maternal HIV disclosure to HIV-uninfected children in rural South Africa: A pilot study of a family-based intervention. *BMC Public Health*, 13, 147.

Rochat, T.J., Arteche, A.X., Stein, A., Mkwanazi, N., Bland, R.M. (2014). Maternal HIV disclosure to young HIV-uninfected children: An evaluation of a family-centred intervention in South Africa. *AIDS*, 28(S3), S331–341.

Rotheram-Borus, M.J., Draimin, B.H., Reid, H.M., Murphy, D.A. (1997). The impact of illness disclosure and custody plans on adolescents whose parents live with AIDS. *AIDS*, 11, 1159–1164.

Rotheram-Borus, M.J., Lee, M.B., Gwadz, M., Draimin, B. (2001). An intervention for parents with AIDS and their adolescent children. *American Journal of Public Health*, 91, 1294–1302.

Rwemisisi, J., Wolff, B., Coutinho, A., Grosskurth, H., WHitworth, J. (2008). 'What if they ask how I got it?' Dilemmas of disclosing parental HIV status and testing children for HIV in Uganda. *Health Policy and Planning*, 23, 36–42.

Sahay, S. (2013). Coming of age with HIV: A need for disclosure of HIV diagnosis among children/adolescents. *Journal of HIV/AIDS and Infectious Diseases* 1, 1–7.

Schrimshaw, E.W., Siegel, K. (2002). HIV-infected mothers' disclosure to their uninfected children: Rates, reasons, and reactions. *Journal of Social and Personal Relationships*, Special Issue: Personal and social relationships of individuals living with HIV and/or AIDS 19, 19–44.

Seidel, G. (1996). Confidentiality and HIV status in Kwazulu-Natal, South Africa: Implications, resistances and challenge. *Health Policy and Planning*, 11(4), 418–427.

Selke, H.M., Kimaiyo, S., Sidle, J.E., Vedanthan, R., Tierney, W.M., Shen, C., Denski, C.D., Katschke, A.R., Wools-Kaloustian, K. (2010). Task-shifting of antiretroviral delivery from health care workers to persons living with HIV/AIDS: Clinical outcomes of a community-based program in Kenya. *Journal of Acquired Immune Deficiency Syndromes*, 55, 483–490.

Simoni, J.M., Davis, M.L., Drossman, J.A., Weinberg, B.A. (2000). Mothers with HIV/AIDS and their children: Disclosure and guardianship issues. *Women and Health*, 31, 39–54.

Simoni, J.M., Pantalone, D.W. (2004). Secrets and safety in the age of AIDS: Does HIV disclosure lead to safer sex? *Topics in HIV Medicine*, 12, 109–118.

Stein, J.A., Riedel, M., Rotheram-Borus, M.J. (1999). Parentification and its impact on adolescent children of parents with AIDS. *Family Process*, 38, 193–208.

Stokols, D. (1996). Translating social ecological theory into guidelines for community health promotion. *American Journal of Health Promotion*, 10, 282–298.

Tasker, M. (1992). *How can I tell you? Secrecy and disclosure with children when a family member has AIDS*. Bethesda, MD: Association for the Care of Children's Health.

Tenzek, K.E., Herrman, A.R., May, A.R., Feinerd, B., Allenb, M. (2013). Examining the impact of parental disclosure of HIV on children: A meta-analysis. *Western Journal of Communication*, 77, 323–339.

Thomas, B., Nyamathi, A., Swaminathan, S. (2009). Impact of HIV/AIDS on mothers in Southern India: A qualitative study. *AIDS and Behavior*, 13, 989–996.

Tiendrebeogo, G., Hejoaka, F., Belem, E.M., Compaore, P.L., Wolmarans, L., Soubeiga, A., Ouangraoua, N. (2013). Parental HIV disclosure in Burkina Faso: Experiences and challenges in the era of HAART. *SAHARA J*, 10 Suppl 1, S46–59.

Tompkins, T.L. (2007). Disclosure of maternal HIV status to children: To tell or not to tell … That is the question. *Journal of Child and Family Studies*, 16, 773–788.

Tompkins, T.L., Henker, B., Whalen, C.K., Axelrod, J., Comer, L.K. (1999). Motherhood in the context of HIV infection: Reading between the numbers. *Cultural Diversity and Ethnic Minority Psychology*, 5, 197–208.

UNAIDS (2013). *Toward an AIDS-free generation: Children and AIDS sixth stocktaking report*. Geneva: UNAIDS.

UNAIDS (2014). *The Gap Report*. Geneva: UNAIDS.

Vallerand, A.H., Hough, E., Pittiglio, L., Marvicsin, D. (2005). The process of disclosing HIV serostatus between HIV-positive mothers and their HIV-negative children. *AIDS Patient Care and STDS*, 19, 100–109.

Werner, H. (1948). *Comparative psychology of mental development*. Chicago: Follett Publishing Company.

WHO (2011). *Guideline on HIV disclosure counselling for children up to 12 years of age*. Geneva: WHO.

Wiener, L., Mellins, C.A., Marhefka, S., Battles, H.B. (2007). Disclosure of an HIV diagnosis to children: History, current research, and future directions. *Journal of Developmental and Behavioral Pediatrics*, 28, 155–166.

Wiener, L.S., Battles, H.B., Heilman, N.E. (1998). Factors associated with parents' decision to disclose their HIV diagnosis to their children. *Child Welfare*, 77, 115–135.

Woodring, L.A., Cancelli, A.A., Ponterotto, J.G., Keitel, M.A. (2005). A qualitative investigation of adolescents' experiences with parental HIV/AIDS. *American Journal of Orthopsychiatry*, 75, 658–675.

Xia, Y.R., Xie, X., Zhou, Z., Defrain, J., Combs, R. (2008). Chinese adolescents' decision-making, parent-adolescent communication and relationships. *Marriage and Family Review* 36, 119–145.

Zea, M.C., Reisen, C.A., Poppen, P.J., Bianchi, F.T., Echeverry, J.J. (2007). Predictors of disclosure of human immunovirus-positive serostatus among Latino gay men. *Cultural Diversity and Ethnic Minority Psychology*, 13, 304–312.

Zhou, Y.R. (2007). 'If you get AIDS … you have to endure it alone': Understanding the social constructions of HIV/AIDS in China. *Social Science and Medicine*, 65, 284–295.

Zhou, Y., Zhan, L., Li, X., Kaljee, L. (2013). Do Chinese parents with HIV tell their children the truth? A qualitative preliminary study of parental HIV disclosure in China. *Child: Care Health and Development*, 39, 816–824.

CHAPTER 11

A family-centred approach to parental illness

Dominik Sebastian Sieh and Anne Visser-Meily

INTRODUCTION

Approximately 10–13% of adolescents grow up with a parent who has a chronic medical condition (CMC). As a result of parental CMCs such as cancer, neuromuscular disease or stroke, young people can experience positive consequences, such as the development of empathy and fewer aggressive feelings. There may also be negative outcomes such as excessive caregiving responsibilities, elevated stress and internalising problems. This chapter contains a review of literature pertaining to CMCs, a critical evaluation of relevant interventions, an 'in practice' section that provides guidance in terms of best practice when addressing the impact of parental CMCs and recommendations for future research. Promoting a family-centred approach is highlighted, as are protective factors for developmental problems in children with chronically ill parents. A newly developed measure, the Screening Instrument for Adolescents of Parents with Chronic Medical Condition (SIAPCMC), is also introduced. The instrument is a short list of questions that can identify adolescents at risk for internalising problems such as anxious and withdrawn behaviour. The SIAPCMC is currently being implemented as a preventive instrument in the Netherlands, serving three objectives: (i) identifying the risk for future internalising problems in children with parental CMC; (ii) facilitating open communication within the family and (iii) suggesting ways of support and interventions for these children.

FAMILY-CENTRED CARE (FCC)

Healthcare should become more family-centred for several reasons. First, disability affects not only the patients involved but also their significant others, e.g. spouses, children and other family members. Many spouses and children of parents with CMC report high levels of burden of care, depressive feelings and low quality of life. Second, support from family members is often pivotal to maintaining participation and quality of life of parents with CMC, and in many cases it is even conditional for the person with a disability to be able to function in society (Kruithof et al., 2013). Support from the family will become even more important in the Western world in the future due to changes and increasing budget cuts in community care (Tummers et al., 2012). More pressure will be put on the family to provide care and professional care will only be provided when the family and social network cannot give it.

Intuitively, the adoption of family-centred care (FCC) for parents with CMC makes sense, considering the general recognition of the significance of the family as the primary social unit – the main educator, supporter and coach of each person. Moreover, FCC models are currently acknowledged to represent best practice in paediatric service (Bamm and Rosenbaum, 2008) and more and more in services for chronic disease like stroke and neuromuscular diseases (Creasy et al., 2015). FCC is not merely focused on augmenting family presence and patient autonomy while decreasing medical paternalism. Instead, it encourages collaboration and partnership among patients, families and the provider. The consideration that families have varied needs has become an important dimension of FCC. Other dimensions of FCC include broadening the explanatory perspective of illness beyond biomedical features, giving attention to the personal meaning of illness and supporting and valuing the relationship between patients and their family members.

LITERATURE REVIEW

A growing number of parents with young children develop a chronic medical condition (CMC). This rise is not only due to the increasing occurrence of auto-immune diseases (Bach, 2008) and improved medical techniques that increase the life expectancy of parents with CMC (such as stroke and cancer), but also due to the fact that parents conceive children at an older age. In turn, older age is associated with heightened vulnerability for CMC (Lubkin and Larsen, 2006; Shifren and Kachorek, 2003). In developed countries, the most common forms of CMC include rheumatoid arthritis, cardiovascular diseases (e.g. stroke), cancer, chronic respiratory diseases and diabetes mellitus. These conditions are the leading cause of mortality in the world, accounting for 63% of all deaths. Such medical conditions involve one or more organ systems impairing health and psychological functioning for at least three months (Brown, 2007; Lubkin and Larsen, 2006).

Worldwide, roughly 10% of children grow up with a parent affected by CMC (Sieh et al., 2010a). CMC affects the entire family (Visser-Meily and Meijer, 2006). About 25% of individuals with CMC have one or more activity limitations (Anderson, 2004). These limitations have an impact on professional, social and family life (Visser-Meily et al., 2005, 2009). Positive family relationships may act as a buffer against adolescent stress, providing resources and possibilities for resilience and growth (Rolland, 1999). However, the family encounters issues in the interpersonal spectrum concerning topics such as averting exhaustion, maintaining autonomy and preserving intimacy in the face of severe impairment or possible death. This in turn can mean that interpersonal relationships are challenged and may not continue to serve as the buffer they used to. Externalising problems like aggression and rule-breaking behaviour are relatively rare among children of parents with CMC (Sieh, 2012). On the contrary, all family members have an elevated risk for internalising problems which refer to problematic behaviour that is directed toward the self (i.e. anxious, depressed and withdrawn behaviour, and somatic complaints). Anxieties, particularly illness-related fears, are common; for example, a child from a parent with CMC may overestimate the chance of becoming ill and feel afraid – even without medical symptoms (Sieh, 2012; Visser-Meily and Meijer, 2006). Worries about the health condition of the chronically ill parent and about becoming ill themselves are widespread among children with parental CMC (Armistead et al., 1995; Lackey and Gates, 2001). Children may generalise anxieties to other areas. For instance, a Dutch study found that almost half of children with parental stroke or Parkinson's reported general fears about the future (Dufour et al., 2006). In comparison with their peers whose parents do not suffer from an illness, children with parental CMC have higher scores for somatisation and life dissatisfaction (Pakenham et al., 2006). In most cases, both spouses and children are required to take care of the parent with CMC. Children frequently have to fulfil caregiving responsibilities that may be inappropriate for their age (Korneluk and Lee, 1998; Meijer et al., 2008). They may feel overwhelmed with the emerging caregiving tasks and may experience emotions of guilt when they spend time away from the parent with CMC. Children may not have sufficient leisure time, feel restricted in daily activities and refrain from school duties (Sieh et al., 2013d). The relevance of research on parental CMC becomes even more evident considering that developmental problems starting early in childhood may persist until adulthood (Lackey and Gates, 2001; Schrag et al., 2004).

In sum, research to date suggests that in general, children can cope well with the parent's chronic illness. In terms of parent-child attachment, coping skills and diurnal salivary cortisol, adolescents with parental CMC do not seem to differ from adolescents without a chronically ill parent (Sieh et al., 2012b, 2013d). However, they report significantly more internalising problems than children from intact families with healthy parents, displaying unfavourable results on many outcome variables, such as caregiving impact, self-report of daily difficulties and stress and grade point average (Sieh et al., 2013d). The low prevalence of externalising problems and positive aspects associated with parental CMC should not be ignored, but instead should receive a central focus. Nonetheless, children who have a parent suffering from a CMC do not form a risk group per definition.

RISK AND PROTECTIVE FACTORS FOR DEVELOPMENTAL PROBLEMS

Most children seem to cope well with parental CMC (Annunziato et al., 2007; Romer et al., 2002). Protective factors may account for the ways in which these children are resistant to developing problems. On the one hand, high levels of stress may increase the chance of internalising problems in adolescents. On the other hand, protective factors such as adequate family functioning and functional coping (e.g. social support seeking and active problem solving) can moderate undesirable levels of stress, decreasing the risk for adolescent problem behaviour. Internalising problems are particularly common among children with parental CMC and should therefore receive more attention in preventive measures (Sieh, 2012).

Numerous risk and protective factors for developmental problems and especially adverse outcome variables in adolescents with parental CMC have been examined. Researchers have investigated demographic characteristics of children and parents, illness characteristics and the psychosocial variables of children, parents and the family as a whole (Korneluk and Lee, 1998; Romer et al., 2002). In particular, illness-related characteristics have been examined extensively. According to Rolland (1998), illness types can be categorised on the basis of the presence of disability (non-disabling versus disabling), its onset (gradual versus acute), its course (progressive, episodic, or constant), its outcome (fatal versus non-fatal) and the stage of the illness (crisis, chronic, or terminal). It may be hypothesised that adolescent stress depends on illness-related factors, resulting in a differentiation into illness type in line with the diagnosis. Research, however, suggests that illness type is of minor importance in the chronic stage of a parental medical condition as it proves to be unrelated to child reports of stress and most other adverse outcomes (Sieh, 2012). Instead, family functioning and psychosocial mediators play a major role in determining adolescent stress scores.

A large meta-analysis of more than 1800 children found that internalising and externalising problem behaviour was pronounced in populations with younger children and younger parents, with a range of conditions (but not parental cancer), in samples defined by low average SES, and in studies which included parents with longer illness duration. Externalising problem behaviour was also increased in studies where there was a higher percentage of ill mothers and single parents (Sieh et al., 2010).

When considering psychosocial factors, though, static determinants (e.g. diagnosis or illness characteristics) and demographic determinants (e.g. children's age and gender) are less predictive of children's developmental problems. The most salient mediators are stress and coping variables but also family characteristics, such as the psychosocial state of the family members separately and in constellation. Child reporting of stress is associated with the child's perception of parent attachment and the parent's perception of parent-child interaction (Sieh et al., 2012a). From a longitudinal study on children with a parent who suffered a stroke (Sieh et al., 2010b), it can be deducted that early prediction of long-term stress in children after parental stroke may be most accurate on the basis of female gender of the child and depressive symptoms in the chronically ill parent. The ill parent's depression and child's report of stress are interrelated (Sieh et al., 2013c). Thus, there is evidence for mediating processes within the family, for example, the child's coping skills do not seem to have a significant effect on internalising problems, but active problem solving is significantly related to self-report of stress in children. The child's perception of stress, daily hassles and quality of parent attachment appear to be marked mediating variables between illness and demographic parameters and adolescent internalising problems (Sieh et al., 2014).

By identifying risk and protective pathways to internalising problems, Sieh developed a screening instrument for adolescents with parental CMC. This is part of a secondary prevention which aims to identify children in need of early intervention before developmental problems persist. In a Dutch study on children of parents with various CMCs, four risk factors proved to predict approximately 60% of the variance in internalising problems; that is, illness duration, feelings of isolation, alienation from the mother and daily hassles affecting personal life (Sieh et al., 2012b). In addition, the unpredictability of parental illness, children's caregiving responsibilities and activity restrictions, child report of stress and active problem solving were significantly related to internalising problems in adolescents. Eight questions that covered these underlying risk and protective factors were formulated and now comprise the Screening Instrument for Adolescents of Parents with CMC (SIAPCMC). A longitudinal study including 149 children showed that the SIAPCMC is a sensitive instrument in the identification of adolescents at risk for future internalising problems, indicating that clinical implementation of the SIAPCMC can commence (Sieh et al., 2013a). The SIAPCMC unravels those characteristics of children which play a significant role in the manifestation of children's internalising problems. The SIAPCMC can identify developmental problems in adolescents aged 10–20 years. Compared to latency-aged children, adolescents are more likely to have a parent at an older age, which may in turn lead to an increased chance of having a parent with a chronic illness. Also, adolescents in particular might have experienced the impact of parental CMC for an extended period. A screening instrument may contribute to the identification of adolescents who require interventions in order to prevent potential problems.

EVALUATION OF RELEVANT INTERVENTIONS

Considering that parental CMC affects the whole family, a family-centred approach is to be advocated, bearing in mind the strengths, vulnerabilities and support needs of individual family members and the wider family system. It is essential to invite children to talk about how the parent's condition affects them in the context of their family, school and leisure time. Insight into the relationship between illness-related stressors and adolescent developmental problems is essential when designing interventions for those adolescents who need help. The percentage of (sub)clinically elevated scores in the internalising spectrum can be up to twice as high as in the normal population (Sieh et al., 2012b). Consequently, children with greater internalising problems should receive support from family or, if needed, from school advisors or health professionals, e.g. psychologists or social workers. A family-centred approach may also be more efficient than individual interventions. For instance, Schulz et al. (2009) tested a caregiver-only intervention which was solely focused on the caregiver versus a dual-target intervention which was focused on both the caregiver and the person with spinal cord injury. Only the dual-target intervention improved the quality of life of the caregiver and the dyad.

In the literature, several family-centred interventions have been used. These differ in their purposes and applications. Some focus on discharge planning (Shyu et al., 2008), whereas others focus on psychoeducational information (Ostwald et al., 2013) or on a training programme for caregivers. Recently, a structured training programme for caregivers of inpatients after stroke was robustly tested and found not to be effective on either patients' or caregivers' outcomes (Forster et al., 2012). This study suggested that timing is important and, additionally, caregivers may need more than a structured training programme to reduce caregiver burden. Needs of the couple or family may not be entirely met. Currently, caregivers are actively involved in rehabilitation, although interventions remain primarily focused on the needs of the patient and have little emphasis on the consequences of the disability on other family members. Family members may benefit more from interventions that deal with how the parent's condition affects each individual and the family as a whole in emotional, relational and behavioural dimensions.

In the Netherlands, healthcare institutions embrace FCC more and more (Witteveen et al., 2014). An example of FCC is a meeting in which the family, supported by the social worker of the rehabilitation team, relevant members of their social network (e.g. children, friends, colleagues) and, if applicable, community case managers will come together to discuss the possible impact of the condition on activities and participation of the family, to set priorities for support and to make action plans on how to achieve these priorities. The social worker and the family prepare for the meeting together. Topics to be addressed and people to be invited are family-specific. The social worker has at least two follow-up appointments with the family, six and 12 weeks after the FCC interventions, to monitor the agreements of FCC and to arrange adoption of the proposed plan of action if applicable. This new approach, entitled Family Focus on Future, is to be tested in a controlled study from 2015–2019 in six rehabilitation centres in the Netherlands (www.dehoogstraat.nl/onderzoek-innovatie/diagnose/beroerte/family-focus-on-future).

PARENTS' CHRONIC MEDICAL CONDITION IN PRACTICE

The fact that children affected by parental CMC display more adverse outcomes than other children highlights their need for assistance when adjusting to chronic illness. Generally speaking, these children express possible problems with emotional and behavioural changes, and school and social activities. Children with parental CMC are characterised by greater internalisation of problems such as feelings of fear, sadness and guilt. Such emotions are often illness-related; for example, children may feel guilty thinking of spending more time with friends instead of caring for their parent (Armistead et al., 1995; Lackey and Gates, 2001; Pakenham et al., 2007). Children frequently are afraid of becoming ill themselves. Idiosyncratic fears involve those of worsening health, increasing impairment and loss or death of the parent (Dearden and Becker, 2000; Sieh et al., 2011). In addition, children with parental CMC may not have sufficient time for school and social activities. As a consequence, they may achieve lower school grades and feel inferior or lonely (Sieh, 2012). Teachers, school psychologists, health practitioners and other professionals who have contact with these children should be alert for signs of developmental problems, mainly in the internalising spectrum (i.e. anxious, depressed and withdrawn behaviour and somatic symptoms). Worsening school performance and social isolation should also be of particular concern. Unfortunately, there are few specific interventions for children with parental CMC; at least, few studies on evidence-based interventions have been published. Existing knowledge, however, still provides the clinical field with a number of recommendations.

We advocate a family-centred approach that considers the impact of parental CMC on the whole family (Visser-Meily et al., 2006). This starts with provision of information about FCC but also integrates FCC into the training and continuing-education programme of health professionals such as doctors, therapists and nurses. Health professionals need awareness training, skills training and changes to practice routines so that FCC becomes a standard for the whole team rather than an exception for particular disciplines, e.g. family therapists whom the family may occasionally be referred to. For instance, professionals can change practice routines by inviting children when discussing the individual rehabilitation plan and thereby make a family-centred rehabilitation plan. It is essential to consider the entire family and the environment of the family: chronically ill parents, spouses, children, the wider family and support system, and financial, material and social resources. Possible targets for family-based interventions ideally focus on the quality of life, interpersonal relationships and adaptational processes of family members. Parents may benefit from education about the role of parenthood or from parenting support in order to feel more secure about how to deal with parental CMC within the family. Approximately a third of a sample of Dutch children with parental CMC had the desire to talk to a professional counsellor. Some children explicitly said that they did not want to talk about the illness; instead, they wished to discuss the impact of the illness on their own life within the family, within the wider social network and the school environment (Sieh, 2009; Sieh et al., 2011). Interventions for children should incorporate the child's coping skills, cognitive processes and perception of stress. Interventions to boost protective factors such as active problem-solving skills, social support and high self-esteem appear to be suitable.

Social and family relationships have an especially important protective function; for example, relationships characterised by mutual trust and social support can reduce the adverse effect of depression in children with parental

HIV (Wang et al., 2012). Another study showed that relationships with peers stimulated resilience and reduced feelings of stigmatisation and feelings of isolation in children of mentally ill parents (Foster et al., 2014). Finally, family psychoeducation combined with stress management may help the process of adapting to parental CMC. Conversely, health practitioners should avoid blunt generalisations, unsubtle confrontational techniques or discussing disease-related matters only.

An improvement to the current approach in rehabilitation medicine, which is still rather patient-centred, would be to place greater consideration on the needs of children and spouses of chronically ill parents. It is recommended that health practitioners pay attention to supporting the needs of the family, while taking care that children do not become estranged from their parents. They may invite children and spouses to a session with the parent who is ill. This is challenging because children are often at school during outpatient visiting times, and therefore are unable to accompany their parent. If children are unable to do so, health practitioners could explore the family situation and make recommendations for the parents to use in the home environment. An example would be that parents discuss caregiving tasks while stressing that their children need to focus primarily on school and friends and that it is important for parents to see their children being happy with peers. Importantly, children should not be excluded from the rehabilitation or treatment of the parent with CMC. They require information about CMC and their needs should be recognised by health practitioners.

Children can be invited to talk about how parental CMC has affected their life. They may be openly asked whether they need information about the diagnosis. Healthcare staff should create an opportunity for children to ask sensitive questions, for instance whether parental CMC may be hereditary, severely impairing, progressive or terminal. Often, the actual chance of becoming ill is much lower than children believe and in many cases, CMCs are not inherited at all. According to Romer et al. (2002), children may suffer from vague fantasies of worst-case scenarios. A study showed that children indicated that they would benefit from information on how to deal with their parent with CMC and what to do in challenging situations, for example when their parent has a seizure (Sieh et al., 2011). Every illness and every illness stage has its own characteristics to which children at different ages react in their own way.

The family research project Children of Somatically Ill Parents (COSIP) from Romer et al. (2002) revealed that parents find it difficult to provide age-appropriate information while avoiding burdening or even overloading their child. Children frequently are ambivalent: they wish to have more information but are afraid to elicit distress in their parents, who may feel confronted with questions about their psychological and health condition or even start worrying about burdening the children. Consequently, professional help may be needed to initiate a dialogue about latent cognitions and emotions, breaking with the 'conspiracy of silence' (Romer et al., 2002). Parents often doubt their ability to recognise when children need help. A good indicator for children's support needs might be that peer friends visit the child at home less often, that the child does not talk about personal problems anymore (Romer et al., 2002), or that their academic performance worsens (Sieh et al., 2013d).

Children should be supported according to their specific individual needs. Consequently, professionals should not rely on standard interventions. About a third of adolescents in a Dutch study indicated that they would benefit from chat sessions with other children in their situation (Sieh, 2009). More than a third of those children wished for additional information about parental CMC, indicating that they would benefit from a website dedicated to children with parental CMC (Sieh et al., 2011). Considering that feelings of isolation are quite common among children with parental CMC, it is essential to check whether there is sufficient contact with peers, whether these children are restricted from engaging in social, leisure and school activities, and whether they are overly involved in caregiving tasks. Approximately a third of the children from that same study reported a wish for support in the household (Sieh, 2009; Sieh et al., 2011). Where possible and affordable, healthcare staff may arrange professional care in the household for those children who report excessive caregiving duties. Romer et al. (2002) suggested that it may be advantageous to discuss narrowly defined responsibilities that children are expected to fulfil. Also, help from non-professional caregivers such as family members, volunteers or neighbours may be warranted and could be initiated by, for example, patient organisations or social workers.

Considering that parent attachment and stress appraisal appears to play a significant role in child adjustment to parental CMC (Sieh, 2012), these factors should be targeted and combined in interventions. Harmonious family relationships can buffer stress in children (Sieh et al., 2014). Family relationships should therefore be boosted. Similarly, physicians should be aware that there is a chance of children feeling alienated from their parents. Family counselling or family workshops aiming to increase cohesion and resilience in families may be useful.

RECOMMENDATIONS FOR FUTURE RESEARCH

Considering the increasing prevalence of and pressure on children growing up with a chronically ill parent (Bach, 2008; Lubken and Larsen, 2006; Tummers et al., 2010), research on the impact of parental CMC remains important. There are several recommendations for future studies. Generally, future research needs to explore positive outcomes in children with a chronically ill parent. In addition, specific interventions for family members in need should be developed and tested for efficacy.

First, researchers should consider the complex family dynamics rather than focusing on individual family members alone. Effectively, the family cluster effect (similarity and statistical dependence between family members due to family membership) explains a high percentage of the variance in the outcomes of family members. It is therefore crucial to examine mutual family relationships in more detail; that is, the degree of cohesion, mutual trust and transparency in communication and how these aspects influence the resilience of families. Future research could examine interpersonal relationships in more depth and focus on how parental CMC affects family interactions over time. Process variables concerning the impact of parental CMC – for example caregiving impact, illness cognitions, illness-related self-efficacy and the degree of social restrictions over time – may be difficult to measure with the instruments that are currently available, so future research should also develop and validate illness-specific instruments.

Second, a longitudinal study would be suited to examine families in the long term. Investigating family dynamics before and after the diagnosis would be interesting, but this is difficult to achieve because CMCs can hardly be predicted, and retrospective measures of prediagnostic family functioning may be unreliable. It would be intriguing to examine how mutual relationships change over time, depending on whether the illness course is acute, progressive or episodic. In specific cases (e.g. parental stroke), this has been done. However, more longitudinal research with larger samples is needed to draw firm conclusions (Sieh et al., 2010b).

Third, future research should take a wider range of protective factors into account. Social support and active problem solving are characteristics of what the coping system involves and these seem to play a key role in successful rehabilitation (Visser-Meily et al., 2009). For example, positive interactions with peers and fellow sufferers may play a buffering role (Pakenham and Bursnall, 2006) and those interactions may mediate the social isolation that children with parental CMC frequently experience. Apart from coping skills and competencies associated with developmental problems (Blackford, 1999; Newman, 2002), future research should pay more attention to specific positive outcomes that are not easily detected with instruments available for the general population. For instance, future studies could incorporate children's prosocial behaviour, sense of contributing to society or sense of purpose, which may result from caregiving. Based on qualitative research (e.g. Lackey and Gates, 2001; Visser et al., 2004), a sense of purpose may be more common among children caring for a parent with CMC than among other children.

Fourth, the SIAPCMC should be further validated. This may be achieved by administering the SIAPCMC to a larger sample, initiating its use in clinical settings. In 2013, Sieh started a new project aiming to validate the SIAPCMC for children of parents with a psychiatric disorder or addiction. Also, a screening instrument like the SIAPCMC could be adjusted to serve as an interactive app. With the SIAPCMC, problems in the personal or family area may become apparent. Depending on the scores, health professionals receive specific recommendations for support and possible interventions. This function may also be built into the application for smartphone users. Furthermore, following children with parental CMC in late adolescence over an extended period may also increase our knowledge of their transition into adulthood. Finally, a randomised controlled trial may be useful to design, offer and test an online treatment versus face-to-face treatment based on cognitive behavioural therapy or family counselling to youth scoring above the cut-off score of the SIAPCMC. Accordingly, adolescents may be randomly assigned to several conditions (no support, professional support, e-health and peer support). In addition, the cost-effectiveness of these treatments can be examined. If continuous, such a follow-up study would have the potential to foster the implementation of the SIAPCMC in the healthcare system. Last but not least, the SIAPCMC should be tested in latency-aged children. If the SIAPCMC does not prove suitable for this age group, an alternative screening instrument should be designed for them.

CONCLUSION

A paradigm shift is taking place within Western European welfare states, focusing on increasing responsibilities for parents with CMC and their children, calling for more voluntary and community-based care. Families are expected not to lean on the government but to take care of themselves, if necessary with the help of the wider family and community. The role of young and adult informal caregivers is increasing. Thus parents with CMC and their partners and children need to manage large elements of their own support. In a situation with an increased risk of physical and emotional strain, especially depressive or burn-out symptoms, these families need to be equipped to be able to cope with the caregiving situation. Children, in particular those with prolonged exposure to stress and caregiving strain and with poor social and family support, are at an increased risk for developing internalising problems. Preventive measures from national and local governments and health professionals are therefore required. A good basis for interventions is a family-centred approach that begins with inviting children and family members to talk about psychosocial consequences of their situation. Families appear to benefit from reinforcement of their support system and from developing problem-solving and other active coping strategies. The family support system ideally consists of relatives, community workers, health professionals and fellow sufferers who work together as a team.

REFERENCES

Anderson, G. (2004). *Chronic conditions: Making the case for ongoing care*. Baltimore, MD: Johns Hopkins University.

Annunziato, R.A., Rakotomihamina, V., Rubacka, J. (2007). Examining the effects of maternal chronic illness on child well-being in single parent families. *Journal of Developmental and Behavioral Pediatrics*, 28, 386–391.

Armistead, L., Klein, L., Forehand, R. (1995). Parental physical illness and child functioning. *Clinical Psychological Review*, 15, 409–422.

Bach, J.F. (2008). Why is the incidence of autoimmune diseases increasing in the modern world? Presented at the Society for Endocrinology. *Endocrine Abstracts*, 13, 9.

Bamm, E.L., Rosenbaum, P. (2008). Family-centered theory: Origins, development, barriers and supports to implementation in rehabilitation medicine. *Archives of Physical Medicine Rehabilitation*, 89, 1618–1624.

Blackford, K.A. (1999). A child's growing up with a parent who has multiple sclerosis: Theories and experiences. *Disability and Society*, 14, 673–685.

Brown, R.T., Fuemmeler, B., Anderson, D., Jamieson, S., Simonian, S., Hall, R.K., Brescia, F. (2007). Adjustment of children and their mothers with breast cancer. *Journal of Pediatric Psychology*, 32, 297–308.

Creasy, K.R., Lutz, J.L., Young, M.E., Stacciarini, J.M.R. (2015). Clinical implications of family-centered care in stroke rehabilitation. *Rehabilitation Nursing*, (epub ahead of print).

Dearden, C., Becker, S. (2000). *Growing up caring: Vulnerability and transition to adulthood: Young carers' experiences*. Leicester: Youth Work Press.

Dufour, M.J., Meijer, A.M., van de Port, I., Visser-Meily, J.M.A. (2006). Daily hassles and stress in the lives of children with chronically ill parents. *Netherlands Journal of Psychology*, 61, 54–64.

Forster, A., Young, J., Nixon, J., Kalra, L., Smithard, D., Patel, A., Knapp, M., Monaghan, J., Breen, R., Anwar, S., Farrin, A. (2012). A cluster randomized controlled trial of a structured training programme for caregivers of inpatients after stroke (TRACS). *International Journal of Stroke*, 7, 94–99.

Foster, K., Lewis, P., McCloughen, A. (2014). Experiences of peer support for children and adolescents whose parents and siblings have a mental illness. *Journal of Child and Adolescent Psychiatric Nursing*, 27, 61–67.

Korneluk, Y.G., Lee, C.M. (1998). Children's adjustment to parental physical illness. *Clinical Child and Family Psychology Review*, 1, 179–193.

Kruithof, W.J., van Mierlo, M.L., Visser-Meily, J.M.A., van Heugten, C.M., Post, M.W. (2013). Associations between social support and stroke survivors' health-related quality of life: A systematic review. *Patient Education Counseling*, 93, 169–176.

Lackey, N.R., Gates, M.F. (2001). Adults' recollections of their experiences as young caregivers of family members with chronic physical illnesses. *Journal of Advanced Nursing*, 34, 320–328.

Lubkin, I.M., Larsen, P.D. (2006). *Chronic illness: Impact and interventions*. London: Jones and Bartlett Publishers.

Meijer, A.M., van Oostveen, S.J.E., Stams, G.J.J.M. (2008). De relatie tussen mantelzorg, ziekte van de ouder en gedragsproblemen bij kinderen [Caring for an ill parent: The relationship between caring, parental disease, and the child's problem behavior]. *Kind en Adolescent*, 29, 208–220.

Newman, T. (2002). 'Young carers and disabled parents: Time for a change of direction? *Disability and Society*, 17, 613–625.

Ostwald, S.K., Godwin, K.M., Cron, S.G., Kelley, C.P., Hersch, G., Davis, S. (2013). Home-based psychoeducational and mailed information programs for stroke-caregiving dyads post-discharge: A randomized trial. *Disability and Rehabilitation*, 36, 55–62.

Romer, G., Barkmann, C., Watson, M., Schulte-Markwort, M., Thomalla, G., Riedesser, P. (2002). Children of somatically ill parents: A methodological review. *Clinical Child and Family Psychology Review*, 7, 17–38.

Pakenham, K.I., Bursnall, S. (2006). Relations between social support, appraisal and coping and both positive and negative outcomes for children of a parent with multiple sclerosis and comparisons with children of healthy parents. *Clinical Rehabilitation*, 20, 709–723.

Pakenham, K.I., Bursnall, S., Chiu, J., Cannon, T., Okochi, M. (2006). The psychosocial impact of caregiving on young people who have a parent with an illness or disability: Comparisons between young caregivers and non-caregivers. *Rehabilitation Psychology*, 51, 113–126.

Pakenham, K.I., Bursnall, S., Chiu, J., Cannon, T. (2007). Social support, appraisal, and both positive and negative outcomes in young caregivers. *Journal of Health Psychology*, 12, 89–102.

Rolland, J.S. (1999). Parental illness and disability: A family systems framework. *Journal of Family Therapy*, 21, 242–266.

Romer, G., Barkmann, C., Watson, M., Schulte-Markwort, M., Thomalla, G., Riedesser,

P. (2002). Children of somatically ill parents: A methodological review. *Clinical Child and Family Psychology Review*, 7, 17–38.

Schrag, A., Morley, D., Quinn, N., Jahanshahi, M. (2004). Impact of Parkinson's disease on patients' adolescent and adult children. *Parkinsonism and Related Disorders*, 10, 391–397.

Schulz, R., Czaja, S.J., Lustig, A., Zdaniuk, B., Martire, L.M., Perdomo, D. (2009) Improving the quality of life of caregivers of persons with spinal cord injury: A randomized controlled trial. *Rehabilitation Psychology*, 54, 1–15.

Shifren, K., Kachorek, L.V. (2003). Does early caregiving matter? The effects on young caregivers' adult mental health. *International Journal of Behavioral Development*, 27, 338–346.

Shyu, Y.I., Chen, M.C., Chen, S.T., Wang, H.P., Shao, J.H. (2008). A family caregiver-oriented discharge planning program for older stroke patients and their caregivers. *Journal of Clinical Nursing*, 17, 2497–2508.

Sieh, D.S. (2009). Gezinnen met een chronisch zieke ouder [Families with a chronically ill parent]. *Tijdschrift van de Artsenvereniging Jeugdgezondheidszorg Nederland*, 17, 22–23.

Sieh, D.S. (2012). The impact of parents' chronic medical conditions on children. Unpublished doctoral dissertation, University of Amsterdam.

Sieh, D.S., Meijer, A.M., Oort, F.J., Visser-Meily, J.M.A., van der Leij, D.A.V. (2010a). Problem behavior in children with a chronically ill parent: A meta-analysis. *Clinical Child and Family Psychology Review*, 3, 384–397.

Sieh, D.S., Meijer, A.M., Visser-Meily, J.M.A. (2010b). Risk factors for stress in children after parental stroke. *Rehabilitation Psychology*, 55, 391–397.

Sieh, D.S., Visser-Meily, J.M.A., Meijer, A.M. (2011). Jonge mantelzorger heeft behoefte aan aandacht [Young caregiver needs attention]. *Jeugd en Co Kennis*, 5, 18–26.

Sieh, D.S., Dikkers, A.L.C., Visser-Meily, J.M.A., Meijer, A.M. (2012a). Stress in adolescents with a chronically ill parent: Inspiration from Rolland's family systems-illness model. *Journal of Developmental and Physical Disabilities*, 6, 591–606.

Sieh, D.S., Visser-Meily, J.M.A., Oort, F.J., Meijer, A.M. (2012b). The diurnal salivary cortisol pattern of adolescents from families with single, ill and healthy parents. *Journal of Psychosomatic Research*, 27, 288–292.

Sieh, D.S., Oort, F.J., Visser-Meily, J.M.A., Meijer, A.M. (2013a). Determining risk and protective factors for problem behavior: The screening instrument for adolescents of parents with chronic medical condition. *Child Indicators Research*, 6, 345–361.

Sieh, D.S., Visser-Meily, J.M.A., Oort, F.J., Meijer, A.M. (2012b). Risk factors for problem behavior in adolescents of parents with a chronic medical condition. *European Child and Adolescent Psychiatry*, 21, 459–471.

Sieh, D.S., Visser-Meily, J.M.A., Meijer, A.M. (2013c). The relationship between parental depressive symptoms, family type, and adolescent functioning. *PLoS One*, *8(11): e80699*.

Sieh, D.S., Visser-Meily, J.M.A., Meijer, A.M. (2013d). Differential outcomes of adolescents with chronically ill and healthy parents. *Journal of Child and Family Studies*, 22, 209–218.

Sieh, D.S., Oort, F.J., Visser-Meily, J.M.A., Meijer, A.M. (2014). Mediators for internalizing problem behavior in adolescents with a chronically ill parent. *Journal of Developmental and Physical Disabilities*, 24, 67–82.

Tummers, J.F., Schrijvers, A.J., Visser-Meily, J.M.A. (2010). Review of the economic evidence on integrated care for stroke patients. *International Journal of Integrated Care*, 12, 1–15.

Visser-Meily, J.M.A., Meijer, A.M. (2006). Stroke, consequences for the family and recommendations for rehabilitation. In D.M. Devore (Ed.), *Parent-child relations: New research* (pp. 157–174). Hauppauge, NY: Nova Science Publishers.

Visser, A., Huizinga, G.A., van der Graaf, W.T., Hoekstra, H.J., Hoekstra-Weebers, J.E. (2004). The impact of parental cancer on children and the family: A review of the literature. *Cancer Treatment Review*, 30, 683–694.

Visser-Meily, A., Post, M., Meijer, A.M., Maas, C., Ketelaar, M., Lindeman, E. (2005). Children's adjustment to a parent's stroke: Determinants of health status and psychological problems, and the role of support from the rehabilitation team. *Journal of Rehabilitation Medicine*, 37, 236–241.

Visser-Meily, A., Post, M., Gorter, J.W., Berlekom, S.B.V., van den Bos, T., Lindeman, E. (2006). Rehabilitation of stroke patients needs a family-centred approach. *Disability and Rehabilitation*, 28, 1557–1561.

Visser-Meily, J.M.A., Post, M.W.M., van de Port, I., Maas, C.J.M., Forstberg-Wärleby, G., Lindeman, E. (2009). Psychosocial functioning of spouses of patients with stroke from initial inpatient rehabilitation to 3 years post-stroke: Course and relations with coping strategies. *Stroke*, 40, 1399–1404.

Wang, B., Li, X., Barnett, D., Zhao, G., Zhao, J., Stanton, B. (2012). Risk and protective factors for depression symptoms among children affected by HIV/AIDS in rural China: A structural equation modeling analysis. *Social Science and Medicine*, 74, 1435–1443.

Witteveen, E.M.J., Post, M.W.M., Visser-Meily, J.M.A. (2014). Participatiesamenleving: Naasten direct betrekken bij de revalidatie [Participating society: How to directly involve kin during rehabilitation]. *Nederlandse Tijdschrift voor Revalidatiegeneeskunde*, 1, 42–43.

CHAPTER 12

Measuring the impact of parental illness

Laura Kelly, Crispin Jenkinson and David Morley

INTRODUCTION

The challenges of assessing the impact of parental illness on children are multifaceted. Perhaps the most prominent of these challenges is the age of the child in question, as this has implications regarding who the most appropriate person is to accurately reflect the impact on the child of their parent's condition. For example, establishing whether it is appropriate to discuss with the child directly or to ask a proxy respondent, such as a parent, sibling, close family member, clinician or teacher are fundamental considerations. Selecting an appropriate methodology, which may be guided by the child's age, is a further, significant challenge. A range of options might be considered, from traditional observation to now more widely used techniques such as interview- or questionnaire-based assessment. The picture is a complex one but, if a range of guiding principles is considered, a successful assessment can be made.

This chapter focuses on how some of the challenges mentioned above might best be addressed. A brief discussion of age-related considerations is presented, which includes the issue of selecting the most appropriate respondent. This is followed by a discussion of the principles of sound scientific measurement that require consideration when selecting or developing an appropriate tool for assessing the impact of parental illness. As the most commonly incorporated methodology, the discussion is intentionally focused on questionnaire-based assessment, and is followed by a range of further considerations in their development and administration, with examples of measures previously used in this field of research.

AGE-RELATED CONSIDERATIONS

Childhood and adolescence are periods of development during which there are immense changes mentally, physically and socially. Effective assessment of a child's well-being therefore requires careful consideration of the age and developmental stage of the child and the associated cognitive and emotional changes (Reinfjell et al., 2006). Broadly, it has been proposed that such changes fall into three transitional periods, from infancy through to adolescence. Between the ages of 1 and 4, children develop abilities to experience shame, empathy, pride, moral anger and disapproval, anxiety over harm, loss and sadness over loss. Between the ages of 5 and 11, children start to experience guilt, envy, self-doubt and vicarious pride or shame. After age 11, cognitive maturation allows the developing adolescent child to experience love, uncertainty, depression and hopelessness (Kagan, 2001). Importantly, these cognitive and emotional changes also need be considered within a range of social contexts that are likely to influence a child's well-being at a particular point in the lifespan, such as their school, peer group or community (Matza, 2004). Arguably, one of the most significant social contexts is likely to be the family, and particularly its potential disruption when parental illness enters the family system/unit.

PROXY ASSESSMENT, DIRECT OBSERVATION OR SELF-REPORT?

The trajectory of children's development outlined above raises the significant question of who is most likely to accurately reflect the impact of parental illness on the child. Younger children may find it difficult to provide accurate and reliable accounts of their experiences or simply not be at a developmental stage where specific emotional or cognitive impacts might be expressed. It is therefore important to consider who might be the most suitable person to provide information for assessment. In some cases, it may be more appropriate for the child's parent(s) to assess the child's well-being. This so-called 'proxy assessment' generally takes the form of parents completing an instrument based on their inferences of the child's subjective experiences. An additional technique is to make an assessment based on direct observations of the child's behaviour via an observer-reported outcome (ObsRO) measure. Whilst ObsROs are generally looked upon more favourably than proxy assessment as there is less room for subjective, and potentially inaccurate, interpretation of the child's experiences (FDA, 2009, Matza et al., 2013), they have yet to be widely employed.

Using either of the methods outlined above to assess the well-being of older, more cognitively advanced children is to be discouraged if they are at a developmental stage with the capacity to complete an instrument for themselves (FDA, 2009). Indeed, there is significant evidence suggesting that proxy ratings can be problematic. For example, discrepancies in agreement have been found between proxy- and child-completed questionnaire scores (Rajmil et al., 2013; Upton et al., 2008). Research suggests that the response styles and reasoning methods employed by children and parents are fundamentally different. Children appear to employ a more extreme form of response choice (i.e. the highest or lowest response option), and to base their response on a single experience (Chambers and Johnston, 2002; Davis et al., 2007). In addition, there is evidence that the accuracy of proxy reports might be domain-specific and that, for example, parents may be better judges of physical functioning and symptoms than they are of more covert dimensions such as pain and emotional and social functioning (Verrips et al., 2000). Consequently, wherever possible, assessment of a child's well-being should be achieved by self-report (Ravens-Sieberer et al., 2006).

PRINCIPLES OF SCIENTIFIC MEASUREMENT

There are a number of key considerations to be taken into account when selecting or developing instruments to assess the impact of parental illness on a child. Having considered the merits of who should complete an instrument, it is equally important to consider the measurement properties of a selected instrument. Regardless of the respondent group, an instrument should be easy to administer and have measurement properties which indicate that it is valid, reliable and sensitive to change (EMA, 2004; FDA, 2009; Janssens et al., 2015; Mokkink et al., 2010). A lack of evidence supporting these characteristics may render all subsequent analyses invalid (Nunnally and Bernstein, 1994). A range of measurement (or 'psychometric') criteria that should be used to assess the suitability of an instrument are outlined in this chapter. Before outlining these recommended properties, a brief overview of instrument development is provided for the purposes of context.

Instrument development

Health-related instruments have typically been developed using statistical methods in order to understand how questionnaire items are interrelated. It is increasingly acknowledged, however, that the conceptual underpinnings of a measure must be explicit and empirically based (Bowling, 2005; FDA, 2009; Kerr et al., 2010; McColl, 2005; Reeve et al., 2013; Streiner et al., 2015). To achieve this, health-related scales should be rooted in qualitative research so that the child's perspective is incorporated from the early stages of instrument design. Statistical methods can then be used to assess the structure and grouping of items among a larger sample size. A mixed-methods approach is therefore considered good practice when developing an instrument (DeWalt et al., 2007; Kerr et al., 2010; Ring et al., 2010).

Qualitative methods are best used to develop a pool of candidate questionnaire items which are relevant and applicable to the concept of interest. Methods, such as in-depth interviews or focus groups, must be carried out within the intended population group, or those likely to be representing them if they are young children, to gain an understanding of their subjective views. A review of existing literature may help to inform researchers of topics to be included in an interview guide while allowing participants the opportunity to raise issues or concerns not found in the literature or through consulting healthcare professionals.

Many of the aspects of developing an item pool to assess the impact of parental ill-health on a child will be similar to research carried out with adults; however, some additional considerations should also be taken into account with children (Matza et al., 2013). Interviewers must be aware of the child's developmental stage and be careful to avoid using complicated language that may be confusing or discouraging. Using familiar terminology may be aided through discussing the interview process beforehand with the child's parents to gauge the child's developmental stage. Interviewers should also be aware that the child's attention span may be limited and that there is potential for the child to lose interest easily.

Interviews should take place in an environment which reduces the potential for the child to feel intimidated by or apprehensive about the researcher's presence. Where possible, it is recommended that the child be interviewed without the presence of their parents to reduce the chance of bias and avoid parents answering questions (Matza et al., 2013). It can also be useful to interview a selection of relevant people in addition to the child, including the child's parent(s) or guardians and relevant clinicians to get a full picture of the potential impact of parental ill health in a specific context. For a fuller account of interviewing children see Arbuckle and Abetz-Webb (2013). Interview data can subsequently be analysed to inform a conceptual basis for the instrument and guide researchers to use appropriate wording in the draft questionnaire items, which may be tested further for their applicability to the population of interest.

Having constructed a draft questionnaire relevant to the impact of parental illness on a child, various statistical approaches can be used to reduce the number of items to a more manageable size and examine the structure among the questionnaire items (Hinkin, 1998; Norman and Streiner, 2000). The most common methodological approaches are factor analysis, a technique used to aid selection of items and to guide the allocation of questions to domains (Pett et al., 2003), and, more recently, Rasch analysis, a statistical technique that places questions on a unidimensional continuum of 'difficulty' in a certain area (a so called 'latent trait') and is used to eliminate questions that do not fall within the latent trait (Bond and Fox, 2007).

Instrument properties

When assessing the merits of an instrument's properties, it is important to note the population and context in which the instrument was initially developed. Caution should be taken when selecting instruments for use in different research contexts to which they were developed; for example, with a different developmental age group or parental condition. Where measures are to be used in different cultures than those in which they were developed, it is essential that they remain meaningful and appropriate to the new cultural group. Furthermore, while it is important that initial validation studies demonstrate that an instrument meets the standards outlined below, assessing the acceptability of an instrument and its measurement properties is a continuous process. Using an instrument in subsequent studies can build further evidence to support its validity, reliability and responsiveness.

Reliability

When considering the measurement properties of an instrument, it is important to ensure that there is a consistency with which participants respond to questions (or 'items') within a given scale. This can be supported through demonstrating that responses to items within a scale are free from random error and that responses to items are interrelated (Jenkinson and McGee, 1998; Portney and Watkins, 2009). This is known as a scale's internal reliability (or internal consistency). This is typically examined using the Cronbach's alpha statistic which has a recommended value of 0.7 or above (De Vaus, 2013). It is also good practice to examine how strongly an item in a scale correlates to the scale as a whole after omitting that item from the total. This value is referred to as the item-to-total correlation (Portney and Watkins, 2009). Items with coefficient values of below 0.3 give some indication that they may be measuring a separate construct and their removal is likely to improve the scale's reliability (Kline, 2000).

Best practice also encourages the assessment of the stability of scores over time (test-retest reliability) (FDA, 2009; Kline, 2000; Reeve et al., 2013). This is based on the premise that, providing there has been no underlying change in the construct being measured, test scores should be the same (or very similar) when completed by a respondent on two or more occasions (Hays and Revicki, 2005; Jenkinson and McGee, 1997). To examine test-retest reliability, an instrument is typically administered at two time points with an interval that is sufficiently distant to ensure the respondent cannot simply replicate their answers from memory and short enough so that the underlying construct has not changed for that respondent (Streiner et al., 2015). Changes in scores between the two time points may occur for a variety of reasons, such as: the construct being assessed has in fact changed, contextual issues have changed (for example, the responder feels ill, tired, bored or anxious about an unrelated event), the respondent has been influenced by having already completed the questionnaire on the first occasion, or the instrument cannot measure the construct with a good degree of precision (Streiner et al., 2015). The test-retest reliability of an instrument within a given population is typically assessed using the Intra Class Coefficient (ICC) statistic (Streiner et al., 2015). Participant scale scores at two time points are correlated and values of greater than 0.7 indicate good test-retest reliability (Kline, 2000).

A third aspect of reliability which may be considered is the inter-rater reliability of an instrument. Inter-rater reliability assesses the consistency of responses when two or more respondents complete a questionnaire (McColl, 2005). Inter-rater reliability can be particularly relevant in the context of assessing the impact of parental ill health on children where both parents complete the questionnaire. It can also be used to assess agreement with child and parent responses. The kappa statistic, where a value of 0.70 or higher agreement is considered acceptable, is most frequently used (Eiser and Morse, 2001).

Validity

Determining the reliability of an instrument informs the user about the precision of measurement; however, it tells them little about how well the instrument is measuring the intended construct. Using a range of approaches to examine the validity of an instrument helps to inform the user whether it is the intended construct which is, in fact, being assessed. When assessing the suitability of an instrument, four overall components of validity may be assessed.

Face validity examines the extent to which the questionnaire items superficially make sense and whether they can be easily understood (Jenkinson and McGee, 1997). Although this can seem trivial, checking the questionnaire makes sense within the respondent group for child-completion questionnaires as children may interpret items very differently when compared to parents, clinicians or children of a different developmental group. Testing the face validity of the questionnaire can be carried out at the early stages of the item-development process by seeking opinions from experts in the field and the intended population to see if there is general agreement that the instrument appears suitable.

Content validity ensures all aspects of the construct being measured are represented by the items (Bowling, 2005). Like face validity, content validity can be supported during the early stages of item development. A clear conceptual framework should inform items, and be followed by a period of evaluating respondents' understanding of the items to determine whether their interpretations are relevant to the construct being measured (Bowling, 2005; Brod et al., 2009; Speight and Barendse, 2010). Evidence of content validity is therefore ideally obtained through the use of existing literature and concept elicitation using qualitative methods among the target group. As discussed previously, if the intended population group is children, it may also be beneficial to interview parents and clinicians. Cognitive debriefing interviews can then be used to explore respondents' understanding of questionnaire items and their perceived relevance to the concept (FDA, 2009; Willis, 1999; Willis, 2005). Items which are not found to be directly related to the concept of interest during item testing with potential responders should be removed or amended. Terminology can be interpreted differently among various populations and their involvement at these early stages can ensure that items and response scales are meaningful to different response groups (EMA, 2004; FDA, 2009; Lohr, 2002).

Construct validity is typically assessed by comparing respondents' scores on the instrument being examined with scores from other similar instruments which are thought to measure a similar construct. Two aspects of construct validity can be tested. Convergent validity tests an *a priori* hypothesis that a relationship exists between the new scale(s) and another established 'reference' measure (FDA, 2009; Hinkin, 1998). Discriminant validity is essentially the opposite of convergent validity, which confirms a prior hypothesis stating two instruments are not related (Jenkinson and McGee, 1998). Known-groups validity can also be used to test construct validity. Groups which are hypothesised to have different scores are compared typically using t-tests or analysis of variance (Hays and Revicki, 2005). For example, the well-being of children of parents with multiple sclerosis could be compared with the well-being of children of healthy parents, as has been assessed in previous research (Packenham and Cox, 2014, 2015; Yahav et al., 2005, 2007). Other tests that can be carried out to assess construct validity using Rasch analysis include testing for differences in item functioning across factors such as age and gender to ensure question responses are not influenced by such attributes (so called 'differential item functioning') and confirmatory tests of unidimensionality (Janssens et al., 2015).

Finally, *criterion validity* refers to the ability of an instrument to correspond to other instruments which are considered 'gold standards' (Jenkinson et al., 2011). In the area of health measurement by questionnaire, the notion of a 'gold standard' only truly applies when creating shorter-form measures of existing instruments, and involves comparing results on a shortened version of a questionnaire with results obtained from the parent or longer-form instrument (Jenkinson and McGee, 1998).

Responsiveness

In order for an instrument to be useful when assessing the construct of interest, it must be sensitive enough to detect any changes in health and have the ability to provide both meaningful and interpretable data. Sensitivity to change, or 'responsiveness', is concerned with demonstrating an instrument's ability to detect changes in respondent scores; for example, between an individual's mean scores before and after a treatment or event (Jenkinson et al., 2011). Where any differences occur, however, it is not simply adequate to demonstrate statistically different scores; differences should be meaningful to the person who is completing the questionnaire. This is referred to as the minimum important difference (MID) and is a guide with which to interpret whether an observed change is important from the child's, parent's or clinician's perspective (Revicki et al., 2006, 2008). When establishing MID values, anchor-based methods may be used to evaluate changes in scores for groups of respondents whose health status is known to have changed. Mean differences in scores between those with improved or worsening health can then inform what may be deemed a MID in a given population group. The extent of change by which MIDs are calculated can be measured by clinical endpoints, the use of health-transition questions or through using scores from a previously existing, well-established instrument (Revicki et al., 2006).

Distribution-based methods may also be used to quantify responsiveness. Distribution-based methods are statistical techniques, the most common being the effect-size statistic, a standardised measure of the magnitude of change calculated by dividing the mean change in scores by the baseline standard deviation (Jenkinson et al., 2011; Kazis et al., 1989). The following magnitude of effect sizes has been suggested to assess change: 0.2 indicates a small change, 0.5 indicates a moderate change and 0.8 indicates a large change (Cohen, 1977). However, these are general guides to interpretation and for many instruments specific guidance is provided on the meaning of effect sizes. Other distribution-based approaches may also be used. Examples include the standardised response mean (calculated by dividing the mean change in scores by the standard deviation of the change in scores) (Liang et al., 1990) and the responsiveness statistic, calculated by dividing the mean change in scores by the standard deviation of change in respondents who remain stable over time (Guyatt et al., 1987). Distinct from a MID, the minimal detectable change (MDC) is a distribution-based indication of the degree of change required to be confident that the change is outside the level of possible measurement error, usually the 90% confidence level (Haley and Fragala-Pinkham, 2006). Despite the various approaches discussed, it is recommended that a number of methods (anchor-based methods supported by distribution-based methods) are employed to assess the responsiveness of an instrument. This supports data triangulation and further confidence in a single or small range of MID estimates (Cella et al., 2002; Jenkinson et al., 2011; Revicki et al., 2007, 2008; Yost and Eton, 2005).

Further to the procedures outlined above, those selecting an instrument to administer should also be aware of simple descriptive data which may indicate limited scaling properties. For example, scale distributions may indicate evidence of floor and ceiling effects (Jenkinson, 1997; Nunnally and Bernstein, 1994) and extreme endorsement frequencies are not considered acceptable in psychometric measurement (Streiner et al., 2015). Precision of measurement can also be examined using Rasch analysis to establish equal interval scaling (Janssens et al., 2015).

ADDITIONAL CONSIDERATIONS

Response options

Likert response scales are commonly used in instruments relating to the impact on a child of parental illness. Likert response options are placed on an ordinal scale ranging from complete absence of the domain of interest (e.g. never feeling sad) to the highest possible level (e.g. always feeling sad). Those administering questionnaires should, however, be mindful of the child's reading ability (Streiner et al., 2015) and that younger children may be more likely to use the more extreme response options than those in an older age grouping (Juniper, 1997; Rebok et al., 2001). The appropriateness of using a particular response scale should therefore be examined within the age group of interest (Matza et al., 2013). For younger children it may be more appropriate to illustrate any degree of agreement or frequency of an event using pictorial representations; for example, circles of increasing size (Rebok et al., 2001) or smiley faces ranging from happy to sad (Chaplin et al., 2008).

Recall period

Identifying a suitable 'recall period' or period of time that a child can remember will also be somewhat age-dependent. Younger children may have some difficulty recalling long periods of time (for example, one month) and may be more comfortable recalling more recent events which occurred in the last week (Matza et al., 2004). Indeed, it is impossible to specify a blanket optimal recall period as this will largely depend on the respondent's ability to recall the events in question (FDA, 2009; Matza et al., 2013). Cognitive testing should therefore be used to thoroughly test the time period that children can comfortably recall.

Instrument length

Instruments for use among children should be relatively short and the number of questionnaire items should be carefully considered (Matza et al., 2004). As children's attention span can vary across age groups, it is important to test the number of items to be administered and the time taken to complete them within the intended age group before wide-scale administration. Unsurprisingly, it is generally thought that younger children find longer questionnaires more challenging to complete when compared to their older counterparts (Matza et al., 2004, 2013).

Formatting

The design and layout of an instrument should cater to the age group and cognitive abilities of the intended respondents. This may include paying particular attention to the layout of items and response scales and using a suitable size font for young children (Matza et al., 2004).

Administration

Clearly, the age of the child will have a significant bearing on how assessment is undertaken or the measure is administered. Younger children may require the assistance of, for example, a parent to sit with them and assist with both completion and focus (Matza, 2004). Alternatively, interviewer-administered measures can be incorporated to deal with limitations in reading and attention span (Matza et al., 2013). Older children, however, should wherever possible be encouraged to complete measures on their own.

Additionally, it is important to acknowledge a child's independence during administration. Young people should be allowed undisturbed time alone in which to complete questionnaires, and their confidentiality should be respected, just as one would with adult participants (Erling, 1999). As with the wider literature on outcomes measurement, electronic-based data capture is becoming increasingly prominent with children and has significant potential to be incorporated in the assessment of parental illness. Studies suggest that children and young people prefer both computer and internet administration over traditional survey methods such as pen and paper completion. (Ravens-Sieberer et al., 2000; Mangunkusumo et al., 2005).

Cross-cultural issues

It is good practice to consider language and cultural differences across countries. In addition to factors which need to be taken into account with adult measures, such as cultural references and norms, it is particularly important to be aware that differences in educational systems may influence the ability of children to understand and accurately respond to items (Matza et al., 2013). Family roles and relationships may also differ between countries and consideration should be given to whether the items within instruments are appropriate and meaningful for that context. Other considerations may be specific to the parent's health condition and the implications within that society; for example, the support available to the patient and family, societal attitudes and health insurance. As well as typical checks and balances which may be carried out to assess the cultural and linguistic suitability of adult measures, cognitive interviews must be used to assess the appropriateness of items for specific age groups within a new country.

CLOSING COMMENTS

This chapter has presented some key concepts relevant to the assessment of children's response to parental illness. A number of considerations have been introduced which, together, provide a basis upon which to make a sound assessment of how a parental condition might affect a child's well-being. The following appendix provides examples of a range of measures that have been incorporated in the assessment of parental illness. Whilst by no means an exhaustive list of all measures incorporated in research to date, it should give the reader a broad sense of the range and type of assessment tools that are currently available.

APPENDIX

Attachment Q Sort (AQS; Waters, 1995; Waters and Deane, 1985): The AQS is an observational assessment (conducted by a trained researcher) of the strength of attachment between children aged 1–5 and their primary caregiver (typically the mother). The assessment incorporates a Q-sort ranking methodology whereby participants rank a series of statements or observations that provide insight into the field of investigation. The AQS contains 90 observations that can take approximately 90–120 minutes to complete. The measure demonstrates moderate inter-rater reliability (Vaughn and Waters, 1990) and convergent validity (van Ijzendoorn et al., 2004) and has been used in studies assessing the impact of parental depression (e.g. Forman et al., 2007; van Doesum et al., 2008).

Birleson Depression Self Rating Scale (DSRS; Birleson, 1981; Birleson et al., 1987): The DSRS is regarded as a reliable and valid tool in the assessment of adolescent depression, demonstrating high internal consistency (Ivarsson and Gillberg, 1997; Ivarsson et al., 1994). The instrument has been validated in a number of studies with children ranging between the ages of 8 and 18 (e.g. Fundudis et al., 1991; Ivarsson et al., 1994, 2002) and totals 18 items, answered on a three-point Likert scale. The DSRS has been incorporated in studies to assess, for example, parental PD, MS and stroke (Morley et al., 2005, 2011; Schrag et al., 2004b).

Child Behaviour Checklist (CBCL; Achenbach, 1991, 1999; Achenbach and Rescorla, 2001): The CBCL is a checklist parents complete to detect emotional and behavioural problems in children and adolescents. The instrument is for use among children aged 6–18 and consists of 113 statements that parents rank on a three-point response scale. A recent review indicates that the measure demonstrates favourable validity and reliability (Deighton et al., 2014). The CBCL has been used to investigate, for example, emotional and behavioural problems in children of parents who have MS (Diareme et al., 2006), adolescents' responses to parental breast cancer (Edwards et al., 2008), and children's response to obsessive-compulsive disorder (Black et al., 2003). However, the length of the measure limits its practicality in some studies and settings. A self-report version of the CBCL, the Youth Self Report (YSR; Achenbach and Rescorla, 2001), has also been used in the assessment of parental illness and is included in this appendix.

Child Behaviour Questionnaire (CBQ; Rothbart et al., 2001): The CBQ is a parent/caregiver report measure developed for use in children aged 3–7 years. The original measure comprised 195 items over three dimensions of temperament: Extraversion/Surgency, Negative Affectivity and Effortful Control. Short-form, 94- and 36-item versions have since been developed

(Putnam and Rothbart, 2006). The measures demonstrate adequate validity and reliability (Putnam and Rothbart, 2006; Rothbart et al., 2001) and have been used in, for example, the assessment of parental depression (Forman et al., 2007; Godfrey, 2013).

Child Depression Inventory (CDI; Kovacs, 1985): The CDI measures depressive symptoms in children and adolescents aged 7–17 years. The long- and short-form instruments contain 27 items and 10 items respectively. A parent version consisting of 17 items is also available. The instrument demonstrates sound internal consistency and test-retest reliability (Finch Jr et al., 1987; Saylor et al., 1984), alongside good construct validity (Doerfler et al., 1988). The CDI has been used by rehabilitation teams to investigate the support given to young children of parents with stroke (Visser-Meily et al., 2005).

KIDSCREEN (Ravens-Sieberer et al., 2005, 2007, 2010): A number of versions of the generic KIDSCREEN instrument exist for children aged 8–18. The instrument was developed using Rasch methods and is available in 52-, 27- and 10-item versions and in proxy and self-complete format. Items have a five-point Likert response scale where higher values indicate superior health-related quality of life (HRQoL). The KIDSCREEN-10 summary index has been used to assess HRQoL in children affected by parental cancer (Bultmann et al., 2014; Krattenmacher et al., 2013). While the proxy version is believed to have acceptable psychometric properties (Ravens-Sieberer et al., 2010), parents have been shown to underestimate the burden of parental cancer in adolescents (Krattenmacher et al., 2013).

KINDL-R (Ravens-Sieberer and Bullinger, 1998a, 1998b): Three self-report versions of the 24 item KINDL instrument exist to assess HRQoL in three different age groups; ages 4–7 (interview format), 8–12 and 13–16. Parent/proxy versions are available for the two younger age groups. In addition, a computer-assisted version, CAT-SCREEN, has been developed (Ravens-Sieberer et al., 2000). The instruments demonstrate sound reliability alongside evidence of concurrent and divergent validity, but not content validity (Hullmann et al., 2011). The KINDL has been used in studies to assess, for example, the HRQoL of children with parents who have leprosy (Yamaguchi et al., 2013) and mental health problems (Pollak et al., 2008).

Inventory of Parent and Peer Attachment (IPPA; Armsden and Greenberg, 1987): Developed to measure child/adolescent attachment to parents, this instrument explores communication, trust, and alienation. The instrument contains 28 items, each with a five-point Likert scale response option, and has been widely used due to the high reliability of the scale (Benson et al., 2006). The measure has been incorporated in studies that have assessed, for example, the impact of parental chronic illness (Sieh et al., 2013, 2012) and maternal HIV/AIDS (Marelich et al., 2012; Murphy et al., 2008, 2012).

Parental Illness Impact Scale – Revised (PIIS-R; Morley et al., 2010; Schrag et al., 2004a), a 51-item instrument designed specifically to assess the impact of parental illness. The measure comprises 37 items answered on a five-point Likert scale assessing eight domains of well-being: Burden of Daily Help, Emotional Impact, Social Impact, Communication and Understanding, Impact on Personal Future, Friends' Reactions, Parent/Child Relationship, and Global Well-Being. The PIIS-R incorporates 14 dichotomous items focusing on the needs of children regarding provision of information and sources of support, and a visual analogue scale (VAS). The instrument has been shown to possess sound reliability and validity (Morley et al., 2010). The PIIS-R has been used in the assessment of parental Parkinson's, MS and stroke (Morley et al., 2005, 2011; Schrag et al., 2004b).

Rosenberg Self-Esteem Scale (RSES; Rosenberg, 1989): A short 10-item questionnaire that measures feelings of self-deprecation and self-worth. The instrument has been widely used in adolescent populations aged 11 and above. Response categories comprise a four-point agree-disagree Likert scale. The RSES has been shown to demonstrate good reliability (Blascovich and Tomaka, 1991) and has been used in a range of studies assessing the impact of parental illness, including PD, MS and stroke (Morley et al., 2005, 2011), and leprosy (Yamaguchi et al., 2013).

Youth Activities of Caregiving Scale (YACS; Ireland and Pakenham, 2010): This instrument was designed to assess youth caregiving tasks in the context of family illness or disability. The YACS was developed following a review of relevant literature and consultation with young carers and researchers in the field. The instrument consists of 30 items measuring four domains with good reliability. The instrument also has evidence supporting good convergent and predictive validity. However, it would benefit from testing using a larger sample size. The instrument has been used in children with parents of MS and a parent version is now available (Pakenham and Cox, 2012).

Young Carers of Parents Inventory (YCOPI; Pakenham et al 2006; Cox and Pakenham, 2014). The YCOPI consists of two parts; the 5 factor YCOPI-A, which assesses young caregiver's experiences across multiple caregiving contexts, and the 4 factor YCOPI-B that specifically assesses caregiving in the context of parental illness. The measure demonstrates sound reliability and validity (Pakenham et al 2006), as well as sensitivity to change (Cox and Pakenham, 2014). The YCOPI has been incorporated in a range of studies including those assessing parental MS (Packenham and Bursnall 2006; Pakenham and Cox, 2012) and parental physical and/or psychological illness

(Ireland and Pakenham, 2010; Sieh et al., 2013; Fraser and Pakenham, 2008, 2009).

Youth Self Report (YSR; Achenbach and Rescorla, 2001): The YSR is a child self-report version of the CBCL which assesses emotional and behavioural problems among adolescents aged 11–18. The instrument contains 118 items with three-point response scales. The YSR consists of two broad dimensions measuring internalisation and externalisation problems. It has also been validated in younger people aged 7–10, with both domains exhibiting high reliability (Ebesutani et al., 2011). The YSR has been utilised in studies researching long-term outcomes in children of mothers identified as being at psychological risk (Wadsby et al., 2007), prevalence of problems among children of parents diagnosed with cancer (Thastum et al., 2009; Visser et al., 2007), emotional reactions to cancer (Gazendam-Donofrio et al., 2011) factors associated with the mental health of adolescents when a parent has cancer (Lindqvist et al., 2007) and children's response to parental amyotrophic lateral sclerosis (Calvo et al., 2015).

REFERENCES

Achenbach, T.M. (1991). *Integrative guide for the 1991 CBCL/4–18, YSR and TRF profiles.* Burlington, VT: Department of Psychiatry, University of Vermont.

Achenbach, T.M. (1999). The Child Behavior Checklist and related instruments. *The use of psychological testing for treatment planning and outcomes assessment* (2nd edn). Mahwah, NJ, US: Lawrence Erlbaum Associates.

Achenbach, T.M., Rescorla, L. (2001). *The manual for the ASEBA school-age forms and profiles.* Burlington, VT: University of Vermont, Research Center for Children, Youth, and Families.

Arbuckle, R., Abetz-Webb, L. (2013). 'Not just little adults': Qualitative methods to support the development of pediatric patient-reported outcomes. *The Patient*, 6(3), 143–159.

Armsden, M.D.S., Greenberg, M.T. (1987). The inventory of parent and peer attachment: Individual differences and their relationship to psychological well-being in adolescence. *Journal of Youth and Adolescence*, 16, 427–453.

Benson, M., McWey, L., Ross, J. (2006). Parental attachment and peer relations in adolescence: A meta-analysis. *Research in Human Development*, 3, 33–43.

Birleson, P. (1981). The validity of depressive disorder in childhood and the development of a self-rating scale: A Research Report. *Journal of Child Psychology and Psychiatry*, 22, 73–88.

Birleson, P., Hudson, I., Buchanan, D.G., Wolff, S. (1987). Clinical evaluation of a self-rating scale for depressive disorder in childhood (Depression Self-Rating Scale). *Journal of Child Psychology and Psychiatry*, 28, 43–60.

Black, D.W., Gaffney, G.R., Schlosser, S., Gabel, J. (2003). Children of parents with obsessive compulsive disorder: A 2-year follow up study. *Acta Psychiatrica Scandinavica*, 107, 305–313.

Blascovich, J., Tomaka, J. (1991). Measures of self-esteem. In J. Robinson, P. Shaver, L. Wrightsman (Eds) *Measures of personality and social psychological attitudes* (pp. 115–160). New York: Academic Press.

Bond, T.G., Fox, C. (2007). *Applying the Rasch Measurement Model: Fundamental measurement in the human sciences.* London: Lawrence Erlbaum Associates.

Bowling, A. (2005). *Measuring health: A review of quality of life measurement scales.* Maidenhead: Open University Press.

Brod, M., Tesler, L.E., Christensen, T.L. (2009). Qualitative research and content validity: Developing best practices based on science and experience. *Quality of Life Research*, 18, 1263–1278.

Bultmann, J.C., Beierlein, V., Romer, G., Möller, B., Koch, U., Bergelt, C. (2014). Parental cancer: Health-related quality of life and current psychosocial support needs of cancer survivors and their children. *International Journal of Cancer*, 135(11), 2668–2677.

Calvo, V., Bianco, F., Benelli, E., Sambin, M., Monsurrò, M.R., Femiano, C., Querin, G., Soraru, G., Palmieri, A. (2015). Impact on children of a parent with ALS: A case-control study. *Frontiers in Psychology*, 6, 288.

Cella, D., Eton, D.T., Lai, J.S., Peterman, A.H., Merkel, D.E. (2002). Combining anchor and distribution-based methods to derive minimal clinically important differences on the Functional Assessment of Cancer Therapy (FACT) anemia and fatigue scales. *Jounal of Pain and Symptom Management*, 24, 547–561.

Chambers, C., Johnston, C. (2002). Developmental differences in children's use of rating scales. *Journal of Pediatric Psychology*, 27, 27–36.

Chaplin, J.E., Koopman, H.M., Schmidt, S.; DISABKIDS Group. (2008). DISABKIDS smiley questionnaire: The TAKE 6 assisted health-related quality of life measure for 4 to 7-year-olds. *Clinical Psychology and Psychotherapy*, 15(3), 173–180.

Cohen, J. (1977). *Statistical power for the behavioural sciences.* New York: Academic Press.

Cox, S.D., Pakenham, K.I. (2014). Confirmatory factor analysis and invariance testing of the Young Carer of Parents Inventory (YCOPI). *Rehabilitation Psychology*, 59(4), 439–452.

Davis, E., Nicolas, C., Waters, E., Cook, K., Gibbs, L., Gosch, A., Ravens-Sieberer, U. (2007). Parent-proxy and child self-reported health-related quality of life: Using qualitative methods to explain the discordance. *Quality of Life Research*, 16, 863–871.

Deighton, J., Croudace, T., Fonagy, P., Brown, J., Patalay, P., Wolpert, M. (2014). Measuring mental health and wellbeing outcomes for children and adolescents to inform practice and policy: A review of child self-report measures. *Child and Adolescent Psychiatry and Mental Health*, 8, 14.

De Vaus, D.A. (2013). *Surveys in social research* (6th edn). London: Routledge.

DeWalt, D.A., Rothrock, N., Yount, S., Stone, A.A; PROMIS Cooperative Group. (2007).

Evaluation of Item Candidates: The PROMIS Qualitative Item Review. *Medical Care*, 45 (5 Suppl 1), S12–21.

Diareme, S., Tsiantis, J., Kolaitis, G., Ferentinos, S., Tsalamanios, E., Paliokosta, E., Anasontzi, S., Lympinaki, E., Anagnostopoulos, D.C., Voumvourakis, C., Romer, G. (2006). Emotional and behavioural difficulties in children of parents with multiple sclerosis: A controlled study in Greece. *European Child and Adolescent Psychiatry*, 15(6), 309–318.

Doerfler, L.A., Felner, R.D., Rowlison, R.T., Raley, P.A., Evans, E. (1988). Depression in children and adolescents: A comparative analysis of the utility and construct validity of two assessment measures. *Journal of Consulting and Clinical Psychology*, 56(5), 769–772.

Ebesutani, C., Bernstein, A., Martinez, J.I., Chorpita, B.F., Weisz, J.R. (2011). The youth self report: Applicability and validity across younger and older youths. *Journal of Clinical Child and Adolescent Psychology*, 40, 338–346.

Edwards, L., Watson, M., St James-Roberts, I., Ashley, S., Tilney, C., Brougham, B., Osborn, T., Baldus, C., Romer, G. (2008). Adolescent's stress responses and psychological functioning when a parent has early breast cancer. *Psycho-Oncology*, 17, 1039–1047.

Eiser, C., Morse, R. (2001). Quality-of-life measures in chronic diseases of childhood. *Health Technology Assessment*, 5(4), 1–157.

EMA. (2004). Reflection paper on the regulatory guidance for the use of health-related quality of life (HRQL) measures in the evaluation of medicinal products. London: European Medicines Agency.

Erling, A. (1999). Methodological considerations in the assessment of health-related quality of life in children. *Acta Paediatrics*, 428 (Suppl), 106–107.

FDA (2009). *Guidance for industry: Patient-reported outcome measures: Use in medical product development to support labeling claims*. Silver Spring, MD: US Department of Health and Human Services Food and Drug Administration.

Finch Jr, A.J., Saylor, C.F., Edwards, G.L., McIntosh, A.J. (1987). Children's Depression Inventory: Reliability over repeated administrations. *Journal of Clinical Child Psychology*, 16, 339–341.

Forman, D.R., O'Hara, M.W., Stuart, S., Gorman, L.L., Larsen, K.E., Coy, K.C. (2007). Effective treatment for postpartum depression is not sufficient to improve the developing mother–child relationship. *Development and Psychopathology*, 19(02), 585–602.

Fraser, E., Pakenham, K.I. (2008). Evaluation of a resilience-based intervention for children of parents with mental illness. *Australian and New Zealand Journal of Psychiatry*, 42, 1041–1050.

Fraser, E., Pakenham, K.I. (2009). Resilience in children of parents with mental illness: Relations between mental health literacy, social connectedness and coping, and both adjustment and caregiving. *Psychology, Health and Medicine*, 14, 573–584.

Fundudis, T., Berney, T.P., Kolvin, I., Famuyiwa, O.O., Barrett, L., Bhate, S., Tyrer, S.P. (1991). Reliability and validity of two self rating scales in the assessment of childhood depression. *British Journal of Psychiatry*, 159(S11), 36–40.

Gazendam-Donofrio, S.M., Hoekstra, H.J., van der Graaf, W.T., van de Wiel, H.B., Visser, A., Huizinga, G.A., Hoekstra-Weebers, J.E. (2011). Adolescents' emotional reactions to parental cancer: Effect on emotional and behavioral problems. *Journal of Pediatric Psychology*, 36, 346–359.

Godfrey, E.B. (2013). System justification, mental health, and behavior among disadvantaged mothers and their children. *Basic and Applied Social Psychology*, 35(4), 382–395.

Guyatt, G., Walter, S., Norman, G. (1987). Measuring change over time: Assessing the usefulness of evaluative instruments. *Journal of Chronic Diseases*, 40(2), 171–178.

Haley, S.M., Fragala-Pinkham, M.A. (2006). Interpreting change scores of tests and measures used in physical therapy. *Physical Therapy*, 86(5), 735–743.

Hays, R.D., Revicki, D. (2005). Reliability and validity (including responsiveness). In P.M. Fayers, R.D. Hays (Eds) *Assessing quality of life in clinical trials: Methods and practice*. Oxford: Oxford University Press.

Hinkin, T.R. (1998). A brief tutorial on the development of measures for use in survey questionnaires. *Organizational Research Methods*, 1, 104–121.

Hullmann, S.E., Ryan, J.L., Ramsey, R.R., Chaney, J.M., Mullins, L.L. (2011). Measures of general pediatric quality of life: Child Health Questionnaire (CHQ), DISABKIDS Chronic Generic Measure (DCGM), KINDL-R, Pediatric Quality of Life Inventory (PedsQL) 4.0 Generic Core Scales, and Quality of My Life Questionnaire (QoML). *Arthritis Care and Research*, 63(S11), S420–S430.

Ireland, M.J., Pakenham, K.I. (2010). The nature of youth care tasks in families experiencing chronic illness/disability: Development of the Youth Activities of Caregiving Scale (YACS). *Psychology and Health*, 25, 713–731.

Ivarsson, T., Gillberg, C. (1997). Depressive symptoms in Swedish adolescents: Normative data using the Birleson Depression Self-Rating Scale (DSRS) *Journal of Affective Disorders*, 42(1), 59–68.

Ivarsson, T., Lidberg, A., Gillberg, C. (1994). The Birleson Depression Self-Rating Scale (DSRS). Clinical evaluation in an adolescent inpatient population. *Journal of Affective Disorders*, 32(2), 115–125.

Ivarsson, T., Gillberg, C., Arvidsson, T., Broberg, A.G. (2002). The Youth Self-Report (YSR) and the Depression Self-Rating Scale (DSRS) as measures of depression and suicidality among adolescents. (2002). *European Child and Adolescent Psychiatry*, 11, 31–37.

Janssens, A., Rogers, M., Thompson Coon, J., Allen, K., Green, C., Jenkinson, C., Tennant, A., Logan, S., Morris, C. (2015). A systematic review of generic multidimensional patient-reported outcome measures for children, part II: Evaluation of psychometric performance of English-language versions in a general population. *Value in Health*, 18, 334–345.

Jenkinson, C. (1997). Assessment and evaluation of health care and medical care: An introduction and overview. In C. Jenkinson (Ed.) *Assessment and evaluation of health care and medical care: A methods text* (pp. 1–5). Buckingham: Open University Press.

Jenkinson, C., McGee, H.M. (1997). Patient assessed outcomes: Measuring health status and quality of life. In C. Jenkinson (Ed.) *Assessment and evaluation of health and medical care: A methods text* (pp. 64–84). Buckingham: Open University Press.

Jenkinson, C., McGee, H.M. (1998). *Health status measurement: A brief but critical introduction.* Oxford: Radcliffe Medical Press.

Jenkinson, C., Dawson, J., Morris, C. (2011). Aspects of methodology relevant to patient-reported outcome measures (PROMs). In C. Jenkinson, M. Peters, M. Bromberg (Eds) *Quality of life measurement in neurodegenerative and related conditions.* Cambridge: Cambridge University Press.

Juniper, E.F. (1997). Quality of life in adults and children with asthma and rhinitis. *Allergy*, 52, 971–977.

Kagan, J. (2001). Emotional development and psychiatry. *Biological Psychiatry*, 49(12), 973–979.

Kazis, L.E., Anderson, J.J., Meenan, R.F. (1989). Effect sizes for interpreting changes in health status. *Medical Care*, 27, S178–189.

Kerr, C., Nixon, A., Wild, D. (2010). Assessing and demonstrating data saturation in qualitative inquiry supporting patient-reported outcomes research. *Expert Review of Pharmacoeconomics and Outcomes Research*, 10, 269–281.

Kline, P. (2000). *A psychometric primer.* London: Free Association Books.

Kovacs, M. (1985). The Children's Depression Inventory (CDI). *Psychopharmacology Bulletin*, 21, 995–998.

Krattenmacher, T., Kühne, F., Führer, D., Beierlein, V., Brähler, E., Resch, F., Klitzing, K.v., Flechtner, H.H., Bergelt, C., Romer, G., Möller, B. (2013). Coping skills and mental health status in adolescents when a parent has cancer: A multicenter and multi-perspective study. *Journal of Psychosomatic Research*, 74, 252–259.

Liang, M.H., Fossel, A.H., Larson, M.G. (1990). Comparisons of five health status instruments for orthopedic evaluation. *Medical Care*, 28, 632–642.

Lindqvist, B., Schmitt, F., Santalahti, P., Romer, G., Piha, J. (2007). Factors associated with the mental health of adolescents when a parent has cancer. *Scandinavian Journal of Psychology*, 48, 345–351.

Lohr, K.N. (2002). Assessing health status and quality-of-life instruments: Attributes and review criteria. *Quality of Life Research*, 11, 193–205.

Mangunkusumo, R.T., Moorman, P.W., Van Den Berg-de-Ruiter, A.E., Van Der Lei. J., De Koning, H.J., Raat, H. (2005). Internet-administered adolescent health questionnaires compared with a paper version in a randomized study. *Journal of Adolescent Health* 36(1), 70.e1–70.e6.

Marelich, W.D., Murphy, D.A., Payne, D.L., Herbeck, D.M., Schuster, M.A. (2012). Self-competence among early and middle adolescents affected by maternal HIV/AIDS. *International Journal of Adolescence and Youth*, 17(1), 21–33.

Matza, L.S., Swensen, A., Flood, E., Secnik, K., Leidy, N. (2004). Assessment of health-related quality of life in children: A review of conceptual, methodological, and regulatory issues. *Value in Health*, 7, 79–92.

Matza, L.S., Patrick, D.L., Riley, A.W., Alexander, J.J., Rajmil, L., Pleil, A.M., Bullinger, M. (2013). Pediatric patient-reported outcome instruments for research to support medical product labeling: Report of the ISPOR PRO good research practices for the assessment of children and adolescents task force. *Value in Health*, 16, 461–479.

McColl, E. (2005). Developing questionnaires. In P. Fayers, R. Hays (Eds.) *Assessing quality of life in clinical trials* (2nd edn). Oxford: Oxford University Press.

Mokkink, L.B., Terwee, C.B., Patrick, D.L., Alonso, J., Stratford, P.W., Knol, D.L., Bouter, L.M., de Vet, H.C. (2010). The COSMIN checklist for assessing the methodological quality of studies on measurement properties of health status measurement instruments: An international Delphi study. *Quality of Life Research*, 19, 539–549.

Morley, D., Selai, C. Jahanshahi, M., Thompson, A. (2005). Assessing the impact of parental illness on adolescent and adult children. *Quality of Life Research* 14(9), 1987.

Morley, D., Selai, C., Schrag, A., Thompson, A., Jahanshahi, M. (2010). Refinement and validation of the Parental Illness Impact Scale. *Parkinsonism and Related Disorders*, 16(3), 181–185.

Morley, D., Selai, C., Schrag, A., Jahanshahi, M., Thompson, A. (2011). Adolescent and adult children of parents with Parkinson's disease: Incorporating their needs in clinical guidelines. *Parkinson's Disease*, 2011, 951874.

Murphy, D.A., Greenwell, L., Resell, J., Brecht, M.L., Schuster, M.A. (2008). Early and middle adolescents' autonomy development: Impact of maternal HIV/AIDS. *Clinical Child Psychology and Psychiatry*, 13(2), 253–276.

Murphy, D.A., Marelich, W.D., Lanza, H.I., Herbeck, D.M. (2012). Effects of maternal HIV on children's psychosocial adjustment with peers and with their mother. *Vulnerable Children and Youth Studies*, 7(4), 357–370.

Norman, G., Streiner, D. (2000). *Biostatistics: The bare essentials*. Hamilton, Ontario: B.C. Decker Inc.

Nunnally, J., Bernstein, I.H. (1994). *Psychometric theory*. New York: McGraw-Hill.

Pakenham, K.I., Bursnall, S. (2006). Relations between social support, appraisal and coping and both positive and negative outcomes for children of a parent with multiple sclerosis and comparisons with children of healthy parents. *Clinical Rehabilitation*, 20, 709–723.

Pakenham, K.I., Bursnall, S., Chiu, J., Cannon, T., Okochi, M. (2006). The psychosocial impact of caregiving on young people who have a parent with an illness or disability: Comparisons between young caregivers and non-caregivers. *Rehabilitation Psychology*, 51, 113–126.

Pakenham, K.I., Cox, S. (2012). The nature of caregiving in children of a parent with multiple sclerosis from multiple sources and the associations between caregiving activities and youth adjustment over time. *Psychology and Health*, 27, 324–346.

Pakenham, K.I., Cox, S. (2014). The effects of parental illness and other ill family members on the adjustment of children. *Annals of Behavioural Medicine*, 48(3), 424–437.

Pakenham K.I., Cox, S. (2015). The effects of parental illness and other ill family members on youth caregiving experiences. *Psychology and Health*, 30(7), 857–878.

Pett, M.A., Lackey, N.R., Sullivan, J.J. (2003). *Making sense of factor analysis: The use of factor analysis for instrument development in health care research*. London: Sage.

Pollak, E., Bullinger, M., Jeske, J., Wiegand-Grefe, S. (2008). How do mentally ill parents evaluate their children's quality of life? Associations with the parent's illness and family functioning. *Praxis der Kinderpsychologie und Kinderpsychiatrie*, 57, 301–314.

Portney, L., Watkins, M. (2009). *Foundations of clinical research: applications to practice.* New Jersey: Pearson Education.

Putnam, S.P., Rothbart, M.K. (2006). Development of short and very short forms of the Children's Behavior Questionnaire. *Journal of Personality Assessment*, 87(1),102–112.

Rajmil, L., López, A.R., López-Aguilà, S., Alonso, J. (2013). Parent-child agreement on health-related quality of life (HRQOL): A longitudinal study. *Health and Quality of Life Outcomes*, 11, 101.

Ravens-Sieberer, U., Bullinger, M. (1998a). Assessing health-related quality of life in chronically ill children with the German KINDL: First psychometric and content analytical results. *Quality of Life Research*, 7, 399–407.

Ravens-Sieberer, U., Bullinger, M. (1998b). News from the KINDL-Questionnaire: A new version for adolescents. *Quality of Life Research*, 7, 653.

Ravens-Sieberer, U., Erhart, M., Wille, N., Wetzel, R., Nickel, J., Bullinger, M. (2006). Generic health-related quality assessment in children and adolescents: Methodological considerations. *Pharmacoeconomics*, 24, 1199–1220.

Ravens-Sieberer, U., Heilmann, M., Walleser, S. (2000). Assessment of quality of life in young children with a Computer Assisted Touch Screen Program (CAT-Screen): Reliability, validity and feasibility. 7th Annual Conference of the International Society for Quality of Life Research (ISOQOL). *Quality of Life Research*, 9, 298.

Ravens-Sieberer, U., Gosch, A., Rajmil, L., Erhart, M., Bruil, J., Duer, W., Auquier, P., Power, M., Abel, T., Czemy, L., Mazur, J., Czimbalmos, A., Tountas, Y., Hagquist, C., Kilroe, J., Kidscreen Group E. (2005). KIDSCREEN-52 quality-of-life measure for children and adolescents. *Expert Review of Pharmacoeconomics and Outcomes Research*, 5, 353–364.

Ravens-Sieberer, U., Auquier, P., Erhart, M., Gosch, A., Rajmil, L., Bruil, J., Power, M., Duer, W., Cloetta, B., Czemy, L., Mazur, J., Czimbalmos, A., Tountas, Y., Hagquist, C., Kilroe, J; European KIDSCREEN Group. (2007). The KIDSCREEN-27 quality of life measure for children and adolescents: Psychometric results from a cross-cultural survey in 13 European countries. *Quality of Life Research*, 16, 1347–1356.

Ravens-Sieberer, U., Erhart, M., Rajmil, L., Herdman, M., Auquier, P., Bruil, J., Power, M., Duer, W., Abel, T., Czemy, L., Mazur, J., Czimbalmos, A., Tountas, Y., Hagquist, C., Kilroe, J; European KIDSCREEN Group. (2010). Reliability, construct and criterion validity of the KIDSCREEN-10 score: A short measure for children and adolescents' well-being and health-related quality of life. *Quality of Life Research*, 19, 1487–1500.

Rebok, G., Riley, A., Forrest, C., Starfield, B., Green, B., Robertson, J., Tambor, E. (2001). Elementary school-aged children's reports of their health: A cognitive interviewing study. *Quality of Life Research*, 10, 59–70.

Reeve, B.B., Wyrwich, K.W., Wu, A.W., Velikova, G., Terwee, C.B., Snyder, C.F., Schwartz, C., Revicki, D.A., Moinpour, C.M., McLeod, L.D., Lyons, J.C., Lenderking, W.R., Hinds, P.S., Hays, R.D., Greenhalgh, J., Gershon, R., Feeny, D., Fayers, P.M., Cella, D., Brundage, M., Ahmed, S., Aaronson, N.K., Butt, Z. (2013). ISOQOL recommends minimum standards for patient-reported outcome measures used in patient-centered outcomes and comparative effectiveness research. *Quality of Life Research*, 22, 1889–1905.

Reinfjell, T., Diseth, T., Veenstra, M., Vikan, A. (2006). Measuring health-related quality of life in young adolescents: Reliability and validity in the Norwegian version of the Pediatric Quality of Life Inventory 4.0 (PedsQL) generic core scales. *Health and Quality of Life Outcomes*, 4, 61.

Revicki, D.A., Cella, D., Hays, R.D., Sloan, J.A., Lenderking, W.R., Aaronson, N.K. (2006). Responsiveness and minimal important differences for patient reported outcomes. *Health and Quality of Life Outcomes*, 4, 70.

Revicki, D.A., Erickson, P.A., Sloan, J.A., Dueck, A., Guess, H., Santanello, N.C; Mayo/FDA Patient-Reported Outcomes Consensus Meeting Group. (2007). Interpreting and reporting results based on patient-reported outcomes. *Value in Health*, 10(S2), S116–124.

Revicki, D., Hays, R.D., Cella, D., Sloan, J. (2008). Recommended methods for determining responsiveness and minimally important differences for patient-reported outcomes. *Journal of Clinical Epidemiology*, 61, 102–109.

Ring, L., Gross, C.R., McColl, E. (2010). Putting the text back into context: Toward increased use of mixed methods for quality of life research. *Quality of Life Research*, 19, 613–615.

Rosenberg, M. (1989). *Society and the adolescent self-image*. Middletown, CT: Wesleyan University Press.

Rothbart, M.K., Ahadi, S.A., Hershey, K.L., Fisher, P. (2001). Investigations of temperament at three to seven years: The Children's Behavior Questionnaire. *Child Development*, 72, 1394–1408.

Saylor, C.F., Finch, A.J. Jr., Spirito, A., Bennett, B. (1984). The Children's Depression Inventory: A systematic evaluation of psychometric properties. *Journal of Consulting and Clinical Psychology*, 52, 955–967.

Schrag, A., Morley, D., Quinn, N., Jahanshahi, M. (2004a). Development of a measure of the impact of chronic parental illness on adolescent and adult children: The Parental Illness Impact Scale (Parkinson's disease). *Parkinsonism and Related Disorders*, 10(7), 399–405.

Schrag, A., Morley, D., Quinn, N., Jahanshahi, M. (2004b). Impact of Parkinson's disease on patients' adolescent and adult children. *Parkinsonism and Related Disorders*, 10(7), 391–397.

Sieh, D.S., Visser-Meily, J.M., Oort, F.J., Meijer, A.M. (2012). Risk factors for problem behavior in adolescents of parents with a chronic medical condition. *European Child and Adolescent Psychiatry*, 21(8), 459–471.

Sieh, D.S., Visser-Meily, J.M., Meijer, A.M. (2013). Differential outcomes of adolescents with chronically ill and healthy parents. *Journal of Child and Family Studies*, 22(2), 209–218.

Speight, J., Barendse, S.M. (2010). FDA guidance on patient reported outcomes. *BMJ*, 340, c2921.

Streiner, D., Norman, G., Cairney, J. (2015). *Health measurement scales: A practical guide to their development and use* (5th edn). Oxford: Oxford University Press.

Thastum, M., Watson, M., Kienbacher, C., Piha, J., Steck, B., Zachariae, R., Baldus, C., Romer, G. (2009). Prevalence and predictors of emotional and behavioural functioning of children where a parent has cancer. *Cancer*, 115(17), 4030–4039.

Upton, P., Lawford, J., Eiser, C. (2008). Parent-child agreement across child health-related quality of life instruments: A review of the literature. *Quality of Life Research*, 17, 895–913.

van Doesum, K.M., Riksen-Walraven, J.M., Hosman, C.H., Hoefnagels, C. (2008). A randomized controlled trial of a home-visiting intervention aimed at preventing relationship problems in depressed mothers and their infants. *Child Development*, 79(3), 547–561.

van Ijzendoorn, M.H., Vereijken, C.M.J.L., Bakermans-Kranenburg, M.J., Riksen-Walraven, J.M. (2004). Assessing attachment security with the attachment Q sort: Meta-analytic evidence for the validity of the observer AQS. *Child Development*, 75(4), 1188–1213.

Vaughn, B.E., Waters, E. (1990). Attachment behavior at home and in the laboratory: Q-sort observations and strange situation classifications of one-year-olds. *Child Development*, 61(6), 1965–1973.

Verrips, G., Vogels, A., Den Ouden, A., Paneth, N., Verloove-Vanhorick, S. (2000). Measuring health related quality of life in adolescents: Agreement between raters and between methods of administration. *Child: Care, Health and Development*, 26, 457–469.

Visser-Meily, A., Post, M., Meijer, A.M., Maas, C., Ketelaar, M., Lindeman, E. (2005). Children's adjustment to a parent's stroke: Determinants of health status and psychological problems, and the role of support from the rehabilitation team. *Journal of Rehabilitation Medicine*, 37, 236–241.

Visser, A., Huizinga, G.A., Hoekstra, H.J., van der Graaf, W.T., Hoekstra-Weebers, J.E. (2007). Temperament as a predictor of internalising and externalising problems in adolescent children of parents diagnosed with cancer. *Supportive Care in Cancer*, 15, 395–403.

Wadsby, M., Svedin, C.G., Sydsjö, G. (2007). Children of mothers at psychosocial risk growing up: A follow up at the age of 16. *Journal of Adolescence*, 30, 147–164.

Waters, E., Deane, K. (1985). Defining and assessing individual differences in attachment relationships: Q-methodology and the organization of behavior in infancy and early childhood. In I. Bretherton and E. Waters (Eds.), Growing points of attachment theory and research. *Monographs of the Society for Research in Child Development*, 50 (Serial No. 209), 41–65.

Waters, E. (1995). The attachment Q-set. In E. Waters, B.E. Vaughn, G. Posada, K. Kondo-Ikemura (Eds). Caregiving, cultural and cognitive perspectives on secure base behavior and working models. *Monographs of the Society for Research in Child Development*, 60 (Serial No. 244), 234–246.

Willis, G.B. (1999). Cognitive Interviewing: A 'How To' Guide. *Short course presented at the 1999 Meeting of the American Statistical Association*. Durham, NC: Research Triangle Institute.

Willis, G.B. (2005). Cognitive interviewing: A tool for improving questionnaire design, London: Sage Publications.

Yahav, R., Vosburgh, J., Miller, A. (2005). Emotional responses of children and adolescents to parents with multiple sclerosis. *Multiple Sclerosis*, 11(4), 464–468.

Yahav, R., Vosburgh, J., Miller, A. (2007). Separation-individuation processes of adolescent children of parents with multiple sclerosis. *Multiple Sclerosis*, 13(1), 87–94.

Yamaguchi, N., Poudel, K.C., Jimba, M. (2013). Health-related quality of life, depression, and self-esteem in adolescents with leprosy-affected parents: Results of a cross-sectional study in Nepal. *BMC Public Health*, 13, 22.

Yost, K.J., Eton, D.T. (2005). Combining distribution- and anchor-based approaches to determine minimally important differences: The FACIT experience. *Evaluation and the Health Professions*, 28, 172–191.

Index